W9-BHE-426

HEALTH

POLICY

ISSUES

An Economic

Perspective

FOURTH EDITION

HEALTH

POLICY

ISSUES

An Economic

Perspective

FOURTH EDITION

Paul J. Feldstein

Health Administration Press, Chicago, Illinois
AUPHA Press, Washington, DC

AUPHA
HAP

Library of Congress Cataloging-in-Publication Data

Feldstein, Paul J.
    Health policy issues : an economic perspective / Paul J. Feldstein. — 4th ed.
      p. cm.
    Includes bibliographical references and index.
    ISBN-13: 978-1-56793-274-4
    ISBN-10: 1-56793-274-6 (alk. paper)
    1. Medical economics—United States. 2. Medical policy—Economic aspects—United States. 3. Medical care—United States—Cost control. 4. Medical care, Cost of—United States. I. Title.
RA410.53F455 2007
338.4'73621—dc22

2006052580

The paper used in this publication meets the minimum requirements of American National Standard for Information Sciences—Permanence of Paper for Printed Library Materials, ANSI Z39.48-1984. ♾™

Acquisitions editor: Janet Davis; Project manager: Gregory Sebben; Cover design: Shawnna Rovinsky

Health Administration Press
A division of the Foundation of the
   American College of Healthcare Executives
1 North Franklin Street, Suite 1700
Chicago, IL 60606-3529
(312) 424-2800

To my health care executive MBA students,
who are such a pleasure to teach

Contents

Detailed Contents

List of Figures

List of Tables

Preface

BEING AN ECONOMIST, I believe an economic approach is very useful, not only for understanding the forces pressing for change in health care but also for explaining why the health system has evolved to its current state. Even the political issues surrounding the financing and delivery of health services can be better understood when viewed through an economic perspective, that is, the economic self-interest of participants.

For these reasons, I believe an issue-oriented book containing short discussions on each subject and using an economic perspective is needed. The economic perspective used throughout is that of a "market" economist, namely one who believes markets—in which suppliers compete for customers on the basis of price and quality—are the most effective mechanisms for allocating resources. Of course, at times markets fail or lead to outcomes that are undesirable in terms of equity. Market economists generally believe government economic interventions, no matter how well-intentioned or carefully thought out, can neither replicate the efficiency with which markets allocate resources nor fully anticipate the behavioral responses of the economic agents affected by the intervention. In cases of market failure, market economists prefer solutions that fix the underlying problem while retaining basic market incentives rather than replacing the market altogether with government planning or provision.

Health care reform has been an ongoing process for decades. At times, legislation and regulation have brought about major changes in the financing and delivery of medical services. At other times, competitive forces have restructured the delivery system. Both legislative and market forces will continue to influence how the public pays for and receives its medical services. Any subject affecting the lives of so many and requiring such a large portion of our country's resources will continue to be a topic of debate, legislative change, and market restructuring. I hope this book will help to clarify some of the more significant issues underlying the politics and economics of health care.

For this fourth edition, in addition to revising and updating each of the chapters, tables, and figures, several new chapters have been added. These chapters address several of the more topical issues in health care. One new chapter discusses the future role of hospitals. Another discusses market competition; has it been tried, and has it failed to improve the health care system? A previous chapter on a Medicare prescription drug benefit has been omitted, and in its place is a new chapter on the public policy dilemma facing the pharmaceutical industry.

Given the large number of chapters and topics covered, and given that not all chapters will be assigned to students, some overlap naturally occurs in subject matter.

To help the reader focus on important points related to each issue, a list of discussion questions appears at the end of each chapter. A glossary is also included.

For instructors, an Instructor's Manual and PowerPoint slides are available. The Instructor's Manual includes a brief overview of each chapter and a list of the key topics covered. Also included are discussion points related to the Discussion Questions that appear at the end of each chapter. Additional questions and answers have been provided for instructor use. The Instructor's Manual and PowerPoints reside in a secure area on the Health Administration Press (HAP) web site and are available only to adopters of this book. For access information, e-mail hap1@ache.org.

I thank Glenn Melnick, Thomas Wickizer, Jerry German, Jeff Hoch, and several anonymous reviewers for their comments. For this fourth edition I also thank Elzbieta Kozlowski and Mary Alice Pike for the collection of data, construction of the figures and tables, and preparation of the manuscript.

Paul J. Feldstein
Irvine, California

Chapter 1

The Rise in Medical Expenditures

THE RAPID GROWTH in medical expenditures since 1965 is as familiar as the increasing percentage of our gross domestic product (GDP) devoted to medical care. Less well-known are the reasons for this continual rise in medical expenditures. The purpose of this introductory chapter is twofold: to provide a historical perspective to the medical sector and to explain the rise in medical expenditures within an economic framework.

BEFORE MEDICARE AND MEDICAID

Until 1965, spending in the medical sector was predominantly private—80 percent of all expenditures were spent by individuals out of pocket or by private health insurance on their behalf. The remaining expenditures (20 percent) were paid by the federal government (8 percent) and the states (12 percent) (see Table 1.1). Personal medical expenditures were $35 billion and represented approximately 6 percent of our GDP, that is, six cents of every dollar spent was for medical services.

EFFECTS OF MEDICARE AND MEDICAID

In 1965, two major government programs, Medicare and Medicaid, were enacted, dramatically increasing the role of government in financing medical care. Medicare covers the aged and consists of two parts: Part A is for hospital care and is financed by a separate (Medicare) payroll tax on the working population. Part B covers physicians' services and is financed by federal taxes (currently 75 percent) and by a premium paid by the aged, which covers only 25 percent of the program's costs. (In December 2003, a new Medicare prescription drug benefit was enacted.) Medicaid is for

Table 1.1: Personal Health Services Expenditures, by Source of Funds, 1965 and 2005

Source of Funds	1965 $ In billions	1965 %	2005 $ In billions	2005 %
Total	34.7	100.0	1,661.4	100.0
Private	27.6	79.5	914.5	55.0
Out of pocket	18.1	52.2	249.4	15.0
Insurance benefits	8.7	25.1	596.7	35.9
All other	0.8	2.3	68.4	4.1
Public	7.1	20.5	746.9	45.0
Federal	2.8	8.1	568.5	34.2
State and local	4.3	12.4	178.4	10.7

Source: Centers for Medicare & Medicaid Services, Office of the Actuary, National Health Statistics Group. 2007. [Online information.] http://www.cms.hhs.gov/NationalHealthExpendData/downloads/tables.pdf.

the categorically or medically needy, which includes indigent aged and families with dependent children who receive cash assistance. Each state administers its program, and the federal government pays, on average, more than half of the costs. As a result of Medicare and Medicaid, the federal government became a major payer of medical services.

In 2005, 45 percent of total medical expenditures were paid by the government; the federal share was 34 percent and the states contributed 11 percent. The private share declined to 55 percent; of that, 15 percent was paid out of pocket (compared with 52 percent out of pocket in 1965). The rapid increase in total health expenditures is illustrated in Table 1.2, which shows expenditures on the different components of medical services over time. Figure 1.1 shows where health care dollars come from and how they are distributed among the different health care providers.

In the United States, $1.987 trillion, or 16 percent of the GDP, was spent on medical care in 2005, and these expenditures are rising at about 8 percent (2000–2005) per year. The rate of increase in medical expenditures has increased since 2000, when it was about 5.5 percent (1994–2000). An important reason for the slowdown in medical expenditures in the earlier period was the growth of managed care, with its emphasis on utilization management, and price competition among providers that

Table 1.2: National Health Services Expenditures, Selected Calendar Years, 1965–2005 (Billions of Dollars)

	1965	1970	1980	1990	2000	2005
Total national health expenditures	$42.2	$74.9	$253.9	$714.0	$1,353.3	$1,987.7
Health services and supplies	37.3	67.1	234.0	666.7	1,264.5	1,860.9
Personal health care	34.7	62.9	215.3	607.5	1,140.0	1,661.4
Hospital care	13.8	27.6	101.0	251.6	417.1	611.6
Physician and clinical services	8.3	14.0	47.1	157.5	288.6	421.2
Dental services	2.8	4.7	13.3	31.5	62.0	86.6
Other professional care	0.5	0.7	3.6	18.2	39.1	56.7
Home health care	0.1	0.2	2.4	12.6	30.5	47.5
Nursing home care	1.4	4.0	19.0	52.6	95.3	121.9
Drugs, medical nondurables	5.9	8.8	21.8	62.8	151.0	234.8
Durable medical equipment	1.0	1.6	3.8	11.2	19.3	24.0
Other personal health care	0.8	1.3	3.3	9.6	37.1	57.2
Program administration and net cost of private health insurance	2.0	2.8	12.2	39.2	81.2	143.0
Government public health activities	0.6	1.4	6.4	20.0	43.4	56.6
Research and construction	4.9	8.1	20.9	50.7	94.0	126.8
Research	1.5	2.0	5.4	12.7	25.6	40.0
Construction	3.3	5.8	14.5	34.7	63.2	86.8
National health expenditures per capita	211	356	1,102	2,813	4,790	6,697

Source: Centers for Medicare & Medicaid Services, Office of the Actuary, National Health Statistics Group. 2007. [Online information.] http://www.cms.hhs.gov/ NationalHealthExpendData/downloads/tables.pdf.

were included in managed care provider networks. Since 2000, managed care's cost-containment approaches have been weakened as a result of public dissatisfaction with managed care, lawsuits against managed care organizations (MCOs) for denial of care, government legislation, and a tight labor market that led employers to offer their employees more

Figure 1.1: The Nation's Health Services Dollar, 2005

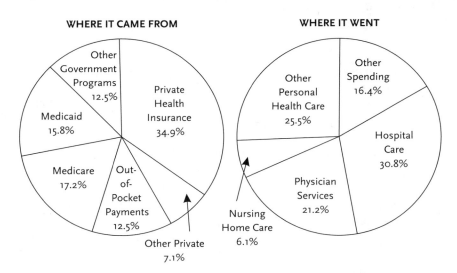

Note: "Other personal health care" includes dental care, vision care, home health care, drugs, medical products, and other professional services. "Other spending" includes program administration, net cost of private health insurance, government public health, and research and construction.

Source: U.S. Department of Health and Human Services, Centers for Medicare & Medicaid Services. 2007. [Online information.] http://www.cms.hhs.gov/ NationalHealthExpendData.

health plan choices. As a result, medical expenditures have been rising at a more rapid rate.

The government estimates that national health expenditures will rise at a higher rate in the coming decade as the first of the baby boomers become eligible for Medicare and new technology that improves quality, but at a higher cost, continues to be introduced. By 2015, national health expenditures are expected to double to $4 trillion.

Medical expenditures consist of prices multiplied by quantity of services. The rise in medical expenditures can be explained by looking at the factors that lead to changes in medical prices and quantities. In a market system, prices and output of goods and services are determined by the interaction of buyers (the demand side) and sellers (the supply side) in a market. We can analyze changes in prices and output by examining how various interventions change the behavior of buyers and sellers. One such intervention is Medicare, which lowered the out-of-pocket price the aged had to pay for medical care. The result was a dramatic increase in the demand for hospital and physician services by the aged, leading to rapid increases in prices and, to a lesser amount, an increase in use of those services. Total expenditures increased because the higher prices multiplied by the greater quantity equaled a higher level of expenditures.

When costs, which underlie the supply of any service, increase, prices also increase. For example, as hospitals tried to attract more nurses to care for the increased number of aged patients, they had to raise nurses' wages, and this increase was then passed on to payers in higher hospital prices. Similarly, government payments for the poor under Medicaid increased their demand for medical services. The result of increased demand for care and higher costs of providing that care was rapidly rising expenditures.

At the same time the government was subsidizing the demands of the aged and poor, the demand for medical services by the employed population was increasing. Stimulating the growth in private health insurance during the late 1960s and 1970s was the growth in incomes, the high marginal (federal) income tax rates (up to 70 percent), and the high inflation rate in the economy. The high inflation rate was pushing more people into higher marginal tax brackets. Receiving additional income in the form of wages, and then paying federal, state, and Social Security taxes, would have left employees with less disposable income to spend, up to 50 percent less if they were in a 50 percent marginal income tax bracket. Instead of having the employer pay wage increases in after-tax cash, which could be taxed at 50 percent, employees often chose to have the employer spend those same dollars, before tax, to buy additional health insurance. Thus, employees could have their out-of-pocket medical expenses paid with before-tax dollars rather than after-tax dollars. This tax subsidy for employer-paid health insurance stimulated the demand for medical services in the private sector and further increased medical prices.

Demand increased most rapidly for those medical services that were covered by government and private health insurance. As of 2005, only 3.3 percent of hospital care and 10.0 percent of physician services were paid out of pocket by the patient; the remainder was paid by some third party. Patients had little incentive to be concerned with the price of a service when they were not responsible for paying a significant portion of the price. As the out-of-pocket price declined, the use of services increased.

The aged, who represent 12.4 percent of the population and use more medical services than any other age group, filled 40 percent of hospital beds. Use of physician services by the aged, the poor, and those with insurance also increased.

Advances in medical technology led to a further stimulus in demand for medical treatment. New methods of diagnosis and treatment were developed; those with previously untreatable diseases could now have access to technology that offered hope of a recovery from illness. New diseases, such as acquired immunodeficiency syndrome (AIDS), led to further demands on the medical system. These dramatic increases in third-party payments (both public and private), an aging population, and new technologies led to increases in both prices and quantities of medical services.

Providers (hospitals and physicians) responded to these increased demands for care. However, the method by which they responded unnecessarily increased the cost of providing medical services. When Medicare was enacted, hospitals were paid their costs plus 2 percent for serving Medicare patients. Hospitals, which were predominantly not-for-profit, consequently expanded their capacity, invested in the latest technology, and duplicated facilities and services available in nearby hospitals. Hospitals had few incentives to be efficient, as their costs were reimbursed. Hospital prices rose faster than any other medical service. Similarly, physicians had little cause for concern over hospital costs. Physicians wanted their hospitals to have the latest equipment so that they would not have to refer their patients elsewhere (and possibly lose them); they would hospitalize patients for diagnostic workups and keep them in the hospital longer, as it was less costly for the patient covered by hospital insurance. Outpatient services, which were less costly than hospital care, were generally not covered by third-party payers.

In addition to the lack of incentives for patients to be concerned with the cost of their care and the similar lack of incentives for providers to supply that care efficiently, the government imposed restrictions on the delivery of services. Under both Medicare and Medicaid, the government was not permitted to contract with organizations such as health maintenance organizations (HMOs) to deliver care for an annual capitation payment. Organized medicine was instrumental in having the concept of *free choice of provider* included in both Medicare and Medicaid. Organizations such as HMOs that preclude their enrollees from choosing any physician in the community would violate the free choice of physician rule and were thus unable to receive capitation payments from the government. Numerous state restrictions on HMOs further inhibited their development. These restrictions made contracting with less-expensive closed panels of providers impossible for the government (and difficult for private insurers).

The effect of increased demand and limited patient and provider incentives to search for lower-cost approaches, together with restrictions on the delivery of medical services, resulted in rapidly rising prices, increased use of services, and, consequently, greater medical expenditures.

GOVERNMENT RESPONSE TO RISING COSTS

As expenditures under Medicare and Medicaid increased, the federal government faced limited options: It could (1) raise the Medicare payroll tax and income taxes on the nonaged to continue funding these programs, (2) require the aged to pay higher premiums for Medicare and increase their deductibles and copayments, or (3) reduce payments to hospitals and physicians. Each of these approaches would cost the administration and Congress political support from some constituency, such as employees, the aged, or health care providers. The least politically costly options appeared to be to increase taxes on the nonaged and to pay hospitals and physicians less.

Federal and state governments used additional regulatory approaches to control these rapidly rising expenditures. Medicare utilization review programs were instituted, and controls were placed on hospital investment in new facilities and equipment. These government controls proved ineffective as hospital expenditures continued their rapid rise throughout the 1970s. The government then limited physician fee increases under Medicare and Medicaid; as a consequence, many physicians refused to participate in these programs. Access to care by the aged and the poor decreased. As physicians refused to participate in Medicare, many Medicare patients had to pay higher out-of-pocket fees to be seen by physicians.

In 1979, President Carter's highest domestic priority was to enact expenditure limits on Medicare hospital cost increases; a Congress controlled by his own political party defeated him.

The 1980s

By the beginning of the 1980s, political consensus on what should be done to control increases in Medicare hospital and physician expenditures was lacking, and private health expenditures continued to rise rapidly. Yet by the mid-1980s, strong cost-containment pressures were being imposed on both the Medicare and private medical sectors.

Several events in the early 1980s brought major changes to the medical sector. The HMO legislation enacted in 1974 began to have its effect in the 1980s. In 1974, President Nixon had wanted a health program that would not increase federal expenditures. The result was the HMO Act of 1974, which legitimized HMOs and removed restrictive state laws retarding the development of federally approved HMOs. Unfortunately, many HMOs decided not to seek federal qualification because imposed restrictions would have caused their premiums to be too high to be price competitive with traditional health insurers. These restrictions were removed by the late 1970s, and the growth of HMOs began in the early 1980s.

To achieve savings in Medicaid, in 1981 the Reagan administration removed the free choice of provider requirement for Medicaid enrollees; states were able to require their Medicaid populations to participate in closed provider panels. The states were then able to contract with HMOs and accept bids from hospitals for care of their Medicaid patients. (The "free choice" requirement remained in place for the aged until the mid-1980s, when the aged were permitted to voluntarily join HMOs.)

Federal subsidies to expand the number of medical school spaces, which were enacted in 1964, began to affect the supply of physicians: The number of active physicians expanded from 146 per 100,000 civilian population in 1965 to 195 per 100,000 in 1980; it reached 229 per 100,000 by 1990 and 275 per 100,000 in 2004 (Division of Survey and Data Resources 1991, 2006). The increased supply of physicians created excess capacity among physicians, dampened increases in their fees, made it easier for HMOs to attract physicians, and, therefore, made it easier for the HMOs to expand.

A new Medicare hospital payment system was phased in during 1983. Hospitals were no longer to be paid according to their costs; fixed prices were established for each diagnostic admission (referred to as diagnosis-related groups, or DRGs), and each year Congress set an annual limit on the increase in these fixed prices per admission. DRG prices changed hospitals' incentives. Because hospitals could keep the difference between their costs and the fixed DRG prices, they now had an incentive to reduce their costs for caring for Medicare patients and to discharge them earlier. The length of stay per admission fell, and occupancy rates declined. Hospitals also became concerned with physician practice behavior that increased the hospitals' costs of care.

In addition to the government policy changes of the early 1980s, important events were also occurring in the private sector. The new decade started with a recession, and as the United States began to recover, the dollar was very strong relative to other currencies. To survive the recession and remain competitive internationally, the business sector looked to reduce labor costs. Because health insurance was the fastest-growing labor expense, business began to pressure health insurers to better control both the use and cost of medical services. Competitive pressures forced insurers to increase the efficiency of their benefit packages by including lower-cost substitutes to inpatient care, such as outpatient surgery. Patient price sensitivity was increased by increasing deductibles and copayments. Use of the hospital was decreased by requiring the patient to receive prior authorization before being admitted and having the patient's length of stay reviewed while in the hospital. These actions greatly reduced hospital admission rates and lengths of stay. The number of admissions in community hospitals in 1975 was 152 per 1,000 population. By 1990 it had fallen to 123 per 1,000 and has continued to decline, reaching 113 in 2005 (American Hospital Association 2007; U.S. Census Bureau 2006).

As a result of the federal DRG payment system, the above private programs, and a shift to the outpatient sector facilitated by changes in technology (both anesthetic and surgical techniques), hospital occupancy rates declined from 76 percent in 1980 to about 67 percent in 2005. Hospitals had excess capacity. At the same time, increases in the supply of physicians created downward pressures on fees.

The preconditions for price competition were in place: There was excess capacity among suppliers, and health care purchasers were interested in reducing their employees' medical expenses. The last necessary condition for price competition occurred in 1982 when the U.S. Supreme Court upheld the applicability of the antitrust laws to the medical sector. Successful antitrust cases were brought against the American Medical Association for its restrictions on advertising, against a medical society that threatened to boycott an insurer over physician fee increases, against a dental organization that boycotted an insurer's cost-containment program, against medical staffs that denied hospital privileges to physicians because they belonged to an HMO, and against hospitals whose mergers threatened to lessen price competition in their communities.

The applicability of the antitrust laws, excess capacity among providers, and employer and insurer interest in lowering medical costs brought about profound changes in the medical marketplace. Traditional insurance plans lost market share as managed care plans, which controlled utilization and limited access to hospitals and physicians, grew. Preferred provider organizations (PPOs) were formed and included only physicians and hospitals that were willing to discount their prices. Employees and their families were offered price incentives in the form of lower out-of-pocket payments to use these less-expensive providers. Large employers and health insurers began to select PPOs based on their prices, use of services, and outcomes of their treatment.

Although the federal government agreed to pay HMOs a capitated amount for enrolling Medicare patients in the mid-1980s, fewer than 10 percent of the aged voluntarily participated. In 1992, the federal government also changed the method of paying physicians under Medicare. A national fee schedule (resource-based relative value system, or RBRVS) was adopted, and volume-expenditure limits were established to limit the total rise in physician Medicare payments. Furthermore, physicians could no longer choose to accept the Medicare fee for some Medicare patients but not others. Physicians now had to participate for all their Medicare patients or none. Medicare patients represent such a significant portion of a physician's practice that few physicians decided not to participate; consequently, they accepted Medicare fees. Thus, the main approach used by the federal government to contain Medicare expenditures continues to be the use of price controls and expenditure limits on payments to hospitals and physicians for services provided to Medicare patients.

The 1980s brought about a disruption in the traditional physician–patient relationship. Insurers and HMOs used utilization review to control patient demand, emphasize outcomes and appropriateness of care, and limit patients' access to higher-priced physicians and hospitals by not including them in their provider networks; they also used case management for catastrophic illnesses, substituted less-expensive settings for more costly inpatient care, and affected patients' choice of drugs through the use of formularies.

The use of cost-containment programs and the shift to outpatient care lowered hospital occupancy rates. The increasing supply of physicians, particularly specialists, resulted in excess capacity. Hospitals in financial trouble closed, and others merged. Hospital consolidation increased. It was not until years later that hospitals' excess capacity was removed and increases in demand for care began to exceed the available supplies of hospitals and physicians. Until then, hospitals and physicians continued to be subject to intense competitive pressures.

A change in employee incentives has been an important stimulant to competition among HMOs and insurers. As employers required employees to pay the additional cost of more expensive health plans, employees chose the lowest-priced plan. Health plans competed for enrollees primarily on the basis of their premiums and provider networks.

The 1990s

As managed care spread throughout the United States during the 1990s, the rate of increase in medical expenditures lessened. Dramatic reductions in the use of hospitals were seen, and both hospitals and physicians gave large price discounts to be included in an insurer's provider panel. These cost-containment approaches lowered the rate of increase in medical expenditures. However, as price competition reduced medical costs, some of the methods by which this competition did so came under attack. The public wanted greater access to care, particularly referrals to specialists. Congress and states began to impose restrictions on MCOs, such as mandating minimum lengths of stay in the hospital for normal deliveries.

THE CURRENT PERIOD

The forces that are increasing demand and the costs of providing care are causing medical expenditures and insurance premiums to once again increase more rapidly. The population is aging (the first of the baby boomers retire in 2011), technological advances can improve early diagnosis, and new methods of treatment are becoming available, all of which result in increased demands for medical services. Government regulations at both the federal and state levels mandating minimum care requirements and freer access to specialists increase costs. *New technology is believed to be the most important force behind rising expenditures.* For example, the number of persons receiving organ transplants has increased dramatically, as has the diffusion of new equipment. The cost of providing medical services is also increasing as more highly trained medical personnel are needed to handle the increased technology and as wage rates increase so as to attract more nurses and technicians to the medical sector.

Thus, although the medical sector has become more efficient and price competitive, increased demand and higher costs of providing medical services are causing medical expenditures to increase more rapidly. The past approaches to achieving large cost reductions—decreased hospital use and price discounts—will not produce similar savings in the future.

Instead, health plans and medical groups will have to develop more innovative, less costly ways of managing patient care.

Several of the newer approaches for cost containment include high-deductible health plans, evidence-based medicine, and disease management programs. Shifting more of their medical costs to consumers is referred to as "consumer-driven health care" (CDHC). In return for lower health insurance premiums, consumers pay higher deductibles and copayments. Consumers are then presumed to evaluate the costs and benefits of spending their own funds on health care. Alternatively, instead of relying on consumer incentives to reduce medical costs, health insurers are using evidence-based medicine, which relies on the analysis of large data sets to determine the effect on cost and medical outcomes of different physician practice patterns. Similarly, insurers are using disease management programs to provide chronically ill patients with preventive and continuous care, which not only improves the quality of care but also reduces costly hospitalizations.

More recently, health insurers have started pay-for-performance programs. Physicians and other health care providers are paid more if they provide high quality of care, usually based on process measures developed by medical experts.

Innovative approaches to reducing health care costs are more likely to occur in a system that has price incentives to do so, such as health insurers competing for enrollees, than in a regulated system. Any regulatory approach that arbitrarily seeks to reduce the rate of increase in medical expenditures will have to result in reduced access to both medical care and new technology.

SUMMARY

Although the United States spends more on health care than any other country, a scarcity of funds to provide for all of our medical needs and population groups, such as the uninsured and those on Medicaid, still exists. Therefore, choices must be made. The first choice that we as a society must make is how much of our scarce resources should be spent on medical care? What approach should be used for making this choice? Should the decision be left to individuals to determine how much of their incomes they want to spend on health care? Or should the government decide what percentage of the GDP goes to health care?

The second choice that must be made is, what is the best way of providing medical services? Would competition among health plans, or government regulation and price controls, achieve greater efficiency in providing medical services?

Third, how rapidly should medical innovation be introduced? Should regulatory agencies evaluate each medical advance and determine whether its benefits exceed its costs, or should the evaluation of those costs and benefits be left to the separate health plans competing for enrollees?

Fourth, how much should be spent on those who are medically indigent, and how should their care be provided? Should the medically indigent be enrolled in a separate medical system, such as Medicaid, or should they be provided with vouchers to enroll in competing health plans?

These choices can be better understood when we are more aware of the consequences of each approach to deciding these choices, such as which groups benefit and which groups bear the costs. Economics clarifies the implications of different approaches to making these choices.

DISCUSSION QUESTIONS

1. What are some of the reasons for the increase in demand for medical services since 1965?

2. Why has employer-paid health insurance been an important stimulant of demand for health insurance?

3. How did hospital payment methods in the 1960s and 1970s affect hospitals' incentives for efficiency and investment policy?

4. Why were HMOs and managed care not more prevalent in the 1960s and 1970s?

5. What have been the federal government's choices to reduce the greater-than-projected Medicare expenditures?

6. What events occurred during the 1980s in both the public and private sectors to make the delivery of medical services price competitive?

REFERENCES

American Hospital Association. 2007. *Hospital Statistics*. Chicago: AHA.

Division of Survey and Data Resources. 1991. *Physician Characteristics and Distribution in the United States*. Chicago: American Medical Association.

———. 2006. *Physician Characteristics and Distribution in the United States*. Chicago: American Medical Association.

U.S. Census Bureau. 2006. *Statistical Abstract of the United States*. Washington, DC: U.S. Census Bureau.

Chapter 2

How Much Should We Spend on Medical Care?

THE UNITED STATES spends a greater portion of its GDP on medical care than any other country. We are spending 16 percent of GDP, and all expectations are that this percentage will continue to increase. Can we afford to spend that much of our scarce resources on medical care? Why do we view growth in expenditures in other areas, such as automobiles, so much more favorably than expenditures on medical services? Increased medical expenditures create new health care jobs, do not pollute the air, save rather than destroy lives, and alleviate pain and suffering. More directly than any other industry, the medical sector serves those who are sick. Why should society not be pleased that more resources are flowing into a sector that cares for the aged and the sick? Spending on medical care would seem to be a more appropriate use of a society's resources than spending those same funds on faster cars, alcohol, or other consumption items, yet increased expenditures on these other industries do not cause the concern that arises when medical expenditures increase.

Is the concern over rising medical costs merely a result of the belief that we are not receiving value for our money, namely that the additional medical services and technologies are not worth what they cost in relation to other uses of those resources? Or is there a more fundamental difference of opinion regarding the proper rate of increase in medical expenditures?

To understand why increased expenditures on medical services are a cause for concern, we must discuss what is an "appropriate" or "right" amount of expenditure. Only then can we evaluate whether we are spending "too much" on medical care. Furthermore, if we determine that too much is being spent, we would have a greater understanding as to the types of public policy necessary to achieve the right expenditure level.

CONSUMER SOVEREIGNTY

The right amount of health expenditure is based on a set of values and on the concept of economic efficiency. Given the limited resources available, these resources should be directed to their highest-valued uses, as perceived by consumers. Consumers decide how much to purchase based on their perception of the value they expect to receive and on how much they have to pay for it, knowing that an expenditure on one good or service means forgoing other goods and services. Consumers differ greatly in the value they place on medical care and in how much they are willing to forgo other goods and services to spend more on health care. In a competitive market, consumers receive the full benefits of their purchases and in turn pay the full costs of receiving those benefits. When the benefits received from the last unit equal the cost of consuming that last unit, the quantity consumed is said to be optimal. If more or fewer services were consumed, the benefits received would be either less or greater than the cost of that service.

Consumer sovereignty can best be achieved in a competitive market system, which is able to accommodate consumers who have different values with regard to medical services and who differ in their willingness to pay for those services. Through their expenditures, consumers communicate their values in terms of the goods and services they wish to consume. By these expenditures, producers are directed to use scarce resources to produce the goods consumers desire. If producers are to survive and profit in competitive markets, they must be efficient in their use of resources and produce the goods consumers are willing to pay for; otherwise, more efficient and responsive producers will replace them.

Some people believe, however, that consumer sovereignty should not be the basis for how much is spent on medical care. More than in other areas, patients lack information and have limited ability to judge needs for medical treatment. Another factor is the concern about the quality of care patients receive and how much care is appropriate.

Unfortunately, no perfect alternative exists. At one extreme, if medical care was free to all and physicians (paid on a fee-for-service basis or salaried) decided on the quantity of medical care, the result would be "too much" care. Physicians are likely to prescribe services as long as some benefit is perceived, no matter how small, particularly because the physician would not be responsible for the cost of that care. The inevitable consequence of a free medical system is a government-imposed expenditure limit. Although physicians would still be responsible for determining who would receive care and for which diagnoses, "too little" care would likely be provided; this occurs in government-controlled health systems such as those in Canada and Great Britain. Queues are established to ration the available medical care, and waiting times and age become criteria for allocating the available medical resources.

No government that funds health care spends sufficient resources to provide all the care that is demanded at the going price. As does an individual making purchases, the government makes trade-offs between the benefits received from additional health expenditures and the cost of those expenditures. However, the benefits and costs to the government are different from those consumers use in their decision-making processes. The benefits to the government represent the additional political support gained by further health expenditures; the cost is the lost political support of having to raise taxes to fund these programs or shifting funds from other, politically popular, programs.

Let us therefore assume that consumer sovereignty will continue to be the guiding principle regarding how much is spent on medical expenditures. This does not mean, however, that this country is currently spending the right amount on medical services. To understand this, we must discuss the concept of economic efficiency.

ECONOMIC EFFICIENCY
Efficiency in Providing Medical Services
If medical services were produced in an inefficient manner, medical expenditures would be excessive. For example, rather than treating a patient for ten days in the hospital, that medical treatment might possibly be provided using fewer hospital days and a number of visits in the patient's home by a visiting nurse, with the same level of patient satisfaction and treatment outcome. Similarly, a treatment might be provided in an outpatient setting rather than in the hospital. Unless appropriate incentives exist for the providers of medical services to be efficient, economic efficiency in providing medical services is unlikely to be achieved.

Previously, when hospitals were paid on a cost-plus basis, their incentive was to increase their costs. Since the early 1980s, both the government and the private sector have been pressing for increased efficiency of the delivery system. Cost-based payment for hospitals under Medicare has given way to payment based on fixed prices in the form of DRGs. Price competition among hospitals and physicians has increased as insurance companies are themselves competing on the basis of premiums in the sale of group health insurance. The PPOs, HMOs, and managed care systems have increased their market share at the expense of traditional insurers. Hospitalization rates have declined as utilization review mechanisms have increased, and the trend toward implementing case management for catastrophic illness and monitoring providers for appropriateness of care and medical outcomes is also increasing.

Although few would contend that the provision of medical services is as efficient as it could be, the proportion of waste in the health system is becoming smaller over time. With the growth of cost containment and managed care, inefficiency has been declining rather than increasing. Even if administrative costs for private health insurance were drastically reduced by 50 percent (which would have saved $48 billion in 2004), the profits of the pharmaceutical drug companies were reduced by 50 percent ($20 billion), and all physician incomes were reduced by 25 percent ($44 billion), these savings of approximately $112 billion represent less than one year's annual percentage increase in total medical expenditures. Inefficiency in providing medical services, although important, is not the main cause for concern over the rise in medical expenditures.

Efficiency in the Use of Medical Services

Inefficiencies in the use of medical services occur when individuals do not have to pay the full cost of their choices; they consume "too much" medical care because their use of services is based on the out-of-pocket price they pay, and that price is less than the cost of producing the service. Consequently, the cost of providing the service exceeds the benefit the patient receives from consuming additional units of the service. The resources devoted to producing these additional services could be better used in producing other services, such as education, that would provide greater benefits.

The effect of paying less than the full price of a service is easily visualized with respect to some other consumer product, such as automobiles. If the price of automobiles was greatly reduced for consumers, they would purchase more automobiles (and more costly ones). Resources used to produce these additional automobiles must come from resources used to produce other goods. Similarly, lowering the price the person has to pay results in increased use of medical services. Studies have shown that patients who pay less out of pocket have more hospital admissions, make more physician visits, and use more outpatient services than patients who pay higher prices (Feldstein 2005). This relationship between price and use of medical services also holds for patients classified by health status.

Use inefficiency is important in medical care because the price of medical care has been *artificially* lowered for many consumers of medical services. The government subsidizes the purchase of medical care for both the poor and the aged under Medicaid and Medicare. Those who are eligible under these programs use more services than if they had to pay the full price themselves. Although the purpose of these programs was to increase the use of medical services by the poor and the aged, the artificially low prices also result in inefficient use, for example, when a patient uses the more expensive emergency department rather than a physician's office in a nonemergent situation.

A greater concern with use inefficiency concerns the working population. Employer-purchased health insurance is not considered to be taxable income for employees. If the employer gave the same amount of funds directly to the employee in the form of higher wages, the employee would have to pay federal and state income tax as well as Social Security tax on that additional income. Because employer-purchased health insurance is not subject to these taxes, the government effectively subsidizes the purchase of health insurance and hence additional medical services. Employees do not pay the full cost of health insurance. All other purchases made by consumers are made with after-tax dollars. Thus, the price of health insurance (and medical services) is effectively reduced relative to other purchases.

The greatest beneficiaries of this tax subsidy for the purchase of health insurance are those in higher income tax brackets. For example, rather than receive additional income as cash, which is then subject to high taxes (in the 1970s, the highest federal income tax bracket was 70 percent), employees choose to have more of their increased wages paid in the form of increased health insurance coverage. Instead of spending after-tax dollars on vision and dental services, employees can purchase these services more cheaply when they are paid for with before-tax dollars in the form of health insurance.

As a result, "too much" health insurance is purchased; the price of insurance is reduced by the employee's tax bracket. Employees increase their health insurance because they do not have to pay the full cost of that coverage. As a consequence, the additional insurance coverage is worth less to the employee than its full cost.

With the purchase of additional health insurance, the out-of-pocket price consumers paid for medical services declined, resulting in an increase in use of all medical services covered by health insurance. As employees and their families became less concerned with the real cost of medical services, few constraints limited the rise in medical expenditures. Had this inefficiency in use of medical services (as a result of the tax subsidy for purchasing health insurance) been less, medical expenditures would have risen more slowly.

Inefficiencies in the use and provision of medical services are legitimate reasons for concern over how much is spent on medical care. Public policy should attempt to eliminate these government-caused inefficiencies. However, there are other, less-valid reasons for concern over the rise in medical expenditures.

GOVERNMENT AND EMPLOYER CONCERNS OVER RISING MEDICAL EXPENDITURES

The payers of medical expenditures, namely government and employers, are concerned about rising medical costs. Both the federal and state governments are large payers of medical expenditures. State governments pay half the costs of caring for the medically indigent in their states; the federal government pays the remaining half. Medicaid expenditures have risen more rapidly than any other state expenditure and have caused states to reduce other politically popular programs so they will not be forced to increase taxes. At the federal level the government is also responsible for Medicare (acute medical services for the aged). The hospital portion of this program is financed by a specific Medicare payroll tax, which has been increased numerous times, and the physician portion of the program (Part B) is financed from general income taxes. Expenditures under both programs have risen rapidly.

As shown in Table 2.1, federal health spending as a proportion of total federal spending is increasing rapidly, from 12.4 percent of total federal expenditures in 1985, to 20.3 percent in 1995, to 24.7 percent in 2005, and to a projected 28.1 percent in 2011. As baby boomers begin to retire and become eligible for Medicare in 2011, Medicare expenditures are expected to increase dramatically. Unless the federal government can reform Medicare and reduce its growth rate, the Medicare payroll tax on the working population will be sharply increased to prevent the

Table 2.1: Federal Spending on Health, Fiscal Years 1965–2011 (Billions of Dollars)

	1965	1975	1985	1995	2005	2011*
Total federal spending	118.2	332.3	946.5	1,515.9	2,472.2	3,240.0
Federal health spending	3.1	29.5	117.1	307.1	610.4	910.5
Medicare	n/a	12.9	65.8	159.9	298.7	493.7
Medicaid	0.3	6.8	22.7	89.1	181.7	264.4
Veterans Administration	1.3	3.7	9.5	16.4	28.8	30.1
Other	1.5	6.1	19.1	41.7	101.2	122.3
Federal health spending as a percentage of total federal spending	2.6%	8.9%	12.4%	20.3%	24.7%	28.1%

*Projected data.

Source: The White House, Office of Management and Budget. 2007. "Budget of the United States Government: Historical Tables Fiscal Year 2007." [Online information.] http://origin.www.gpoaccess.gov/usbudget/fy07/pdf/hist.pdf.

Medicare trust fund from going bankrupt. Funding Medicare Part B and the new prescription drug benefit (Part D) will require increased income taxes, a very large federal deficit, or reductions in other popular federal programs.

Thus, even if there were no inefficiencies in the use or provision of medical services, increases in Medicare and Medicaid expenditures would still exceed what the government is willing to finance. If the government were the purchaser of 45 percent of all automobiles, the government would also become concerned with the price, use, and expenditures on automobiles. The pressure on government to continue funding Medicaid and Medicare through increased taxes or larger budget deficits is driving government to seek ways to limit medical expenditure increases.

Similarly, unions and their employers are concerned with the rise in employee medical expenditures for reasons other than inefficiencies in the provision or use of services. The business sector's spending on health insurance premiums has risen rapidly over time, both as a percentage of total employee compensation and as a percentage of business profits. Health insurance is part of an employee's total compensation. Employers are only interested in the total cost of an employee, not in the form in which the employee takes it, whether wages or health benefits. Thus, the employee bears the cost of rising health insurance premiums because a rise in health insurance premiums results in lower cash wages. Large unions with generous health benefits want to reduce the rise in medical expenditures because they have seen more of their gains in compensation spent to finance health insurance payments rather than to increase employee wages.

Large employers were also seriously affected by the Financial Accounting Standards Board ruling stating that, starting in 1993, employers who promised medical benefits to their retirees are required to list this unfunded liability on their balance sheets. Employers previously paid their retiree medical expenses only as they occurred and did not set aside funds, as is done with pensions. By having to acknowledge these liabilities on their balance sheets, the net worth of many large corporations, such as the automobile companies, declined by many billions of dollars. General Motors (GM), for example, has an unfunded retiree medical benefits liability of $77 billion. Furthermore, because these companies have to expense a portion of these future liabilities each year (not only for their present retirees but also for their future retirees), they have to report lower earnings per share. If the government were to reduce the rate of increase in medical expenditures, the net worth of companies with large unfunded retiree liabilities would increase, as would their earnings per share.

We must be aware that different reasons for concern over rising medical expenditures exist. Which concern should drive public policy—the desire by government not to raise revenues to fund its share of medical services, unions' and employers' interest in lowering employee and retiree medical expenses, or society's desire to achieve the appropriate rate of increase in medical expenditures? The interests of government, unions, and large employers have little to do with achieving an appropriate rate of growth in medical expenditures. Instead, their own political and economic burdens drive their proposals for limiting increases in medical expenditures.

APPROACHES TO LIMITING INCREASES IN MEDICAL EXPENDITURES

This country should strive to reduce inefficiencies in both the provision and use of medical services. Inefficiencies in the provision of services, however, are becoming smaller as managed care plans are forced to compete on price for enrollees. Vigilant application of the antitrust laws is needed to ensure that health care markets remain competitive and providers, such as hospitals, do not monopolize their markets. Inefficiencies in the use of services are declining as managed care plans control use of services through utilization management and patient cost sharing. As these inefficiencies are reduced, the growth in medical expenditures will approximate the "correct" rate of increase.

The public would naturally like to pay lower insurance premiums and less out-of-pocket costs for their medical care and still have unlimited access to health care and to the latest in medical technology. As in other sectors of the economy, however, choices must be made.

Unfortunately, some politicians believe they will receive the public's political support by proposing arbitrary limits on increases in medical expenditures and premiums, mandated discounts on drug prices for the aged, and managed care regulations that require that enrollees have freer access to specialists and other health care providers.

Medical expenditures have consistently increased faster than the rate of inflation, sometimes several times faster and other times just several percentage points greater than the inflation rate. Figure 2.1 shows the annual percentage change in health expenditures and inflation since 1965.

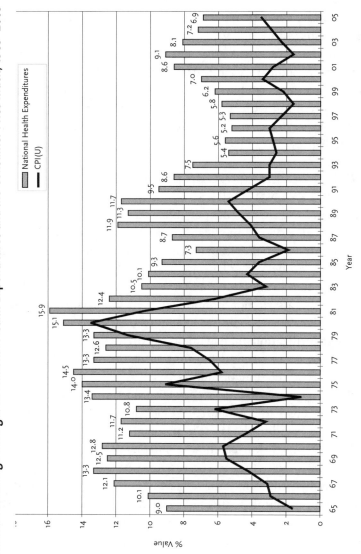

Figure 2.1: Annual Percentage Changes in National Health Expenditures and the Consumer Price Index, 1965–2005

Note: CPI(U) = consumer price index for all urban consumers.

Sources: DOL, Bureau of Labor Statistics. 2007. [Online information.] http://www.bls.gov/cpi/home.htm; U.S. Department of Health and Human Services; Centers for Medicare & Medicaid Services. 2007. [Online information.] http://www.cms.hhs.gov/NationalHealthExpendData/.

During the 1990s, expenditure increases moderated as managed care enrollment increased. Expenditures have increased more rapidly in recent years as a result of the backlash against managed care in the late 1990s and the consequent relaxation of managed care's cost-containment methods. As the population ages and new technology is developed, medical expenditures are expected to continue rising much faster than the inflation rate. If further regulations are imposed on how MCOs are able to achieve cost savings, expenditures and premiums will increase still faster.

What would be the consequences of holding expenditure and premium increases below what would otherwise occur in an efficient but aging and technologically advanced medical system?

The United States is undergoing important demographic changes; it is aging, and as it does so the population requires more medical services, both for relieving suffering and curing illnesses. Furthermore, the most important reason for the rapid rise in medical expenditures has been the tremendous advances in medical science. Previously incurable diseases can now be cured, other diseases can be diagnosed at an earlier stage, and for still others, although no cure is available, life can be prolonged, as with expensive drugs for AIDS patients. Limiting the growth in medical expenditures to an arbitrarily low rate will decrease investment in new technologies and limit the availability of medical services.

The cost-containment methods currently available can achieve some reduction in the rate of increase in medical expenditures; these would require imposing higher out-of-pocket payments; or, through the use of MCOs, requiring physicians to accept evidence-based medicine guidelines and disease management protocols; or restricting enrollees to use only participating physicians, specialists, and hospitals. The middle class, however, appears unwilling to make even these trade-offs; they want both lower expenditures and unlimited access. (Politicians are responding to these concerns by indicating their willingness to regulate broader access to providers and services without, however, indicating the higher premiums that would result.) Yet to really lower the rate of increase in expenditures and provide universal access to all will require more than just the cost-containment measures mentioned. Services and technology will have to become less available to many (Fuchs 1993).

Unfortunately, some politicians have led the public to believe these trade-offs are not necessary; they claim that by eliminating waste in the health system, universal coverage can be achieved and everyone can have all the medical care they need at a lower cost. Such rhetoric merely postpones the time when the public realizes it must make the unpleasant choice between spending and access to care.

However, once people understand that a trade-off must be made, they are likely to want to make their own choices about how much of their resources should be spent on medical care rather than having government or employer self-interest determine the rate of increase in medical expenditures. After all, who is better able to decide on issues of access and technology—and what those are worth—than the individuals who benefit from and must pay for those services?

SUMMARY

A basic decision that must be made with regard to medical services is who should decide how much is to be spent on medical care. Different countries have made different choices. In some countries the government decides on the allocation of resources to the different medical sectors and controls medical prices. When made by the government, trade-offs between cost and access are likely to be different from the choices made by consumers.

In the United States, except for Medicare and Medicaid, consumers determine the amount of their incomes to be spent on medical services. Although consumer sovereignty has been the guiding principle in allocating resources in the United States, inefficiencies in the medical sector have caused "too much" to be spent on medical services. Consumers have not always received "value for their money." Inappropriate provider incentives (and certain government regulations) have caused medical services to be more costly, and subsidies for the purchase of health insurance (tax-exempt employer-paid health insurance) have caused greater use of services.

The debate over the appropriate amount to be spent on medical services will be clarified once these two issues—the concept of consumer sovereignty and how to improve the efficiency of the current system—are separated.

DISCUSSION QUESTIONS

1. How does a competitive market determine the types of goods and services to be produced, how much it costs to produce those goods, and who receives them?

2. Why do economists believe the value of additional employer-paid health insurance is worth less than its full cost?

3. Why do rising medical expenditures cause concern?

4. What are the reasons for inefficiencies in the demand and provision of medical services?

5. Why are large employers and government concerned about rising medical expenditures?

REFERENCES

Feldstein, P. J. 2005. "The Demand for Medical Care." In *Health Care Economics*, 6th ed., 86–110. Albany, NY: Delmar Publishers.

Fuchs, V. R. 1993. "No Pain, No Gain—Perspectives on Cost Containment." *Journal of the American Medical Association* 269 (5): 631–33.

ADDITIONAL READINGS

Aaron, H. 2003. "Should Public Policy Seek to Control the Growth of Health Care Spending?" *Health Affairs* Web exclusive, January 8, W3-29–W3-36. [Online article; retrieved 11/15/06.] http://content.healthaffairs.org/cgi/reprint/hlthaff.w3.28v1.

Baker, L., H. Birnbaum, J. Geppert, D. Mishol, and E. Moyneur. 2003. "The Relationship Between Technology Availability and Health Care Spending." *Health Affairs* Web exclusive, November 5, W3-537–W3-551. [Online article; retrieved 11/15/06.] http://content.healthaffairs.org/cgi/reprint/hlthaff.w3.537v1.

Pauly, M. 2003. "Should We Be Worried About High Real Medical Spending Growth in the United States?" *Health Affairs* Web exclusive, January 8, W3-15–W3-27. [Online article; retrieved 11/15/06.] http://content.healthaffairs.org/cgi/reprint/hlthaff. w3.15v1.

Chapter 3

Do More Medical Expenditures Produce Better Health?

THE UNITED STATES spends more per capita on medical services and devotes a larger percentage of its GDP to medical care than other countries, yet our health status is not proportionately better. In fact, many countries that have lower per capita medical expenditures than the United States also have lower infant mortality rates and higher life expectancies. Is our medical system less efficient at producing good health than these other countries? Or are medical expenditures less important than other factors that affect health status?

MEDICAL SERVICES VERSUS HEALTH

Medical services are often mistakenly considered to be synonymous with health. When policymakers talk of "health reform," they really mean reform of the financing and delivery of medical services. Medical services consist of diagnosis and treatment of illness, which can lead to an increase in health. But medical services also consist of amelioration of pain and discomfort, reassurance to well people who are worried, and heroic treatments to those who are terminally ill. For example, 24 percent of all medical expenditures, $418 billion in 2003, are spent on just 1 percent of the population.[1] Increased medical expenditures, therefore, may have relatively little effect on a nation's health status.

---

1. Furthermore, in 2003, 49 percent of total medical expenditures were spent on 5 percent of the population. Nearly half of those upon whom a great amount of money was spent were elderly (Yu 2006).

The United States is generally acknowledged to have a technically superior medical system for treating acute illness (for a brief but excellent discussion of criteria to be used for evaluating a country's health system see Fuchs 1992). Financing and payment incentives have all been directed toward this goal. The training of physicians has emphasized treatment rather than prevention of illness. Public policy debates with regard to medical services have been concerned with two issues: (1) equity, namely whether everyone has access to medical services and how those services should be financed; and (2) efficiency, such as whether medical services are efficiently produced. Knowing how to produce a medical treatment more efficiently, however, is not the same as knowing how to produce health efficiently.

In contrast, health policy has been less well-defined. The goal of health policy presumably should be an improvement in health status or increased life expectancy, in which case we should be concerned with the most efficient ways to improve health status. Once the policy objective becomes focused on health and its efficient production, it is obvious that devoting increased resources to medical care is just one way to increase health and is *unlikely* to be the most efficient way to do so.

The more accurate the definition of health, the more difficult health is to measure. Health is a state of physical, mental, and social well-being. More simply, health is defined as the absence of disease or injury. Empirically, negative definitions are used to measure health, such as mortality rates, days lost to sickness, or life expectancy. Definitions of health can be broad, such as the use of age-adjusted mortality rates, or they can be disease specific, such as neonatal infant mortality rates (within the first 27 days of birth) and age-adjusted death rates from heart disease. The advantage of using such relatively crude measures is that they are readily available and are probably correlated with more comprehensive definitions of health. It should be remembered, however, that unavailability of measures of morbidity or quality of life does not mean they are unimportant or should be neglected in any analysis.

HEALTH PRODUCTION FUNCTION

To determine the relative importance of medical expenditures in decreasing mortality rates, economists have used the concept of a *health production function*. Simply stated, a health production function examines the relative contribution of each of the various factors that affect health to determine the most cost-effective way to improve health. For example, mortality rates are affected by the use of medical services, environmental conditions (such as the amount of air and water pollution), education levels (which may indicate knowledge of prevention and ability to use the medical system when needed), and lifestyle behavior (such as smoking, alcohol and substance abuse, diet, and exercise).

Each of these determinants of health has differential effects. For example, medical expenditures may initially cause a large decrease in mortality rates, as when a hospital establishes the first neonatal intensive care unit (NICU) in its community. As additional NICUs are added within that community, the decline in the neonatal infant mortality rate will become smaller. The first low-birth-weight infants admitted to the NICU will be those most likely to benefit from the medical care and continuous monitoring of their conditions. With a larger number of NICU beds, the beds may either be unused or the infants admitted to those beds will not be as critically ill or high risk. Investment in additional NICU beds will have less of an effect on infant mortality.

Figure 3.1 illustrates the relationship between increased medical expenditures and improvements in health status. Increased expenditures produce a curvilinear rather than a constant effect on improved health. The "marginal" (additional) change in health becomes smaller as more is spent on that particular program. As shown in Figure 3.1, an initial expenditure to improve health, moving from A to B, has a much larger marginal benefit (effect) than subsequent investments, such as moving from C to D. The increase from H_1 to H_2 is greater than the increase from H_3 to H_4.

This same curvilinear relationship holds for each of the other determinants of health. Expenditures to decrease air pollution, such as mandating smog-control devices on automobiles, will reduce the incidence of respiratory illness. Additional spending by automobile owners, such as having their smog-control devices tested once a year rather than every three years, will further reduce air pollution. The reduction in respiratory illness, however, will not be as great as the initial expenditure to install smog-control devices. The reduction in respiratory illness from additional expenditures to control air pollution gradually declines.

Everyone would probably agree that additional lives could be saved if more infants were admitted to NICUs (or respiratory illness decreased further with more frequent smog-control inspections). More intensive monitoring might save a patient's life. However, those same funds could be spent on prevention programs to decrease the number of low-birth-weight infants, such as prenatal care programs or education programs that decrease teen pregnancy. *The true "cost" of any program to*

Figure 3.1: Effect of Increased Medical Expenditures on Health

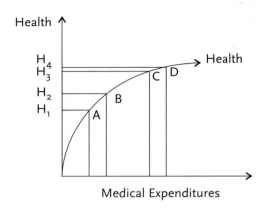

decrease mortality is the number of lives that could have been saved if those same funds had been spent on another program.

Physicians, hospitals, dentists, and other health professionals all want increased government expenditures to decrease the unmet needs among their populations. However, the government cannot possibly spend all that is necessary to eliminate all medical, dental, mental, and other needs. To do so would mean forgoing the opportunity to eliminate other needs, as in welfare and education, because resources are limited. At some point it becomes too costly in terms of forgone opportunities to save all the lives that medical science is capable of saving. Reallocating those same expenditures for apprehending drunk drivers or improving highways might save more lives.

Deciding which programs should be expanded to improve health status requires a calculation of the cost per life saved for each of the programs that affect mortality rates. Based on the curve in Figure 3.1, assume that an additional medical expenditure of $1 million results in a movement from H_3 to H_4, or C to D, saving 20 additional lives. The same $1 million spent on an education program to reduce smoking may result in a movement from H_1 to H_2, or A to B, saving an additional 40 lives from lung cancer. The smoking reduction program therefore results in a lower cost per life saved ($1,000,000/40 = $25,000) than if those same funds were spent on additional medical services ($1,000,000/20 = $50,000). Continued expenditures on smoking cessation programs will result in a movement along the curve. After some point, fewer lung cancer deaths will be prevented (the cost per life saved will therefore increase), and a lower cost per life saved could be achieved by spending additional funds on other programs such as stronger enforcement of drunk driving laws.

Crucial to the calculation of cost per life saved is knowing, first, where the program, such as medical treatments or smoking cessation, is on the curve shown in Figure 3.1 (that is, knowing the marginal benefit of that program) and, second, the cost of expanding that program. Dividing the cost of expanding each program by its marginal benefit enables a comparison of the cost per life saved. The enormous and rapidly increasing medical expenditures in the United States have most likely placed the return to medical services beyond point D. Further improvements in health status from continued medical expenditures are very small. The cost of expanding medical treatments has also become very expensive. Consequently, the cost per life saved through medical services is much higher than for other programs.

IMPROVING HEALTH STATUS COST EFFECTIVELY

Numerous empirical studies have found that further expenditures on medical services are not the most cost-effective way to improve health status. Medical programs have a much higher cost per life saved than nonmedical programs. Researchers have concluded that changing lifestyle behavior offers the greatest promise for lowering mortality rates, at a much lower cost per life saved.

The leading contributors to reductions in mortality rates over the past 30 years have been the decline in the neonatal infant mortality rate (infant deaths within the first 27 days of birth) and the reduction in deaths from heart disease.

Neonatal Infant Mortality Rate

The neonatal mortality rate represents about two-thirds (67 percent in 2004) of the overall infant mortality rate; the decline in the overall mortality rate has been primarily attributable to the decline in the neonatal rate. For a long time the neonatal infant mortality rate has steadily declined; however, starting in the mid-1960s the rate began declining more rapidly. The neonatal mortality rates for whites declined from 16.1 per 1,000 live births in 1965 to 3.8 in 2004, as shown in Figure 3.2. For African Americans the corresponding decline was from 26.5 to 9.0. During that period the availability of NICUs increased, government subsidies were provided for family planning services for low-income women, maternal and infant

Figure 3.2: Neonatal Mortality Rates, by Race, 1950–2004

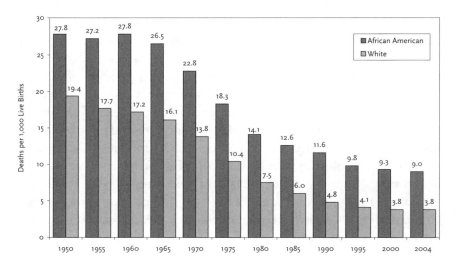

Sources: U.S. Census Bureau. 2006. *Statistical Abstract of the United States,* 1950–2000 data; National Center for Health Statistics. 2006. *Deaths: Preliminary Data for 2004. National Vital Statistics Report* 59 (14), June 28. [Online information.] http://www.cdc.gov/nchs/data/nvsr/nvsr54/nvsr54_19.pdf.

nutrition programs expanded, Medicaid was initiated and paid for obstetric services for those with low incomes, and abortion was legalized. One study found that increased education levels and subsidized nutrition programs were the most important factors in reducing the neonatal mortality rate among whites. The availability of abortion, followed by the availability of NICUs and the increase in education were the most important factors among African Americans.

Simply knowing the reasons for the decline in neonatal mortality, however, is insufficient for deciding how to spend money to reduce neonatal mortality; it is important to know which programs are more cost effective. Joyce, Corman, and Grossman (1988) determined that teenage family planning programs, NICUs, and prenatal care saved 0.6, 2.8, and 4.5 lives, respectively, per 1,000 additional participants. The corresponding costs of adding 1,000 participants to each of these programs (in 1984 dollars) were $122,000, $13,616,000, and $176,000. To determine the cost per life saved by expanding each of these programs, the cost of the program was divided by the number of lives saved. As shown in Table 3.1, the cost per life saved was $203,000 ($122,000/0.6) for teenage family

Table 3.1: Cost per Life Saved Among Three Programs to Reduce Neonatal Mortality (Whites)

	Number of Lives Saved per 1,000 Additional Participants	Cost of Each Program per 1,000 Additional Participants (in Thousands*)	Cost per Life Saved (in Thousands*)
Teenage family planning	0.6	$122	$203
NICUs	2.8	$13,616	$4,778
Prenatal care	4.5	$176	$39

*In 1984 dollars.

Source: Reprinted with permission as it appeared in T. Joyce, H. Corman, and M. Grossman. 1988. "A Cost-Effectiveness Analysis of Strategies to Reduce Infant Mortality." *Medical Care* 26 (April): 348–60. © 1988 J.B. Lippincott Company.

planning, $4,778,000 for NICUs, and $39,000 for prenatal care, which was the most cost-effective program for reducing neonatal mortality. Reducing the potential number of women in high-risk pregnancies and the number of unwanted births (e.g., by providing teenage family planning programs and prenatal care) offers a greater possibility of more favorable birth outcomes than investing in additional NICUs.

Heart Disease Mortality Rate

The leading cause of death in the United States is cardiovascular disease. Between 1970 and 2004, the mortality rate from diseases of the heart declined more rapidly than any other cause of death, from 362 per 100,000 to 223 per 100,000. Improvements in medical technology (such as coronary bypass surgery, coronary care units, angioplasty, and clot-dissolving drugs) as well as changes in lifestyle (such as the reduction in smoking, increased exercise, and changes in diet that lower cholesterol levels) contributed to this decline in mortality from heart disease. One study estimated that the development of new treatment techniques and their increased use over time decreased cardiovascular disease deaths by about one-third. The remaining two-thirds of the reduction in deaths from heart disease are attributed to a reduction in risk factors through

prevention, including new drugs to control hypertension, high cholesterol, and smoking cessation (Cutler and Kadiyala 2003). These lifestyle
changes, however, are not uniform among the population; those with
more education are more likely to undertake them.

The above study, as well as many others that have examined the reduction in heart disease deaths over time, reach similar conclusions,
that *lifestyle changes are more important—and much less expensive—than
medical interventions* (Feldstein 2005).

Causes of Death by Age Group

Perhaps the clearest indication of the importance of lifestyle behavior
as a determinant of mortality is the causes of death by age group. As
shown in Table 3.2, the main causes of death for young adults (aged 15 to
24 years) are accidents (particularly auto), homicides, and suicides. For
those in the middle age groups, human immunodeficiency virus (HIV)
infection, accidents, cancer, heart disease, suicides, and homicides are
the major causes of death. For those in late middle age, cancer and heart
disease are the leading causes of death. After examining data by cause
of death, Victor Fuchs (1974, 46) concluded that medical services have a
smaller effect on health than the way in which people live: "The greatest
potential for reducing coronary disease, cancer, and the other major kill-
ers still lies in altering personal behavior."

RELATIONSHIP OF MEDICAL CARE
TO HEALTH OVER TIME

The above studies have shown that the marginal contribution of medical
care to improved health is relatively small. Improvements in health status can be achieved in a less-costly manner through increased spending
on lifestyle factors. Over time, however, there have been major technologic advances in medical care, such as new drugs to lower cholesterol
and hypertension, diagnostic imaging, less-invasive surgery, transplants,
and treatment for previously untreatable diseases. Few would deny that
these technologic advances have reduced mortality rates and increased
life expectancy.

Cutler and Richardson (1999) reconcile these seemingly conflicting
findings of medical care's relatively low marginal contribution to health
and technologic advances that have clearly increased life expectancy;
they separate medical care's effect at a point in time versus its technologic
contribution over time. The authors illustrate the relationship between

Table 3.2: Leading Causes of Death, by Age Group, 2004

Age Group (Years)	Major Causes of Death	Deaths per 100,000
15–24	All causes	78.9
	Accidents	36.4
	Homicide and legal intervention	11.7
	Suicide	10.1
	Cancer	4.0
	Heart disease	2.3
25–44	All causes	147.8
	Accidents	33.6
	Cancer	21.7
	Heart disease	18.7
	Suicide	13.6
	Homicide and legal intervention	8.5
	HIV infection	7.5
45–64	All causes	621.0
	Cancer	205.5
	Heart disease	141.5
	Accidents	35.8
	Diabetes mellitus	23.0
	Cerebrovascular disease	22.7
	Pulmonary disease	21.7
	Chronic liver disease/cirrhosis	19.5

Source: National Center for Health Statistics. 2006. *Deaths: Preliminary Data for 2004. National Vital Statistics Report* 54 (19), June 28, Table 7.

the total contribution of medical care to health and greater quantities of medical care using Figure 3.3. Comprehensive health insurance combined with fee-for-service physician payment reduces both the patient's and physician's incentive to be concerned with the cost of care, resulting in the medical care system moving to point A in Figure 3.3, where the marginal contribution of medical care to health is very small. Additional medical care expenditures increase health, but at a decreasing rate.

Over time, however, medical advances shift the production function for health upward. The level of health has improved, and the number of

Figure 3.3: Relationship Between Medical Care and Health

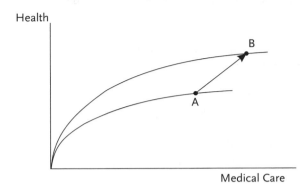

Source: Reprinted from Cutler, D. M., and E. Richardson. 1999. "Your Money and Your Life: The Value of Health and What Affects It." In *Frontiers in Health Policy Research*, vol. 2, ed. A. Garber, pp. 99–132, Figure 5-6. Cambridge, MA: MIT Press.

patients treated has increased, but the marginal contribution of medical care is still low, point B. Too many patients whose need for treatment is doubtful are treated with the new technology or excess capacity occurs as too much of the new technology is made available.

Thus, although the public believes the medical care they receive today is much more valuable than treatments received 30 years ago, the medical care system remains inefficient; the marginal benefit of additional medical care expenditures is low (Skinner, Staiger, and Fisher 2006).

SUMMARY

If expenditures on medical services have been shown to be less cost effective in reducing mortality rates than are changes in lifestyle behavior, why does the United States spend an increasing portion of its resources on medical care?

First, health insurance coverage has been so comprehensive, with low deductibles and small copayments, that individuals faced a very low out-of-pocket price when they went to the hospital or a specialist. Thus, patients used more medical services than if they had to pay a greater portion of the cost. The expression "the insurance will cover it" is indicative of the lack of incentives facing patients and their providers. The public has also had little incentive to compare prices among different providers, as the costs they would incur searching for less-expensive providers would exceed any savings on their already low copayments. It is also not surprising, given these low copayments and the incentives inherent in fee-for-service payments to providers, that enormous resources are spent on those in their last year of life. Rapidly rising medical expenditures and limited reductions in mortality rates are the consequences of this behavior.

Second, the primary objective of government medical expenditures has not been to improve health and decrease mortality rates. Medicare benefits the elderly, and approximately half of Medicaid expenditures are spent for care of the elderly in nursing homes. The purpose of these government expenditures is to help the aged finance their medical needs. Were the government's objective to improve the nation's health, the types of services financed would be very different, as would the age groups who would most benefit from those expenditures. (One should also remember that the aged are perhaps the most politically powerful group in society.)

Although medical expenditures have a relatively small marginal effect on health, it would be incorrect to conclude that the government should limit all medical expenditure increases. To an individual, additional medical services may be worth their additional cost even when they are not subsidized. As incomes increase, people are willing to purchase medical services to relieve anxiety and seek relief of pain, which are not life-saving events but are entirely appropriate personal expenditures. From society's perspective, financing medical services for those with low incomes is also appropriate. As society becomes wealthier, individuals and government are willing to make more non–life-saving medical expenditures. These "consumption" versus "investment" types of medical expenditures are appropriate as long as all recognize them for what they are.

When government attempts to improve the health of those with low incomes, using the concept of a health production function, expenditures will be directed toward the most cost-effective programs, that is, those that result in the lowest cost per life saved. Allocating funds in this manner will achieve a greater reduction in mortality rates for a given total expenditure than any other allocation method.

The health production function concept is increasingly used by employers and MCOs that face financial pressures to reduce their medical costs. Employer use of health risk appraisal questionnaires recognizes that employees' health can be improved less expensively by changes in lifestyle behavior. Incentives given to employees to stop smoking, reduce their weight, and exercise enable employers to retain a skilled workforce longer while reducing medical expenditures. The emphasis by MCOs on reducing per capita medical costs has led them to identify their high-risk groups who can benefit from early preventive measures to reduce costly medical treatments.

The recognition by government, employers, MCOs, and individuals that resources are scarce and that their objective is improved health rather than provision of additional medical services will lead to new approaches to improve health. The concept of a health production function should clarify the trade-offs between different programs and improve the allocation of expenditures.

DISCUSSION QUESTIONS

1. How can a health production function allocate funds to improve health status?

2. Why does this country spend an increasing portion of its resources on medical services, although they are less cost effective than other methods for improving health status?

3. How can employers use the concept of a health production function for decreasing their employees' medical expenditures?

4. Describe a production function for decreasing deaths from coronary heart disease.

5. Describe a production function for decreasing deaths of young adults.

REFERENCES

Cutler, D. M., and S. Kadiyala. 2003. "The Return to Biomedical Research: Treatment and Behavioral Effects." In *Measuring the Gains from Medical Research: An Economic Approach,* edited by K. M. Murphy and R. H. Topel, 110–62. Chicago: The University of Chicago Press.

Cutler, D. M., and E. Richardson. 1999 "Your Money and Your Life: The Value of Health and What Affects It." In *Frontiers in Health Policy Research,* vol. 2, edited by A. Garber, 99–132. Cambridge, MA: MIT Press.

Feldstein, P. J. 2005. "The Production of Health: The Impact of Medical Services on Health." In *Health Care Economics,* 6th ed., 30–47. Albany, NY: Delmar Publishers.

Fuchs, V. R. 1974. *Who Shall Live?* New York: Basic Books, 30–55.

———. 1992. "The Best Health Care System in the World?" *Journal of the American Medical Association* 268 (19): 916–17.

Joyce, T., H. Corman, and M. Grossman. 1988. "A Cost-Effectiveness Analysis of Strategies to Reduce Infant Mortality." *Medical Care* 26 (4): 348–60.

Skinner, J., D. Staiger, and E. Fisher. 2006. "Is Technological Change In Medicine Always Worth It? The Case of Acute Myocardial Infarction." *Health Affairs,* Web exclusive, February 7, 2006, W-34–W-47. [Online article; retrieved 11/15/06.] http://content.healthaffairs.org/cgi/content/abstract/25/2/w34.

Yu, W. W. 2006. Personal communiction. June 5.

Chapter 4

In Whose Interest Does the Physician Act?

PHYSICIANS HAVE ALWAYS played a crucial role in the delivery of medical services. Although only 25 percent of personal medical expenditures are for physician services, physicians control the use of a much larger portion of total medical resources. In addition to their own services, physicians determine admission to the hospital, the length of stay once in the hospital, the use of ancillary services and prescription drugs, referrals to specialists, and even the necessity for services in non-hospital settings such as home care. Any public policies that affect the financing and delivery of medical services must consider physicians' responses to those policies. A physician's knowledge and motivation will affect the efficiency with which medical services are delivered.

The role of the physician has been shaped by two important characteristics of the medical system. The first is the legal system: Only physicians are permitted to provide certain services. Second, both patients and insurers lack the necessary information to make many medically related decisions. The patient depends on the physician for the diagnosis and the recommended treatment and has limited information on the qualifications of the physician or the specialists to whom he is referred. This lack of information on diagnosis, required treatment, and quality of medical providers places patients in a unique relationship to physicians: The physician becomes the patient's agent.

THE PHYSICIAN AS A PERFECT AGENT
FOR THE PATIENT

A major controversy in the medical economics literature involves the agency relationship. In whose best interest does the physician act? If a physician were a *perfect agent* for the patient, he would prescribe the mix of institutional settings and the amount of care in each based on the patient's medical needs, ability to pay for medical services, and preferences. The physician would behave, as would the patient, as if the patient were as fully informed as the physician. Traditional indemnity insurance, once the prevalent form of health insurance, reimbursed the physician on a fee-for-service basis; neither the physician nor the patient was fiscally responsible or at risk for using the hospital and medical services.

Before the 1980s, BlueCross predominantly covered hospital care. Although hospital stays are more costly in terms of resources used, patients paid less to receive a diagnostic workup in the hospital than they would as outpatients. Although this was an inefficient use of resources, the physician acted in the patient's interest and not the insurer's. Similarly, if a woman wanted to stay a few extra days in the hospital after giving birth, the physician would not discharge her before she was ready to return home.

As the patient's agent, the quantity and type of services the physician prescribes would be based on the value of that additional care to the patient and the patient's cost for that care. As long as the value of that care to the patient exceeds the patient's costs for that care, the physician would prescribe it. Considering only the patient's costs and benefits of additional medical services neglected the costs to society of those resources and the costs to the insurance company.

Indemnity insurance and the role of the physician as the patient's agent led the physician to practice what Victor Fuchs (1968) referred to as the *technologic imperative*. Regardless of how small the benefits to the patient or how costly to the insurer, the physician would prescribe the best medical care technically possible. As a consequence, heroic measures were provided to patients in the last few months of their lives, and inpatient hospital costs rose rapidly. Prescribing "low-benefit" care was a rational economic decision because it still exceeded the patient's cost, which was virtually zero with comprehensive insurance.

SUPPLIER-INDUCED DEMAND

The view of the physician as the patient's agent, however, neglects the economic self-interest of the physician. As shown in Figure 4.1, large increases in both the total number of physicians and the number of physicians relative to the population occurred throughout the 1970s and 1980s. The standard economic model, which assumes the physician is a

Figure 4.1: Number of Active Physicians and Physician–Population Ratio, 1950–2004

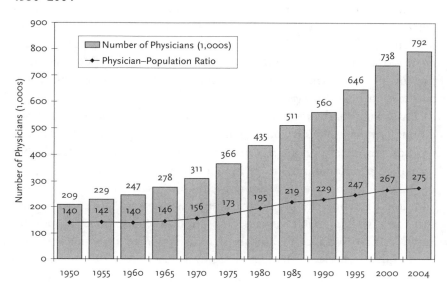

Note: Physician–population ratio is for active physicians and noninstitutionalized civilian population. Active physicians are federal and nonfederal physicians who are involved in patient care or non-patient care (teaching, research administration, or other professional activities) for more than 20 hours a week. Active physicians also include unclassified physicians, that is, physicians whose activity status or present employment setting are not known.

Sources: Division of Survey and Data Resources. *Physician Characteristics and Distribution in the United States*, 1981, 2006 eds. Chicago: American Medical Association, 1982, 2006; U.S. Census Bureau. *Statistical Abstract of the United States,* various editions.

perfect agent for the patient, would predict that an increase in supply, other things being equal, would result in a *decline* in physicians' fees, visits per physician, and, consequently, physician incomes.

Increases in the physician–population ratio, however, did not lead to declines in physician incomes. This observation led to the development of an alternative theory of physician behavior. Physicians are believed to behave differently when their own incomes are adversely affected. In addition to being the patient's agent, physicians are a supplier of a service. Their incomes depend on how much of that service they supply. Do physicians use their information advantage over both patients and insurers to benefit themselves? This model of physician behavior is referred to as *supplier-induced demand*.

The supplier-induced demand theory assumes that if the physician's income falls, the physician will use her role as the patient's agent to prescribe additional services. The physician provides the patient with misinformation to increase the patient's demand for physician services, thereby increasing the physician's income. In other words, the physician becomes an *imperfect agent*.

Physicians might rationalize some demand inducement in that additional services or tests would be beneficial to the patient. However, as more and more services are recommended, the physician must choose between the additional income received and the psychologic cost of knowing those additional services are not really necessary. At some point, the additional revenue the physician receives is not worth the psychologic cost of prescribing such services. The physician must make a trade-off between increased income and the dissatisfaction of knowingly providing too many services. The idea that physicians induce demand only to the extent that they can maintain or achieve a given level of income is referred to as the *target income theory*.

Thus, one might envisage a spectrum of demand inducement depending on the psychologic cost to the physician of greater demand inducement. At one end of the spectrum are those physicians who act solely in their patients' interests; they do not induce demand to increase or even maintain their incomes. At the other end of the spectrum are physicians who attempt to increase their incomes by inducing demand as much as possible; these physicians presumably incur little psychologic cost when they induce demand. In the middle are physicians who induce demand to achieve some target level of income.

The extent to which the physician is willing and able to induce additional demand for medical services is controversial. Few believe the majority of physicians would induce demand as much as possible solely to increase their incomes. Similarly, few would disagree that physicians are able to induce some additional demand. Thus, the choice is mainly between physicians as perfect agents for their patients and the target income model of physician behavior. The issue is how much demand physicians are able to induce.

Demand inducement is limited to some extent by the patient's recognition that the additional medical benefits are not worth the time or cost of returning to the physician. The patient's evaluation of the benefits from additional medical services, however, varies according to the treatment prescribed. Patients may more easily determine that additional office visits are not worth their time and the cost of returning; however, patients have more difficulty evaluating the benefits from certain surgical services. Thus, demand inducement is more likely to occur for those services about which the patient is most ignorant.

Many studies have attempted to determine the extent of demand inducement (see, for example, Feldstein 2005), and the issue is still unresolved. Evidence shows that geographic areas (cities and counties) that have a larger supply of physicians (in relation to the population) also have a greater per capita use of physician services. This relationship, however, may merely indicate that physicians locate where the population has higher insurance coverage and, consequently, a greater demand for their services. One study concluded that primary care physicians are limited in the amount of demand they can induce, although how much demand they may already have induced remains unknown. The positive correlation between the number of surgeons and the number of surgeries has been used as empirical support for the supplier-induced demand theory. Furthermore, studies have found the rate of surgeries for procedures such as tonsillectomies and hysterectomies to be higher when physicians are paid fee-for-service than when they have different income incentives, such as being part of an HMO. Demand inducement appears to be more of a concern with surgeries because patients are less well-informed about whether they need the surgery.

INCREASE IN PHYSICIAN SUPPLY

The large increase in physician supply since the 1960s illustrates the importance of knowing which model of physician behavior, the perfect agent or supplier-induced demand, is more prevalent. As a perfect agent for the patient, the physician would continue to consider only the patient's medical and economic interests when prescribing a treatment, regardless of the fact that his income may decline because the greater supply of physicians may decrease the number of patients seen.

According to the supplier-induced demand model, an increase in the supply of physicians will cause physicians to induce demand to prevent their incomes from falling. Total physician expenditures would also increase as a larger number of physicians, each with fewer patients, attempt to maintain their incomes. Thus, depending on whether one believes in standard economic models or supplier-induced demand, increases in the supply of physicians lead to quite opposite predictions of their effect on physician visits, prices, and incomes.

INSURERS' RESPONSE TO DEMAND INDUCEMENT

Insurers recognize that under fee-for-service payment physicians act as either the patient's agent or to maintain their own income. In either case the value of additional benefits prescribed by a physician is lower than the insurer's cost of those services. Consequently, the premium for indemnity insurance will be higher for a fee-for-service environment than for HMOs, which theoretically attempt to relate the value of additional medical treatment to the resource costs of those additional medical services. As a result of the higher relative premium of indemnity insurance to that of HMOs, more of the insurer's subscribers will switch to HMOs. In recent years, therefore, insurers have developed mechanisms to overcome the information advantage that physicians have over both the insurers and the patients to serve either the patients' or the physicians' interests.

Insurers have, for example, implemented second-opinion requirements for surgery. Once a physician recommends certain types of surgery of doubtful medical necessity, such as back surgery, a patient may be required to receive a second opinion from a list of physicians approved by the insurer. Another approach insurers use is the creation of PPOs. Physicians are selected on the basis of whether they offer lower fees, use fewer medical services, and are considered to be of high quality. A third approach is utilization review. Before a hospital admission a patient must receive the insurer's approval; otherwise, the patient is subject to a financial penalty. The length of stay in the hospital is also subject to the insurer's approval.

These cost-containment approaches by insurers are an attempt to address the imbalances in physician and patient incentives under a fee-for-service system. Furthermore, they ensure that the patient receives appropriate care (when the physician acts to increase her own income) and that the resource costs of a treatment are considered along with its expected benefits.

HMOs

The growth of HMOs and capitation payment provides physicians with incentives to increase their incomes that are opposite from those of the traditional indemnity fee-for-service approach. HMOs typically reward their physicians with profit sharing or bonuses if their enrollees' medical costs are lower than their annual capitation payments. What are the likely effects of these differing models of physician behavior—the perfect agent and the imperfect agent—on an HMO's patients?

In an HMO setting a perfect-agent type of physician would continue to provide the patient with appropriate medical services. Regardless of the effect of profit sharing on his income or pressures from the HMO to reduce use of services, the perfect-agent physician would be primarily concerned with protecting the patients' interests and providing them with the best medical care, so there is little likelihood of underservice. Unlike indemnity insurance, within an HMO the physician would not need to be concerned over whether the patient's insurance covered the medical cost in different settings. HMO patients are also responsible for fewer deductibles and copayments. Thus, the settings chosen for providing the patient's treatment are likely to be less costly for both the patient and the HMO.

The concern that patients would be underserved in an HMO exists with regard to imperfect-agent physicians, those who attempt to increase their incomes. HMO physicians have an incentive to provide fewer services to their patients and to serve a larger number of patients. Those HMO physicians who are concerned with the size of their incomes are more likely to respond to profit-sharing incentives. At times a physician, who may even be salaried, may succumb to an HMO's pressures to reduce use of services and thereby become an imperfect agent. If HMO patients believe they are being denied timely access to the physician, specialist services, or needed technology, they are likely to try to switch HMO physicians or disenroll at the next open enrollment period. Too high a rate of dissatisfaction with certain HMO physicians could indicate that their patients are underserved.

An HMO should be concerned with underservice by its physicians. Although the HMO's profitability will increase if its physicians provide too few services, an HMO that limits access to care and fails to satisfy its subscribers risks losing market share.

The more knowledgeable subscribers are about access to care provided by different HMOs, the greater will be the HMO's financial incentive not to pressure its physicians to underserve its patients and to actually monitor physicians to guard against underservice. Although it is costly in terms of both time and money for individuals to gather information on HMOs and their physicians or on how well their enrollees are served, it is less costly for employers to gather this information, make it available to their employees, and even limit the HMOs from which their employees can choose.

INFORMED PURCHASERS

Informed purchasers are necessary if the market is to discipline imperfect agents, which may be the HMO itself or its physicians. An HMO's reputation is an expensive asset that can be reduced by imperfect-agent physicians underserving their patients. Performance information and competition among HMOs for informed purchasers should prevent these organizations from underserving their enrollees. The financial, reputational, and legal costs of underservice should mitigate the financial incentives to underprescribe in an HMO.

Both indemnity insurers and HMOs lack information on a patient's diagnosis and appropriate treatment needs. Thus, the insurer's (or HMO's) profitability depends on the physician's knowledge and treatment recommendations. Depending on the type of insurance plan and the incentives physicians face, a potential inefficiency exists in the provision of medical services. Physicians may prescribe "too many" or "too few" services. When too many services are prescribed, the value of those additional services to the patient may not be worth the costs of producing them. Too few services are also inefficient in that patients may not realize that the value of the services and technology they did not receive (and for which they were willing to pay) is greater than their physician led them to believe. To decrease the inefficiencies arising from too many services as a result of demand inducement, indemnity insurers who pay physicians on a fee-for-service basis have instituted cost-containment methods.

Medicare, as a fee-for-service insurer for physician services for the aged, has not yet undertaken similar cost-containment methods to limit supplier-induced demand. Until Medicare is able to institute such mechanisms, imperfect-agent physicians will continue to be able to manipulate the information they provide to the aged, change the visit coding to receive higher payment, and decrease the time spent per visit with aged patients.

Monitoring of physician behavior is increasing within HMOs and other managed care insurers. Physicians who were previously in fee-for-service and who increased their incomes by prescribing too many services are being reviewed to ensure that they understand the change in incentives. Once they are aware of the new incentives for increasing their incomes, imperfect-agent physicians must be monitored to ensure that they do not underserve their HMO patients.

The market for medical services is changing. Insurers and large employers are attempting to overcome the physicians' information advantage by profiling physicians according to their prices, use and appropriateness of services provided, and treatment outcomes. These profiles will allow imperfect-agent physicians less opportunity to benefit at the expense of the insurer. Demand inducement, to the extent that it exists, will diminish. One hopes that with improved monitoring systems and better measures of patient outcomes, physicians will behave as perfect agents, providing the "appropriate" quantity and quality of medical services, where the costs as well as the benefits of additional treatment are considered.

Insurers serving millions of enrollees will have very large data sets, which, with information technology, they will be able to use for analyzing different treatment methods along with different physician practice patterns. These data will enable insurers to determine which physicians deviate from accepted medical norms in their treatment patterns.

Not all insurers or employers, however, are engaged in these informational and cost-containment activities. Those who are not will still be at an informational disadvantage to the physician and the HMO. Insurers and employers who are less knowledgeable regarding the services provided to their employees will pay for overuse of services and demand-inducing behavior by fee-for-service providers and underservice by HMO physicians. At some point such purchasers will realize that investing in more information will lower their medical expenditures and improve the quality of care provided.

SUMMARY

Under fee-for-service payment the inability of patients and their insurers to distinguish between imperfect-agent and perfect-agent physicians led to the growth of cost-containment methods. The changes occurring in the private sector and in government physician payment systems must take into account different types of physicians and the fact that, unless appropriately monitored, the response by imperfect-agent physicians will make achieving the intended objectives difficult.

DISCUSSION QUESTIONS

1. Why do physicians play such a crucial role in the delivery of medical services?

2. How might a decrease in physician incomes, possibly as a result of an increase in the number of physicians, affect their role as the patient's agent?

3. What are some of the ways in which insurers seek to compensate for physicians' information advantage?

4. What forces currently limit supplier-induced demand?

5. How do fee-for-service and capitation payment systems affect the physician's role as the patient's agent?

REFERENCES

Feldstein, P. J. 2005. *Health Care Economics*, 6th ed., 97–99, 234–41. Albany, NY: Delmar Publishers.

Fuchs, V. R. 1968. "The Growing Demand for Medical Care." *The New England Journal of Medicine* 279 (4): 190–95.

ADDITIONAL READINGS

De Jaegher, K., and M. Jegers. 2000. "A Model of Physician Behaviour with Demand Inducement." *Journal of Health Economics* 19 (2): 231–58.

Rizzo, J., and D. Blumenthal. 1996. "Is the Target Income Hypothesis Economic Heresy?" *Medical Care Research and Review* 53 (3): 243–66.

Chapter 5

Rationing Medical Services

NO COUNTRY CAN afford to provide unlimited amounts of medical services to everyone. Although few would disagree that there is waste in the current system, all of this country's medical needs could not be fulfilled even if that waste were eliminated and those resources redirected. A large, one-time savings would result from eliminating inefficiencies, but driven by population growth, an aging population, and advances in medical technology, medical expenditures would continue to increase at a rate faster than inflation. As new experimental treatments, such as lung reduction surgery, are developed—no matter how uncertain or small their effect might be—making them routinely available to all those who might conceivably benefit would be very costly. The resources needed to eliminate all of our medical needs, including prescription drugs, mental health, long-term care, dental, and vision, as well as for services that are acute, chronic, and preventive, would be enormous.

The cost of eliminating all medical needs, no matter how small, means forgoing the benefits of spending those resources to meet other needs, such as food, clothing, housing, and education. Forgoing these other needs is the real cost of fulfilling all of our medical needs. As no country can afford to spend unlimited resources on medical services, each society must choose some mechanism to ration or limit access to medical services.

GOVERNMENT RATIONING

Rationing occurs by two methods. The first and most frequently used method is government limits on access to goods and services. In World War II, for example, food, gasoline, and other goods were rationed; their prices were kept artificially low but people could not buy all they wanted at the prevailing price. Similarly, in the 1970s, a gasoline shortage developed when the government kept the price of gasoline below its market price. The available supply was "rationed" by having people wait long hours at gasoline stations, although they were willing, but not permitted, to pay higher prices.

This type of rationing is also used to allocate medical services in other countries such as Great Britain (Aaron and Schwartz 1990). The British government sets low prices for medical services and limits expenditures on those services. Because there is a shortage of services at their prevailing prices, these scarce services are allocated according to a person's age, as when denying kidney transplants to those over a certain age, or according to a queue, in which a person may wait months or even years for certain surgical procedures, such as hip replacements.

In the United States only the state of Oregon proposed such an explicit system of rationing medical services. In contrast to other states, which provide unlimited medical services to a small portion of the poor, the Oregon legislature decided to limit Medicaid recipients' access to expensive procedures, such as organ transplants, and in turn increase Medicaid eligibility to more low-income persons. The state ranked all medical services according to the outcomes that could be expected from treatment (e.g., "prevents death with full recovery") and according to their effect on quality of life. Because the state budget is unlikely to ever be sufficient to fund all medical procedures to all of the poor, those procedures at the lower end of the rankings would not be funded.

RATIONING BY ABILITY TO PAY

Among the general population in the United States such explicit rationing of medical services is not used. Instead, a different type of rationing is used, essentially to distribute goods and services according to those who can afford to pay for them. There are no shortages of services for those who are willing to pay (either out of pocket or through insurance). People with low incomes and without health insurance receive fewer medical services than those who have higher incomes.

Medical services involve a great deal of discretionary use. Empirical studies show that a 10 percent increase in income leads to an approximate 10 percent increase in medical expenditures. As incomes increase, the amount spent on medical services increases proportionally. This relationship between income and medical spending exists not only in this

Figure 5.1: Health Spending and Personal Income in Different Countries, 2003

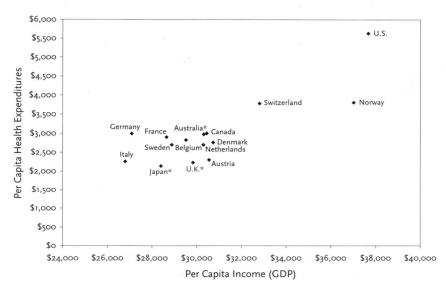

*Per capita health expenditures for 2002.

Note: All values are U.S. dollars measured in GDP purchasing power parities.

Source: Organisation for Economic Cooperation and Development. 2005. *Health at a Glance.* Paris: OECD. Tables A.3.1., A.5.5.

country but also across all countries. As shown in Figure 5.1, the higher the country's income, the greater its medical expenditures.

This observed relationship between income and medical expenditures suggests that as people become wealthier they prefer to spend more on medical care to receive a greater quantity of services and higher-quality services by making greater use of specialists, and they are willing to pay more to avoid waiting to receive those services.

DECISION MAKING BY CONSUMERS OF MEDICAL SERVICES

Thus, understanding why people use medical services requires more than knowing whether they are ill. Also important are their attitudes toward seeking care, the prices they must pay for such care, and their incomes.

Whether rationing is based on ability to pay or on government expenditure limits on medical services, patients are faced with prices they must pay for medical services. These prices may be artificially low, as in Great Britain or Canada, or they may reflect the cost of providing those medical services, as in a market-oriented system like the United States. Regardless of how those prices are determined, they are an essential ingredient for consumer decision making.

Consumers spend (allocate) their money based on the value they place on different needs, how much income they have, and the prices of their different choices. Consumers are faced with an array of choices, each offering additional benefits, but each choice costs a different amount. Consumers choose not just on the basis of the additional benefits they would receive, but also on the cost of achieving those benefits. In this manner prices enable consumers to decide to which services they will allocate their incomes.

Of course, making one choice means forgoing other choices. Similarly, as the prices of some choices increase while others decrease, consumers are likely to rearrange their purchases. An increase in income allows consumers to buy more of everything.

MARGINAL BENEFIT CURVE

Figure 5.2 illustrates the relationship between use of services and the cost to the patient of those services. The marginal benefit curve shows that the additional (marginal) benefit the patient receives from additional visits declines as use of services increases. For example, a patient concerned about her health will benefit greatly from the first physician visit. The physician will take the patient's history, perhaps perform some diagnostic tests, and possibly write a prescription. A follow-up visit will enable the physician to determine whether the diagnosis and treatment were appropriate and provide reassurance to the patient. The marginal benefit of that second visit will not be as high as the first visit. Additional return visits without any indication of a continuing health problem will provide further reassurance, but the value to the patient of those additional visits will be much lower than the initial visits.

How rapidly the marginal benefit curve declines depends on the patient's attitudes toward seeking care and the value she places on that additional care. Not all patients place the same value on medical services. For some, the marginal benefit curve will decline very quickly after the initial treatment; for others, the decline will be very gradual.

Figure 5.2: Relationship Among Prices, Visits, and Marginal Benefit of an Additional Visit

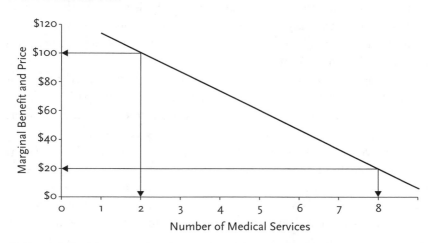

The actual number of patient visits is determined by the cost to the patient for each visit. Given the patient's marginal benefit curve and a price per visit of $100, as shown in Figure 5.2, the marginal benefit to the patient of the first visit exceeds the cost of $100. The patient will demand a total of two visits because the marginal benefit of that second visit equals the cost of that visit. If the patient made more than two visits, the value the patient receives from the third visit would be less than its cost.

Thus, the demand for medical services is determined by the value to the patient (either real or imagined) of those visits and the patient's cost for each visit. When the cost is greater than the value of an additional visit, the patient will not make the additional visit; the patient could receive greater value for his money by spending it on other goods and services.

Health insurance reduces the patient's costs for medical care. Although the insurer pays the physician (or hospital) the full price, the patient pays a reduced out-of-pocket price. For example, if the charge for a physician's office visit is $100 and health insurance pays 80 percent of the charge, the "real" price to the patient is only $20. As the patient's cost for an office visit declines from $100 to $20, the patient will increase the number of visits. The patient will make additional visits until the value received from the last visit is worth only $20.

The patient's decision to use medical services is based solely on a calculation of her own costs (copayment) and the perceived value of those additional visits. Although the real cost of each visit is $100, the patient's cost for additional visits is only $20. The consequence is "too much" medical care; the value to the patient of additional visits is worth less than the full cost of those visits.

In using medical services, the patient usually incurs travel and waiting costs. The importance of these costs differs among patients. Typically, retired persons have low waiting costs, whereas working mothers have high waiting costs. To predict use of services, travel and waiting costs, as well as out-of-pocket payments, must be weighed against the marginal benefit of another visit. A medical system that has high out-of-pocket payments and low waiting costs will affect usage patterns differently than a system that relies on low prices but high waiting costs.

An important empirical question is this: How rapid is the decline in value of additional services to the patient? If the first visit is worth more than $100 to the patient and the second visit is only worth $10, little if any overuse of medical services will occur. If, however, a second visit is worth $100 and the value of subsequent visits declines slowly, the patient will make many visits before the value of a visit falls below $20.

Price Sensitivity

Research on the relationship between the out-of-pocket price paid by the patient and use of medical services indicates that for some medical services the decline in value of additional services is gradual. In general, a 10 percent increase in price of medical services leads to about a 2 percent reduction in use of services (Morrisey 2005). Price sensitivity varies according to type of medical service. Mental health services are quite price sensitive; a 10 percent reduction in price leads to a 10 percent increase in use of services. Hospital services are the least price sensitive. Lowering the price of physician services by 10 percent increases use by about 2 percent. Higher-income groups are generally less price sensitive than lower-income groups. Nursing home services are price sensitive; lowering prices by 10 percent leads to about a 10 percent increase in use. This finding suggests that if long-term care were included as part of national health insurance, large increases in nursing home use and expenditures would result.

The price sensitivity faced by *individual* physicians, hospitals, and other providers is much greater because each provider is a possible substitute for other providers. For example, although a 10 percent overall price decrease leads to a 2 percent increase in overall use of physician services, if an individual physician raises (or lowers) his price by 10 percent, and other physicians do not change their prices, the individual physician will lose (or gain) large numbers of patients, approximately 30 percent. Similarly, greater price sensitivity exists toward any single health plan than toward health insurance in general. When employees have a choice of health plans and have to pay an out-of-pocket premium (copremium) for these plans, their choice of health plan is very price sensitive. One study found that a difference in HMO copremiums of as little as $5 to $10 a month would cause about 25 percent of the HMO's enrollees to switch to the less-costly HMO (Strombom, Buchmueller, and Feldstein 2002).

Moral Hazard

When patients use more medical services because their insurance lowers the out-of-pocket cost of those services, the insurance industry refers to this behavior as *moral hazard*. This term means that having insurance changes a person's behavior; the cost of medical services to the insurance company is increased. Those with insurance (or more comprehensive insurance) use more services, see more specialists, and incur higher medical costs than those who do not have insurance (or less comprehensive insurance), and the value placed on many of these additional services by patients and their physicians is lower than their full costs.

Evidence from the RAND health insurance experiment found that adults who used more medical services because their insurance plan did not require copayments did not have statistically significantly better health status than adults in health plans with lower use rates (Brook et al. 1983).

Indemnity insurance also places an annual limit (referred to as a *stop loss,* for example, $2,500) on a patient's responsibility for out-of-pocket payments. If a patient has a serious illness, that out-of-pocket maximum is reached fairly early in the treatment process. After that point both the patient and her physician (assuming fee-for-service payment) have an incentive to try all types of treatments that may provide some benefit to the patient, no matter how small that benefit. The expression "flat-of-the-curve medicine" came to indicate the use of all medical technology even when the benefit to the patient is extremely small. The only cost to the patient is nonfinancial—the discomfort and risk associated with the treatment. Not surprisingly, medical expenditures for those who are seriously ill are therefore extraordinarily high. Patients in such circumstances have everything available to them that modern medicine can provide.

The problem of moral hazard has plagued health insurers, resulting in excessive use, increased cost of medical care, and increased insurance premiums. Until the 1980s, health insurers primarily controlled moral hazard by requiring patients to pay a deductible and part of the cost themselves by use of a copayment. During the 1980s, insurers began to use more aggressive methods to control overuse of medical services, such as prior authorization for hospital admissions, utilization review once the patient was hospitalized, and second surgical opinions. Unless prior authorization was received, the patient would be liable for part of the hospitalization cost (and often the patient's physician had to spend time justifying the procedure to the insurer). Requirements to obtain a second surgical opinion were an attempt to provide the patient and the insurer with more information as to the value of the recommended surgical procedure.

These cost-containment or rationing techniques are often referred to as *managed care*. Managed care methods also include case management, which minimizes the medical cost of catastrophic medical cases, and preferred physician panels, which exclude physicians who overuse medical services. These provider panels are marketed to employer groups as being less costly, thereby offering enrollees lower out-of-pocket payments and insurance premiums if they restrict their choice of physician to members of the panel.

In addition to changing patient incentives and relying on managed care techniques, moral hazard can also be controlled by changing physicians' incentives. HMOs are paid an annual fee for providing medical services to their enrolled populations. The out-of-pocket price to the enrollee for use of services in an HMO is very low; consequently, usage rates would be expected to be very high. Because the HMO bears the risk that its enrollees' medical services will exceed their annual payments, the HMO has an incentive not to provide "excessive" amounts of medical services. An HMO patient must instead be concerned with receiving too little care. HMO physicians ration care based on the physician's perception of the benefits to the patient and the full costs to the HMO of further treatment. Because HMO enrollees have very low copayments, the onus (and incentives) for decreasing moral hazard, hence rationing care, is placed on the HMO's physicians.

These insurance company and HMO approaches to decreasing moral hazard attempt to match the additional benefit of medical services to their full cost. Copayments and financial penalties for not receiving prior authorization are incentives to change the patient's behavior. In an HMO, the HMO's physicians are responsible for controlling moral hazard.

SUMMARY

Important differences exist between government rationing of services and the rationing (by price) that occurs in a competitive market. In a price-competitive system, patients differ in the value they place on additional medical services; however, those who place a higher value on those services can always purchase more services. As their incomes increase, patients may prefer to spend more of their additional income on medical care than on other goods and services. If an HMO is too slow to adopt new technology or too restrictive on access to medical services provided to its enrollees, those enrollees could switch to another HMO or to indemnity insurance, pay higher premiums, and receive more services.

Under a system of government rationing, if a patient places a higher value on additional medical services than does the government, and the patient is willing to pay the full cost of those services, the patient will still be unable to purchase them.

Medical services must be rationed because society cannot afford to provide all the medical services that would be demanded at zero price. Which rationing mechanism should be used? Having people pay for additional services and voluntarily joining an HMO or an MCO, or allowing the government to decide on the availability of medical resources? The first, or market, approach permits subscribers to match their costs to the value they place on additional services. Only when the government decides on the costs and benefits of medical services will availability be lower than desired by those who value medical services more highly, and those persons not permitted the choice of spending more of their own resources on medical services. Choice of rationing technique, relying on the private sector versus the government, is essential for determining how much medical care will be provided, to whom, and at what cost.

Regardless of which rationing approach is used for allocating resources to medical care, knowledge of price sensitivity is important for public policy and for attaining efficiency. If the government wants to increase the use of preventive services such as prenatal care, mammograms, and dental checkups for underserved populations, would lowering the price (and waiting cost) of such services achieve that goal? If insurers raise the out-of-pocket price for some visits, would that decrease the use of care that is of low value? If stimulating competition among health plans is the goal, how much of a difference in premiums would cause large numbers of employees to switch plans? If consumers are to be able to match the benefits and costs of use of medical services, they must not only have information on each health plan, but they must also face the costs of their decisions; they will be more discriminating in their choice of health plan and use of services.

DISCUSSION QUESTIONS

1. What determines how many physician services an individual demands?

2. What is moral hazard, and how does its existence increase the cost of medical care?

3. In what ways can moral hazard be limited?

4. Assume that medical services are free to everyone but that the government restricts the supply of services so that physician office visits are rationed by waiting time. Which population groups would fare better?

5. How would you use information on price sensitivity of medical services for policy purposes, for example, to increase the use of mammograms?

6. Discuss: The high price sensitivity of health plan copremiums indicates that if employees had to pay the difference between the lowest-cost health plan and any other health plan out of pocket, market competition among health plans would be stimulated.

REFERENCES

Aaron, H., and W. B. Schwartz. 1990. "Rationing Health Care: The Choice Before Us." *Science* 247 (4941): 418–22.

Brook, R. H., J. Ware, W. H. Rogers, E. B. Keeler, A. R. Davies, C. A. Donald, G. A. Goldberg, K. N. Lohr, P. C. Masthay, and J. P. Newhouse. 1983. "Does Free Care Improve Adults' Health? Results from a Randomized Controlled Trial." *New England Journal of Medicine* 309 (23): 1426–34.

Morrisey, M., 2005. *Price Sensitivity in Health Care: Implications for Health Care Policy.* Washington, DC: National Federation of Independent Business.

Strombom, B. A., T. C. Buchmueller, and P. J. Feldstein. 2002. "Switching Costs, Price Sensitivity, and Health Plan Choice." *Journal of Health Economics* 21 (1): 89–116.

Chapter 6

How Much Health Insurance Should Everyone Have?

WHY DO SOME people have health insurance that covers almost all of their medical expenditures, including dental and vision care, while others do not? Why does the government subsidize the purchase of private health insurance for those with high incomes? Has health insurance stimulated the growth in medical expenditures, or has it served as protection against rapidly rising medical expenses? The answers to these questions are important for explaining the rapid increase in medical expenditures, as well as for understanding proposals for health care reform.

The purpose of health insurance is to enable people to get rid of uncertainty and the possibility that they will incur a large medical expense. This possibility of a large loss is converted into a certain, but small, loss by buying health insurance. Insurance spreads risk among a large number of people, and when each person pays a premium the aggregate amount of the premiums covers the large losses of relatively few people.

DEFINITIONS OF INSURANCE TERMS

Before continuing, a number of terms should be defined. *Indemnity insurance* reimburses either the health provider or the patient a fixed amount (or a percentage of the bill) when the insured patient receives a medical treatment. When the insured patient has a *service benefit* policy, the insurer pays the provider for the services needed by the patient. Health insurance policies today typically contain both indemnity and service benefit features. Physician services and out-of-hospital services are usually treated as indemnity insurance, whereas hospital admissions are usually paid for as a service benefit.

The difference between the provider's charge and the insurance payment is for deductibles and copayments. A *deductible* is a given dollar amount that the patient will have to spend before the insurer will pay any medical expenses. Typically, indemnity policies require an insured family to spend between $250 and $500 of their own money before the insurer will start paying part of the medical bills. A deductible lowers the insurance premium because it eliminates the many small medical expenses most families have each year. The insurer is also able to lower its administrative costs by eliminating the claims processing for handling a large number of small claims.

The effect of a deductible on an insurance premium is illustrated in Figure 6.1. As shown, a large percentage of families have relatively small medical expenses, while a small percentage of families have a very large (referred to as *catastrophic*) expense. Eliminating the area designated as a deductible would reduce the overall amount spent on medical care, thereby reducing the insurance premium.

When a patient pays a percentage of the physician's bill, for example, 20 percent, this is referred to as *cost sharing* or a *copayment*. Copayments provide the patient with an incentive to be sensitive to physicians' charges, perhaps by shopping around, as the patient will have to pay part of the bill. The patient will also have an incentive to use fewer services because he will have to balance the value of an additional visit against its cost (copayment). Copayments also reduce the insurer's share of medical expenses, as shown in Figure 6.1. Indemnity policies are typically 80/20 plans, meaning that the insurer pays 80 percent of the bill and the patient pays 20 percent. Indemnity policies also contain a *stop loss*, which places an overall limit on the patient's out-of-pocket expenses. For example, once a patient has paid a deductible and copayments that add up to, say, $2,000, the insurer pays 100 percent of all remaining expenses during that year. Without a stop loss, unlimited copayments could become a financial hardship. Copayments typically apply to use of out-of-hospital services considered to be discretionary.

Only a small percentage of families incur catastrophic claims (see Figure 6.1). The definition of a catastrophic expense depends on the patient's family income, as a $2,000 expense may be catastrophic to some families but not to others. Ideally, the definition of a catastrophic expense should also be related to family income, but few policies do so.

Figure 6.1: Deductibles, Copayments, and Catastrophic Expenses

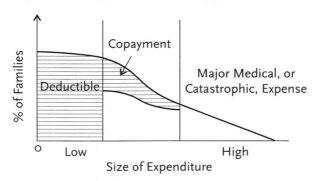

Insurance policies that cover only catastrophic medical expenses may be thought of as high-deductible insurance plans.

The amount of medical expenditures paid out by the insurance company is called the *pure premium*. The pure premium for a group of people with the same risk level (age and sex) represents their expected medical cost, that is, the probability that they will need medical services multiplied by the cost of those services. For example, assuming that the probability of my needing surgery (given my age and sex) is 5 percent and the cost of the surgery, if it were needed, is $50,000, I (and others in my risk group) would have to pay a pure premium of $2,500 a year ($50,000 × 0.05). If I chose not to buy insurance, I would have to put aside $50,000 to pay for that possible medical expense. However, I may not be able to put aside such a large amount—or even larger amounts, for example, the amount needed for a transplant—or I may not want to tie up my funds in that way. Insurance offers me an alternative; it permits me to pay a premium that is equivalent to budgeting for an uncertain medical expense. I can eliminate the uncertainty of a large medical expense by paying an annual premium.

When everyone in a particular group has the same chance of becoming ill and incurring a medical expense, each person is considered to be in the same risk class and is charged the same pure premium. The *actual premium* charged, however, is always greater than the pure premium because the insurer has to recover its administrative and marketing costs and earn a profit. This difference between the pure and actual premium is referred to as the *loading charge*.

INSURANCE-PURCHASING DECISION MAKING

The size of the loading charge often determines why people buy insurance for some medical expenses but not for others. If people could buy insurance at the pure premium, they would buy insurance for almost everything because its price would reflect, on average, what they would likely spend anyway. However, when people are charged more than the pure premium, they must decide whether they want to buy insurance or self-insure, that is, bear the risk themselves. The higher the loading charge relative to the pure premium, the less insurance people will buy. For example, part of the loading charge is related to the administrative cost of processing a claim, which is not too different for a small or a large claim. Small claims therefore have larger loading costs (relative to their pure premium) than do large claims. People are more willing to pay a large administrative cost for a large claim than for a small claim.

In the above example, in which the pure premium is $2,500 a year, even if the insurance company charged me $2,600 a year ($100 more than the pure premium), I would probably buy the insurance rather than bear the risk myself. However, my decision would be different with a smaller expected medical expense. I would rather put aside $200 a year for my family's dental visits than pay the same $100 administrative cost, which would be equal to 50 percent of the pure premium (a $200 pure premium plus a $100 loading charge would equal a premium of $300). In the second case I would rather bear the risk myself than buy insurance.

This discussion suggests that people are more likely to buy insurance for large, unexpected medical expenses than for small medical expenses (for a more complete discussion of the factors affecting the demand for health insurance see Feldstein 2005). This is the pattern typically observed in the purchase of health insurance. A hospital admission and physician expenses connected with that hospital admission, such as the surgeon's and anesthesiologist's fees, are more completely covered by insurance than are expenses for a physician office visit. Thus, *an important characteristic of good insurance is that it covers large catastrophic expenses*. People are less able to afford the catastrophic costs of a major illness or accident than front-end or first-dollar coverage, typically small expenses with relatively high loading charges.

TAX-FREE, EMPLOYER-PAID HEALTH INSURANCE

Surprisingly, however, we also observe that many people have insurance against small claims such as dental visits, physician office visits, and vision services. How can we explain this?

Advantages

The predominant source of health insurance coverage for those under 65 years of age is through the workplace, where 94 percent of all private health insurance is purchased by the employer on behalf of the employee. This occurs because the federal tax code does not consider employer-paid health insurance to be part of the employee's taxable income; it is exempt from federal, state, and Social Security taxes.

Until the early 1980s, marginal tax rates for federal income taxes were as high as 70 percent. Throughout the late 1960s and 1970s, inflation was increasing and pushing employees into higher marginal tax brackets. Social Security taxes have also been steadily rising; as of 2007, the employer and employee each pay 7.65 percent of the employee's wage up to a maximum wage of $97,500. Employees as well as the employer had a financial incentive for providing additional compensation in the form of health insurance benefits rather than cash income. The employer saved its share of Social Security taxes, and employees did not have to pay federal, state, or Social Security taxes on additional health insurance benefits.

For example, assume an employee was in a 30 percent tax bracket, had to pay 5 percent state income tax and 7 percent Social Security tax, already had basic hospital and medical coverage, and was due to receive a $1,000 raise. That employee would be left with only $580 (0.30 + 0.05 + 0.07 = 0.42 subtracted from 100 percent = 0.58 × $1,000) after taxes to purchase dental care and other medical services not covered by insurance for her family. However, if the employer used that $1,000 to purchase additional health insurance to cover these same out-of-pocket payments instead of raising the employee's income, the employee could use the full $1,000 to buy those services she would have had to purchase with after-tax dollars. The employee would be able to pay the $580 with before-tax income and still have $420 available to cover additional out-of-pocket medical expenses.

Higher-income employees had even greater incentives to substitute more comprehensive insurance coverage for wage increases. Imagine someone in a 50 percent tax bracket (before 1980) with the same state and Social Security taxes. A $1,000 raise would leave him with only $380 to purchase dental, vision, and mental health services, whereas the full $1,000 could be spent on those services if it were used to buy additional health insurance.

As employees moved into higher tax brackets, the higher loading charge on small claims was more than offset by using before-tax income to buy health insurance for those small claims. Using the earlier example of dental care, the choice was between spending $200 of after-tax income on dental care or buying dental insurance for $300 ($200 dental expense plus $100 loading charge). Spending $200 on my family's dental care would require me to earn $350 in before-tax income (30 percent federal tax, 5 percent state tax, and 7 percent Social Security tax). However, if my employer used that same $350 to purchase dental benefits for me, the premium, including the $100 loading charge, would be more than covered, leaving $50 to buy even more medical services. Tax-free, employer-purchased health insurance provided a financial incentive to purchase health insurance for small claims.

Another way of viewing the tax subsidy for health insurance is to consider that if an employee saves 40 percent when the employer buys health insurance, the price of insurance to that employee has been reduced by 40 percent. Studies indicate that the purchase of insurance has an approximate proportional relationship to changes in its price (Pauly 1986). Thus, a 40 percent price reduction would be expected to increase the quantity of insurance purchased by 40 percent.

The advantages of tax-free, employer-purchased health insurance stimulated the demand for comprehensive health insurance coverage, particularly among higher-income employees. In some high-income employee groups, such as the United Automobile Workers, deductibles and copayments became smaller and disappeared. More services not traditionally thought of as insurable, such as a dental visit or an eye exam, all small routine expenditures, became part of the employee's health insurance.

Consequences

The greater comprehensiveness of employer-purchased health insurance had important consequences. First, "too many" services were covered by health insurance. Administrative costs increased as insurers had to process many small claims that would have been excluded by a deductible. To process a $20 prescription drug claim cost the same as a much larger medical expense. Second, as insurance became more comprehensive, patients' concern with the prices charged for medical services decreased. Physicians, hospitals, and other health providers could more easily raise their charges because they would be "covered by insurance"—someone else was paying. Similarly, as the amount patients had to pay out of pocket for medical expenses declined, they increased their use of those services, sought more referrals to specialists, and underwent more extensive medical testing.

The growth of health insurance and medical technology was intertwined. Expensive technology, which increases the cost of a medical expense, causes people to buy health insurance to protect themselves from those large, unexpected medical expenses. At the same time, the availability of insurance to pay for expensive technology stimulated its development. When comprehensive insurance removes any concern the insured persons may have about the cost of their care, they (and their physicians acting on their behalf) want access to the latest technology as long as it offers some additional benefit, no matter how small. The benefits of that technology to patients outweigh their out-of-pocket costs of using it. Because insurance was available to pay the costs of expensive technology, such as transplants, financial incentives to develop benefit-producing technology existed. Thus, medical technology was stimulated by, and in turn stimulated, the purchase of health insurance.

Conversely, until recently cost-reducing technology generated little interest because employers could pass on higher insurance costs to employees in the form of reduced wages or to consumers in the form of higher prices. Furthermore, the after-tax value of savings to employees from undertaking stringent cost-containment measures was small. If, for example, insurance premiums could be reduced by $300 by limiting employees' choice of physician, the inconvenience to the employee and his family associated with changing physicians would probably not be worth the after-tax savings of $150.

The lack of concern over the price of medical services and increased use of those services caused medical expenditures to sharply increase, which in turn caused health insurance premiums to rapidly rise. Higher insurance premiums meant smaller wage increases, but this was not obvious to employees because the employer was paying the insurance premium.

Hundreds of billions of dollars in tax revenues have been lost because of employer-paid health insurance. The value of this tax subsidy in 2004 was estimated to be $209 billion a year in forgone federal, Social Security, and state taxes simply because employer-paid health insurance is not considered part of the employee's taxable income (Shields and Haught 2004). These lost tax revenues primarily benefit high-income employees because they are in higher tax brackets. As shown in Figure 6.2, the higher an employee's income, the greater is the value of the exclusion

Figure 6.2: Value of Tax Exclusion for Employer-Paid Health Insurance, by Income Level, 2004

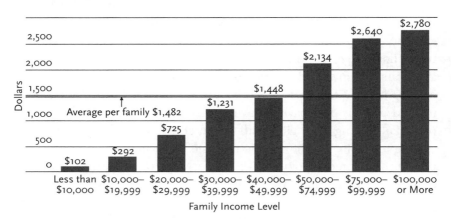

Source: Lewin Group estimates using the Health Benefits Simulation Model.

Reprinted from J. Sheils and R. Haught. 2004. "The Cost of Tax-Exempt Health Benefits in 2004." *Health Affairs* Web exclusive, February 25, W4-109.

from income of employer-purchased health insurance. This $209 billion in lost tax revenues is equivalent to a huge subsidy for the purchase of health insurance to those who can most easily afford it. In contrast, in 2004 the federal government spent $182 billion on Medicaid, a means-tested program for the poor (Congressional Budget Office 2006).

Table 6.1 shows how the value of the exclusion from income of employer-purchased health insurance is distributed across family incomes. Families with incomes of $100,000 or greater in 2004 (26.5 percent of all families) received 50 percent of the federal portion of this tax subsidy for the purchase of health insurance.

Finally, tax-free, employer-paid health insurance reduced employees' incentive to choose lower-cost health plans. Many employers paid the entire premium of any plan selected by the employee (or the employer contributed more than the premium of the lowest-cost plan offered); as there was no visible cost to the employee, the employee's incentive was to choose the most comprehensive plan with the easiest access to physicians and specialists. Previously, health plans did not have financial incentives to compete on premiums.

Table 6.1: Distribution of the Value of the Federal Tax Exclusion for Employer-Paid Health Insurance, by Family Income, 2004

Annual Family Income	Expenditure Amount (Billions of Dollars)	% of Total
$150,000 or more	$25.9	13.7
$100,000–$149,999	24.1	12.8
$75,000–$99,999	40.8	21.6
$50,000–$74,999	44.2	23.4
$40,000–$49,999	17.9	9.5
$30,000–$39,999	17.1	9.1
$20,000–$29,999	12.2	6.5
$10,000–$19,999	5.0	2.7
Less than $10,000	1.3	0.7
Total	188.5	100.0

Source: Lewin Group estimates using the Health Benefits Simulation Model.

Reprinted from J. Sheils and R. Haught. 2004. "The Cost of Tax-Exempt Health Benefits in 2004." *Health Affairs* Web exclusive, February 25, W4-110.

Proposed Limitation of Tax-Free Status

To encourage competition among health plans on the basis of access to services, quality, and premiums, employees have to pay the additional cost of a more expensive health plan out of pocket. The employee would then evaluate whether the additional benefits of that plan are worth its additional costs. Unless a limit is placed on the tax-free employer contribution, many employees will continue to select health plans based on their benefits without regard to their premiums. Competition among health plans based on premiums, reputation, and access to services will not occur until employees have a greater financial stake in their decisions.

Not surprisingly, economists favor eliminating, or at least setting a maximum limit on, the tax-exempt status of employer-paid health insurance. Those with higher incomes would no longer receive a subsidy for their purchase of health insurance. Instead, increased tax revenues would come from those who have benefited most, namely those with higher incomes. These funds could then be used to subsidize health insurance for those with low incomes. Employees using after-tax dollars would be more cost conscious in their use of services and choice of health plans.

Increased price sensitivity by employees (or employers acting on their behalf) has two likely outcomes. First, health insurance coverage would become less comprehensive. It would no longer be worthwhile to buy insurance for small claims that have relatively large loading charges. Consequently, dental and vision services would likely be dropped from insurance policies. Deductibles would be increased on out-of-hospital services, thereby decreasing administrative costs and insurance premiums. Copayments would also be common, both as a means of decreasing the insurance premium and for controlling use of services. Patients would also have a greater incentive (lower copayments) to use a restricted provider panel. Second, those employees who prefer to have comprehensive benefits and not pay large copayments would be more likely to join managed care systems, such as HMOs, in which the decision on use of services is made by the provider rather than the patient.

Whether patients become more price sensitive because of copayments or delegate the decision to restrict use of services to their MCOs, use of services will decline. The basis for making treatment decisions will change. Use of services and choice of health plan will no longer be based only on a consideration of their benefits. Employees (and physicians in MCOs) will also have to consider the costs of their choices.

SUMMARY

Paying an insurance premium enables people to eliminate the uncertainty that arises as to whether they will incur a large expenditure if they become ill. Insurance reduces a person's risk of a large financial loss and is therefore more likely to be bought for protection against large financial losses. Health insurance, however, also provides protection against relatively small losses such as physician office visits and dental care. People buy insurance against such small losses because health insurance is subsidized; employer-paid health insurance is tax exempt. Employees purchase more comprehensive health insurance because of this tax subsidy. The primary beneficiaries of this tax subsidy are those with higher incomes because they are in a higher marginal tax bracket.

Tax-exempt, employer-purchased health insurance has distorted consumers' choices in health care and resulted in diminished consumer incentives to be concerned with the cost of medical services. Reducing or limiting this tax subsidy may not only provide more funds to assist those with lower incomes, but may also make consumers more price sensitive in their choice of health plans and use of medical services.

DISCUSSION QUESTIONS

1. How is a pure premium calculated?

2. What does the loading charge consist of?

3. How does the size of the loading charge affect the type of health insurance purchased?

4. Why does employer-purchased health insurance result in more comprehensive health insurance coverage?

5. What are the arguments in favor of eliminating the tax-exempt status of employer-purchased health insurance?

6. How has health insurance affected the development of medical technology, and how has medical technology affected the growth of health insurance?

REFERENCES

Congressional Budget Office. 2006. *The Budget and Economic Outlook: Fiscal Years 2007 to 2016.* January. [Online publication; retrieved 11/15/06.] http://ftp.cbo.gov/ftpdocs/70xx/doc7027/01-26-BudgetOutlook.pdf.

Feldstein, P. J. 2005. "The Demand for Health Insurance." In *Health Care Economics,* 6th ed., 111–42. Albany, NY: Delmar Publishers.

Pauly, M. V. 1986. "Taxation, Health Insurance, and Market Failure in the Medical Economy." *Journal of Economic Literature* 24 (2): 629–75.

Shields, J., and R. Haught. 2004. "The Cost of Tax-Exempt Health Benefits in 2004." *Health Affairs* Web Exclusive. [Online publication; retrieved 12/27/06.] http://content.healthaffairs.org/cgi/reprint/hlthaff.w4.106v1?maxtoshow=&HITS=10&hits=10&RESULTFORMAT=&author1=Haught&andorexactfulltext=and&searchid=1&FIRSTINDEX=0&resourcetype=HWCIT.

Chapter 7

Why Are Those Who Most Need Health Insurance Least Able to Buy It?

WE HAVE ALL heard stories of individuals who are sick and need, for example, open-heart surgery, but no insurance company will sell them health insurance. Health insurance seems to be available only for those who do not need it. Should health insurance companies be required to sell insurance to those who are sick and need it most? To understand these issues, as well as what would be appropriate public policy, one must understand how insurance premiums are determined and how health insurance markets work.

Seventy percent of private health insurance is purchased through the workplace. The insurance premium paid by an employer on behalf of its employees consists of (1) the loading charge, which represents approximately 10 percent of the premium, and (2) the claims experience of the employee group, which makes up the remaining 90 percent of the premium (see Figure 7.1). The loading charge reflects the insurance company's marketing costs, the administrative costs of handling the insurance claims, and profit. The claims experience of an employee group is the number of claims submitted by members of that group multiplied by the average cost per claim. The claims experience portion of the premium, or *medical loss ratio,* is the total medical expenditures paid out by the insurer on behalf of the group. Differences in premiums among employee groups, as well as the annual rise in employer health insurance premiums, result primarily from differences in claims experience. An *experience-rated* premium is based on the claims experience of the particular group.

When a new group applies for health insurance, the insurer attempts to estimate the likely claims experience of the group. As shown in Figure

Figure 7.1: Determinants of Health Insurance Premiums

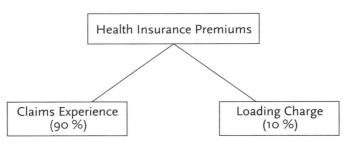

Determinants of Claims Experience

Benefit coverage
State mandates
Demographic characteristics of
    the insured population (age,
    sex, and family status)
Industry
Region
Medical inflation rate
Cost-containment policies
    Copayments
    Deductibles
    Benefit design
    Utilization review
    Case management
    PPOs

Determinants of Loading Charge

Administrative costs
Marketing costs
Reserves
Profits

7.1, the insurer will consider factors that affect the group's medical expenditures, such as the following:

- the types of medical and other benefits provided to the employees and their dependents;
- the types of mandates the state requires to be included in the insurance policy (e.g., hair transplants or coverage for chiropractors);
- the average age of the group (older employees have higher medical expenditures than younger employees);
- the proportion of females (females have higher medical expenditures than males at younger ages and lower expenditures at older ages);

- the industry in which the firm competes (e.g., physicians, nurses, accountants, and lawyers tend to be heavier users of health care than, say, bank tellers);
- the region of the country in which the employees are located (hospital costs and physician fees are higher on the West Coast than in the South); and
- an estimate of the growth rate in medical inflation.

Once an insurer has insured a group long enough to have a history of that group's claims experience, the insurance company will project that claims experience and multiply it by an estimate of the medical inflation rate.

Various approaches can be used to reduce a group's claims experience. For example, increasing the deductible and the coinsurance rate will decrease employees' use of services; expanding insurance benefits to include lower-cost substitutes to inpatient admissions will lower treatment costs; and requiring utilization review of hospital admissions, case management of catastrophic cases, and use of preferred PPOs will lower use rates and provider charges. Thus, the claims experience of a group is related to the characteristics of that group, the medical benefits covered, and the cost-containment methods included in the insurance policy.

The insurer bears the risk of incorrectly estimating the group's medical experience. If the premium charged to that group is too low, the insurer will lose money. In the past, BlueCross and other insurance companies have lost a great deal of money by underestimating claims experience and the medical inflation rate. An insurer cannot merely increase the premiums of the group in the following period to recover its losses because the insurance market is very price competitive. If an insurer says to an employer, "We need to increase our profit this coming year because we lost money on your employees last year," the employer may switch to a competitor or to an HMO.

Even if the claims experience of two employee groups is similar, one group may have a lower insurance premium because it has a lower loading charge. Larger groups have smaller loading charges because administrative and marketing costs, which are generally fixed, are spread over a larger number of employees. Furthermore, insurers earn a lower profit when they insure larger groups because they fear that, if their profit is too high, large groups will decide to self-insure by bearing the risk themselves. Smaller groups, on the other hand, are less likely to be able to bear the risk of self-insurance. If a very large claim were to occur in one year, the financial burden could be too large for a small group to bear. In a larger group, large claims are likely to be offset by premiums from employees making only small or no claims in a given year. In addition to charging small groups a higher rate, an insurer is likely to maintain a higher reserve in case a large claim is made, further increasing the loading charge for small groups. However, the amount of profit the insurer is able to make from a small group is limited by competition from other insurers and HMOs.

MEDICAL LOSS RATIOS

Some provider organizations have viewed the medical loss ratio as an indicator of a health plan's efficiency and even quality of care. The higher the ratio, the more of the premium dollar is paid out for medical services and the lower the administrative expenses are. However, the use of the ratio as any type of evaluative measure is misleading. Higher administrative expenses (hence a lower medical loss ratio) can result from an insurer (1) enrolling a greater mix of small groups, which have higher marketing and administrative costs than fewer large groups; (2) having a smaller enrollment base and therefore having to spread fixed administrative costs over a smaller number of enrollees; and (3) having a larger number of insurance products, which are more costly to administer than a single product. Additional factors are the method used to pay hospitals and physicians (by capitating providers, the administrative and claims processing expense is shifted to the provider, compared with the fee-for-service approach, in which the insurer retains those functions) and the number of cost-containment and quality review activities the insurer undertakes.

For example, a health plan that merely pays out a large percentage of its premiums (high medical loss ratio) is more likely to be inefficient and lower in quality than a health plan that has a higher administrative expense ratio because it reviews the accuracy of claims submitted by providers, conducts reviews of the quality of care provided, and undertakes patient satisfaction surveys.[1]

---

1. Robinson (1997) discusses many of these interpretive problems (and more) with medical loss ratios and demonstrates how medical loss ratios vary greatly within both nonprofit and for-profit health plans, as well as the wide variations that exist in these ratios for the same health plan located in different states.

In a price-competitive health insurance market, a health plan cannot afford to be inefficient in its administrative functions. If it were, its premiums would be higher and it would lose market share. A health plan must undertake a cost-benefit analysis to determine whether each of the administrative functions it performs either saves money (lower claims cost) or provides increased purchaser satisfaction (enrollee satisfaction surveys). To do otherwise places the plan at a competitive disadvantage.

HOW HEALTH INSURANCE MARKETS WORK

This brief description of how insurance premiums are determined serves as background to examine why those who are ill find buying insurance difficult.

Adverse Selection

Assume that an individual without health insurance requires a heart transplant and tries to purchase health insurance. If the insurer does not know that the person requires expensive medical treatment, the person's premium will be based on the claims experience of persons in a similar age (risk) group. This difference in information about the individual's health status between the individual and the insurer can lead to *adverse selection,* that is, a person in ill health will attempt to conceal that information from the insurer so that the insurer will not know of its risk.

For example, if 100 people were in a risk group, each with a 1 percent chance of needing a medical treatment costing $100,000, the pure premium for each (without the loading charge) would be $1,000 (0.01 × $100,000). Each year one member of the group would require a $100,000 treatment. Now, if a person who needs that particular treatment (whose risk is 100 percent) is permitted to join that group at a premium of $1,000 (based on a mistaken risk level of 0.01), that high-risk person receives a subsidy of $99,000, as her premium should have been $100,000 based on her risk level. Because the $1,000 premium was based on a risk level of 1 percent, the insurer collects insufficient premiums to pay for the second $100,000 expense and loses $99,000.

This example does not differ from one in which a man learns that he has a terminal illness and, unbeknownst to the insurer, decides to purchase a $1 million life insurance policy to provide for his wife and children, or from one in which a woman whose home is on fire quickly decides to buy fire insurance. Insurance enables a person to protect against uncertainty.

Once uncertainty no longer exists, however, the person's need for treatment such as a heart transplant is not insurable.

If the insurance company knew that the individual wanted health insurance to cover the costs of a heart transplant, the insurance company would charge a premium that reflected the person's expected claims experience, that is, the person's premium would be equal to the cost of the heart transplant plus a loading charge.

We all favor subsidizing those who cannot afford but need an expensive treatment. Similarly, we favor subsidies to poor families. However, is it not more appropriate for the government, rather than the insurer, to provide those subsidies? When insurers are made to bear such losses, they will eventually be forced out of business unless they can protect themselves from persons who withhold information and claim to be in lower-risk groups.

To protect themselves against adverse selection (insuring high-risk persons for premiums mistakenly based on those with low risks) the insurer could raise everyone's premiums, but then many low-risk subscribers, who would be willing to pay $1,000 but not $2,000 for a 1 percent risk, would drop their insurance. As more low-risk subscribers drop out, premiums for remaining subscribers will increase further, causing still more low-risk subscribers to drop out. Eventually large numbers of low-risk persons would be uninsured, although they would be willing to pay an actuarially fair premium based on their (low) risk group.

Instead, an insurer will attempt to learn as much as the patient about the patient's health status. Examining and testing the person who wants to buy health insurance is a means of equalizing the information between the two parties. Another way in which insurers protect themselves against adverse selection—that is, misclassifying high risks into low-risk groups—is by stating that their insurance coverage will not apply to preexisting conditions, medical conditions known by the patient to exist and to require medical treatment. Similarly, an insurer might use a delay of benefits clause or a waiting period; for example, obstetric benefits may not be covered until a policy has been in effect for ten months. Large deductibles will also discourage high-risk persons because they will realize that they have to pay a large amount of their expenses themselves.

Insurers are less concerned about adverse selection when selling insurance to large groups with low employee turnover. In such groups health insurance is provided by the employer and is a tax-free benefit (subsidized by the government); the total group includes all the low-risk persons as well. Typically, people join large companies more for other attributes of the job than for health insurance coverage. Once in the employer group, employees cannot just drop the group insurance when well and buy it when ill. Thus, for insurance companies adverse selection is more of a concern when individuals or very small groups (with typically higher turnover) want to buy insurance. For example, an insurer might be concerned that the owner of a small firm might hire family members who become ill to receive insurance benefits. Thus, employees with preexisting medical conditions will be denied coverage because insurers will use testing and exclusions to protect themselves against adverse selection.

Some state and local governments have attempted to assist people with preexisting conditions by prohibiting insurers from using tests to determine, for example, whether someone is HIV positive. Rather than subsidize care for such individuals themselves, governments have tried to shift the medical costs to the insurer and its other subscribers. This is an inequitable way of subsidizing care for those with preexisting conditions, as many insured but low-risk subscribers have low incomes. Government use of an income-related tax to provide the subsidy would be fairer. Another consequence of government regulations that shift the cost of those who are ill to insurers and their subscribers is that insurers will rely on other types of restrictions not covered by the regulations, such as delay of benefits and exclusion of certain occupations, industries, or geographic areas, to protect themselves.

Healthy people may not have health insurance for several reasons. An insurance premium that is much higher than the expected claims experience of an individual will make that insurance too expensive. For example, if an employee is not part of a large insured group, he will be charged a higher insurance premium because the insurer suspects he will be a higher risk. The loading charge will also be higher for the self-employed and those in small groups because the insurer's administration and marketing costs are spread over fewer employees, leading to a higher premium. Furthermore, state insurance mandates that require expensive benefits or more practitioners to be included in all insurance sold in that state result in higher insurance premiums; consequently, fewer people are willing to buy such insurance. Many individuals and members of small groups also lack insurance coverage because premiums are too high relative to their incomes. Such persons would rather rely on Medicaid if they become ill. Others can afford to purchase insurance but choose not to; if they become ill, they become a burden on taxpayers because they cannot be refused treatment in emergency departments or by hospitals.

The best way to eliminate the problem of adverse selection is to require everyone to have health insurance. Subsidies to purchase insurance could be provided to those with low incomes and to those who are high risk in relation to their incomes. Under mandatory health insurance most individuals would be good risks when they purchased health insurance and would not wait until they were ill and hence uninsurable; everyone would have health insurance when they needed it. During the transition toward mandatory insurance, the government should establish a high-risk pool (at subsidized premiums) to cover those who are uninsurable because they have preexisting conditions.

Preferred-Risk Selection

Because insurers want to protect themselves against bad risks, they clearly prefer insuring individuals who are better-than-average risks. Although their risks vary, as long as different groups and individuals pay the same premium, insurers have an incentive to engage in *preferred-risk selection*, that is, seek out those who have lower-than-average risks.

As shown in Table 7.1, in 2003, 1 percent of the population incurred 24 percent of total health expenditures (44 percent of those in the top 1 percent are over the age of 65 years). In 1963, 1 percent of the population incurred only 17 percent of total expenditures, which indicates the effect that medical technology has had on increasing medical expenditures. Five percent of the population incurs 49 percent of total expenditures. Given this high concentration of expenditures among a small percentage of the population, an insurer could greatly increase its profits and avoid losses by trying to avoid the most costly patients. An insurer able to select enrollees from among the 50 percent of the population that incurs only 3 percent of total expenditures will greatly profit. The only way to provide insurers with an incentive to take the high-risk, hence costly, patients is to provide insurers with *risk-adjusted premiums*. For example, premiums for persons in older age groups should be higher than for those in lower age groups. Insurers would then have an incentive to minimize the cost of treating these patients rather than search for low-risk enrollees.

When the premium is the same for all risks, insurers attempt to enroll persons with better-than-average risks in several ways. For example, if everyone enrolling with a particular health insurer pays the same annual

Table 7.1: Distribution of Health Expenditures for the U.S. Population, by Magnitude of Expenditures, Selected Years, 1928–2003

% of U.S. Population Ranked by Expenditures	1928	1963	1970	1977	1980	1987	1996	2003
Top 1 percent	—	17%	26%	27%	29%	28%	27%	24%
Top 2 percent	—	—	35	38	39	39	38	33
Top 5 percent	52%	43	50	55	55	56	55	49
Top 10 percent	—	59	66	70	70	70	69	64
Top 30 percent	93	—	88	90	90	90	90	89
Top 50 percent	—	95	96	97	96	97	97	97
Bottom 50 percent	—	5	4	3	4	3	3	3

Sources: Adapted with permission from "The Concentration of Health Care Expenditures, Revisited, Exhibit 1," by M. L. Berk and A. C. Monheit, *Health Affairs*, 20(2), 2001, March/April: 12. Copyright © 2001 Project HOPE-the People-to- People Health Foundation, Inc., All Rights Reserved; Yu, W. W., Agency for Healthcare Research and Quality. 2006. Personal correspondence, June 5.

premium, the HMO would prefer those who have lower-than-average claims experience, are in low-risk industries, and are younger-than-average employees. To encourage younger subscribers the HMO might empha-size services used by younger couples, such as prenatal and well-baby care. Emphasizing wellness and sports medicine programs is also likely to draw a healthier population. Similarly, de-emphasizing tertiary care facilities for heart disease and cancer treatment sends a message to those who are older and at higher risk for those illnesses. Locating clinics and physicians in areas where lower-risk populations reside also results in a favorably biased selection of subscribers.

Medicare beneficiaries can voluntarily decide to join an HMO. Previ-ously, if an aged person decided to change her mind, she could leave the HMO with only one month's notice. (This one-month notice, which was permitted to the aged but not to those in Medicaid HMOs, reflected the greater political power of the aged.) When some HMOs determined that a Medicare patient required high-cost treatment, they were able to encourage patients to disenroll by suggesting that they might ben-efit from more suitable treatment for the condition outside the HMO.

By eliminating these high-cost subscribers, an HMO could save a great deal of money. To discourage some HMOs from using this approach to maintain only the most favorable Medicare risks, the one-month notice by the aged was repealed in 2003.[2]

IMPROVING THE HEALTH INSURANCE MARKET

Biased selection, both adverse and preferred risk, is a problem in the health insurance market that occurs because of differences in information on health status, consumer choice of health plans, and fixed premiums for subscribers whose expected medical expenses differ from those of the average cost per subscriber.

Several proposals have been made for improving the health insurance market,[3] although not all of them will improve its efficiency. One such example is requiring all insurers to *community rate* their subscribers, that is, charge all subscribers the same premium regardless of health status or other risk factors. The cost of higher-risk individuals would be spread among all subscribers. Community rating, however, provides insurers with even stronger incentives to select preferred risks. Furthermore, with uniform premiums, regardless of risk status, insurers and employers would no longer have an incentive to encourage risk-reducing behavior among their subscribers and employees, for example, by providing smoking cessation and wellness programs. Premiums for employee groups could not be reduced relative to other groups who do not invest in such cost-reducing behavior. Skydivers, motorcyclists, and others who engage in risky behavior are subsidized by those who attempt to lower their risks. Rather than reducing the cost of risky behavior to these groups, higher premiums for those who engage in higher-risk activities would provide them with an incentive to reduce such behavior and bear the full cost of their activities.

Additionally, when there is only one choice of health plan, then the higher, community-rated, premium will result in lower-risk individuals dropping their coverage. This is inefficient because lower-risk persons

---

2. This change was a result of the Balanced Budget Act of 1997, which sought to decrease Medicare expenditures. To compensate for this change, the aged were provided with additional preventive benefits.

3. These proposals are directed toward improving the health insurance market for small employee groups and assume that these small groups can afford to purchase health insurance. Financing health care for the poor is discussed in later chapters, as are other aspects of health care reform such as competitive medical systems and malpractice.

are unable to buy insurance at the cost of insuring them. The result will be an increase in the number of uninsured. When there is a choice of community-rated health plans, then those who are low risk will select less costly, but more restrictive, health plans that are less attractive to higher-risk individuals. As low-risk individuals leave these more costly plans and choose plans that are less costly and more restrictive, the more generous plans will contain a higher portion of higher-risk individuals. This appears to have happened in New Jersey (Monheit et al. 2004). Consequently, the premiums in these more costly plans will increase, likely leading to their demise.

Community rating also has serious equity effects. A community-rated system benefits those who are at high risk and penalizes those who are at low risk. Those at lower risk pay higher premiums, and those at higher risk pay lower premiums, than they would under an experience-rated system. Those at higher risk are in effect subsidized by a tax on those who are lower risk. Because these "subsidies" and "taxes" are based on risk rather than income, low-risk individuals who also have low incomes end up subsidizing some higher-risk, higher-income people. Not all high-risk persons are poor, and not all low-risk persons are wealthy.

Several beneficial health insurance market reforms were included in the Health Insurance Portability and Accountability Act (HIPAA) of 1996. Two components of this law are *restrictions on preexisting condition exclusions* and *guaranteed renewability*. According to HIPAA, once an insured employee has met the preexisting condition exclusion, it cannot be applied again to that employee if he decides to switch insurance companies. Previously, employees were reluctant to leave their employers if they had a medical condition that could have resulted in another 12-month preexisting condition exclusion with their new employer's insurance company that would thereby leave them without insurance for one year. Guaranteed renewability requires insurers to renew a group's health insurance within standard "rate bands," that is, upon renewal, premium increases can vary from the average increase in premiums by only plus or minus 20 percent. Previously, an insurer might not renew a small group's insurance if an employee had a costly and continuing medical condition.

These two reforms make insurers sell "real" insurance. A person buys insurance to decrease uncertainty. Job portability is increased when employees do not have to drop their insurance for a year if they decide to change jobs. Furthermore, if an employee (or her family member) within a small group becomes ill and the insurer does not renew her insurance or charges a very high premium, the initial purchase of insurance has not decreased her uncertainty. Unless employees are able to renew their insurance, they will not be protected from a large, unexpected loss.

SUMMARY

Adverse and preferred-risk selection occurs because the premium an individual is charged does not match the risk group he is in. These selection problems would be minimized if premiums were related to risk group, because insurers would not need to reject high-risk persons or search for low-risk persons. (In the case of adverse selection the problem would be eliminated if everyone were required to have health insurance.) Government regulations, such as eliminating testing and mandating community rating for insurers, have indirect effects that may worsen equity, decrease risk-reducing behavior by employers, and lead to offsetting actions by insurers.

Adverse and preferred-risk selection affect subscribers and health insurers. Solving these problems will require an awareness of why biased selection occurs. Proposed solutions should be evaluated on the basis of whether they encourage risk-reducing behavior, include incentives for efficient utilization of medical services, and impose a burden on those with low incomes who may also be low risk. Having health insurers compete on the basis of risk-adjusted premiums will result in insurers competing on the basis of how well they can manage care rather than on how well they can select better risk groups. Finally, health insurance reform should be directed toward eliminating uncertainty, which is what people want when they buy health insurance.

DISCUSSION QUESTIONS

1. What are the different components of a health insurance premium? If an employer wanted to reduce its employees' premiums, which components could be changed?

2. What is adverse selection, and how do insurance companies protect themselves from it? If the government prohibited insurers from protecting themselves against adverse selection, how would it affect insurance premiums?

3. Why do insurers and HMOs have an incentive to engage in preferred-risk selection?

4. What are some methods by which insurers and HMOs try to achieve preferred-risk selection?

5. What is the difference between experience rating and community rating, and what are some consequences of using community rating?

REFERENCES

Monheit, A., J. Cantor, M. Koller, and K. Fox. 2004. "Community Rating and Sustainable Individual Health Insurance Markets in New Jersey." *Health Affairs* 23 (4): 167–75.

Robinson, J. C. 1997. "Use and Abuse of the Medical Loss Ratio to Measure Health Plan Performance." *Health Affairs* 16 (4): 164–87.

ADDITIONAL READING

Feldstein, P. J. 2005. "The Demand for Health Insurance." In *Health Care Economics,* 6th ed., 111–42. Albany, NY: Delmar Publishers.

Chapter 8

Medicare

In 1965, Congress enacted two different financing programs to cover two separate population groups, Medicare for the aged and Medicaid for the poor. As a result, the government's (particularly the federal government's) role in financing personal medical services increased dramatically. As of 2005, federal and state expenditures represented 45 percent of total medical expenditures.

Both Medicare and Medicaid have serious problems. Medicare's impending financial deficits mean that the program will require substantial changes to survive. Medicaid must be improved if it is to serve more than half of those classified as poor, and it faces huge financial liabilities as an aging population requires long-term care. Medicaid is discussed in Chapter 9.

CURRENT STATE OF MEDICARE

Medicare is a federal program that primarily serves the aged. In addition to the aged, those under the age of 65 years who receive Social Security cash payments because they are disabled become eligible for Medicare after a two-year waiting period. People requiring kidney dialysis and kidney transplants, regardless of age, were added to Medicare in the early 1970s. As shown in Figure 8.1, Medicare covers 35.6 million aged and 6.5 million disabled beneficiaries, a total of 42 million beneficiaries. The number of aged is expected to double over the next three decades.

Medicare has four parts, each offering different benefits and using different financing mechanisms. Part A provides hospital insurance (HI), Part B provides supplemental medical insurance (SMI), Part C offers

Figure 8.1: Number of Medicare Beneficiaries, Fiscal Years 1970–2030

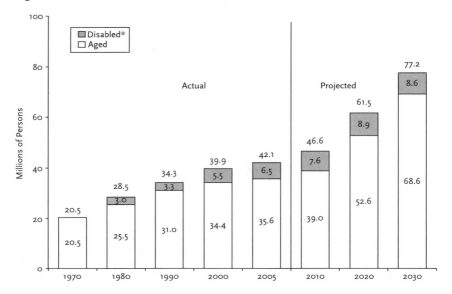

*Includes beneficiaries whose eligibility is based solely on end-stage disease.

Note: Disabled became eligible for Medicare in 1973; therefore, there are no values for disabled before 1974.

Source: Centers for Medicare & Medicaid Services. *2005 CMS Statistics.* [Online information.] http://www.cms.hhs.gov/MedicareMedicaidStatSupp/downloads/ 2005_CMS_Statistics.pdf; Projected data are from Centers for Medicare & Medicaid Services (then the Health Care Financing Administration). 2000. *Medicare 2000: 35 Years of Improving Americans' Health and Security.* Baltimore: CMS.

Medicare beneficiaries a greater variety of health plan choices, and Part D is a new prescription drug benefit.

Part A (HI)

All of the aged are automatically enrolled in Part A when they retire at age 65. Part A covers acute hospital care (up to 90 days for each episode of care), skilled nursing home care after hospitalization (up to 100 days), and hospice care for the terminally ill. If a Medicare patient requires hospitalization, she must pay a deductible that is indexed to increase with health costs each year ($992 as of 2007). Part A is financed by an earmarked Medicare HI payroll tax, which is set aside in the Medicare Hospital Trust Fund. In 1966, this tax was a combined 0.35 percent

(0.175 percent tax on both the employer and the employee) on wages up to $6,600. As Medicare expenditures exceeded projections, both the HI tax and the wage base to which the tax applied were increased. As of 1994, the total HI tax is a combined 2.9 percent on all earned income.

The Medicare Hospital Trust Fund is a "pay-as-you-go" fund; current Medicare expenditures are funded by current employee and employer contributions. The HI taxes from current Medicare beneficiaries were never set aside for their own future expenses but were instead used to pay for those who were Medicare eligible at the time the funds were collected. This is in contrast to a pension fund, in which a person sets aside funds to pay for his own retirement. At times when Medicare actuaries have estimated that the trust fund will become insolvent, that is, when current HI taxes will be insufficient to pay current Medicare expenditures, Medicare HI taxes on employees and employers have been increased.

In 2005, the federal government spent $184 billion on Part A; this amount is estimated to rise to $356 billion by 2015. Medicare's expenditures by type of service are shown in Figure 8.2.

Part B (SMI)

Medicare Part B (SMI) pays for physician services, outpatient diagnostic tests, certain medical supplies and equipment, and (since 1998) home health care (previously included in Part A). Medicare beneficiaries are not automatically enrolled in SMI, which is a voluntary program, but 95 percent of the aged pay the premium ($93.50 a month as of 2007), which represents only 25 percent of the program's costs. The remaining 75 percent of Part B expenditures are subsidized from federal tax revenues. The aged are also responsible for an annual $131 deductible (in 2007) and a 20 percent copayment for their use of Part B services.

For the first time in Medicare, beginning in 2007, the Part B premium will be income related; those aged earning $80,000 to $100,000 will receive a 65 percent premium subsidy, and those earning more than $200,000 will receive only a 20 percent premium subsidy. It is estimated that in 2007 only 3 percent of Part B enrollees will be affected by the reduced premium subsidies.

Unlike the Hospital Trust Fund, when Part B expenditures exceed projections there is no concern with insolvency. The federal subsidy simply becomes larger than expected; Part B expenditures increase the size of the federal deficit. In 2005, the federal subsidy for Part B expenditures

Figure 8.2: Estimated Medicare Benefit Payments, by Type of Service, Fiscal Year 2005

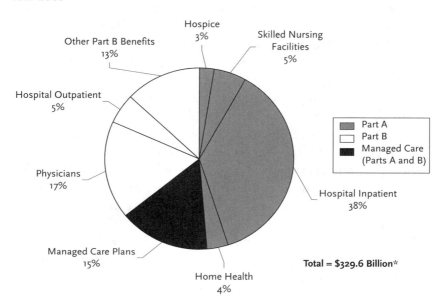

*Excludes administrative expenses and low-income subsidy payments.

Source: Congressional Budget Office. 2006. *Medicare Baseline.* March. [Online information.] http://www.cbo.gov/budget/factsheets/2006b/medicare.pdf.

exceeded $116 billion; this is estimated to rise to $221 billion by 2015. By way of comparison, Medicare's share of the federal budget was 13.5 percent ($333 billion) in 2005 and is expected to rise to 21.0 percent ($808 billion) of all federal expenditures by 2015.

Part C: Medicare Advantage Plans

Since the 1980s, the aged have been able to voluntarily enroll in a managed care plan, such as an HMO or PPO. The managed care plan receives a capitation payment from Medicare based on the total Part A and Part B expenditures for a Medicare beneficiary in that particular geographic area (adjusted for age, sex, and Medicaid and institutional status). In return for this capitation payment the managed care plan provides more comprehensive benefits, such as lower out-of-pocket payments and additional services not covered under Medicare Part B. The managed care plan, which is at risk for providing all the promised benefits in return for the capitation payment, limits the aged enrollees' choice of physicians and hospitals to those in the managed care plan's provider network. Thus, the managed care plan has a financial incentive to reduce inappropriate care and manage the aged's care in a more cost-effective manner.

About 5.7 million, or 13.6 percent, of the aged are enrolled in Medicare managed care plans; the remainder are in traditional fee-for-service Medicare, where the hospitals and physicians are paid on a fee-for-service basis, and the government regulates prices. Since 2003, the aged have to remain in a given health plan for a minimum of one year, whereas previously they were able to switch health plans with one month's notice.

Part D: Outpatient Prescription Drugs

In December 2003 the Medicare Modernization Act was enacted, which provided the aged with a new stand-alone outpatient prescription drug benefit starting in 2006. The drug benefits are provided by private, risk-bearing, plans. The aged use more outpatient prescription drugs than any other age group, and the financial burden of these drugs was often of greater concern than the costs of hospital and physician services, most of which were covered by Medicare. Although the aged are required to pay a $35 monthly premium for the new (voluntary) benefit, the cost of the program is heavily subsidized (75 percent) from federal tax revenues.

The design of the new prescription drug benefit was affected by an overall budgetary limit and legislators' desire that all the aged receive some benefit, that it should not be limited to just those aged with very large drug expenses. As shown in Figure 8.3, after meeting a $250 deductible, the aged must then pay 25 percent of their drug expenses between $250 and $2,500 (so almost all of the aged would receive some benefit). Then, to remain within the budget limit for this new benefit, the aged must pay 100 percent of their drug expenses between $2,500 and $5,100 before the government picks up 95 percent of their remaining drug expenses. The deductibles increase over time, as shown for 2013 in the bottom part of Figure 8.3.

"Medigap" Insurance

About 75 percent of the aged (mostly middle- and high-income aged) also purchase private "Medigap" insurance to cover the HI and SMI out-of-pocket costs not covered by Medicare. These out-of-pocket expenses—the HI and SMI deductibles and the 20 percent SMI copayment—can be a substantial financial burden as Medicare does not have

Figure 8.3: Medicare Prescription Drug Benefit

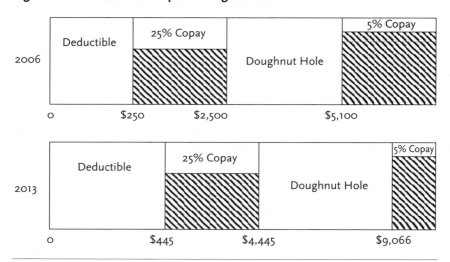

any stop-loss limit for out-of-pocket expenses. (When their out-of-pocket expenses become too great a financial burden, the low-income aged must fall back on Medicaid.) Medigap policies provide the aged with nearly first-dollar coverage, eliminating patients' financial incentives to limit their use of services or join managed care plans.

CONCERNS ABOUT THE CURRENT MEDICARE SYSTEM

Two basic concerns with Medicare are whether its redistributive system is fair and whether it promotes efficiency.

Redistributive Aspects of Medicare

Does Medicare promote equity in terms of who receives and who finances its subsidies? When a person pays the full cost of the benefits she receives, no redistribution occurs. However, when a person pays less than the full costs of his benefits, he receives a subsidy and other population groups must bear the financial burden of that subsidy. Because Medicare is a pay-as-you-go system, its beneficiaries contributed on average much less than the benefits they have received.

Redistribution is based on a societal value judgment that subsidies should be provided to particular groups. Typically, subsidies are expected to go to those with lower incomes and be financed by those with higher incomes.

Medicare's redistributive system raises two concerns. First, Medicare benefits have been the same for all of the aged regardless of income. Medicare pays on average only half of the aged's medical expenses. Medicare has relatively high deductibles and no limit on out-of-pocket expenditures, and nonacute services, such as long-term care, are not covered. Furthermore, those aged requiring home care or nursing home services unrelated to an illness episode must typically rely on their own funds to cover such expenses. Thus, out-of-pocket payments for excluded benefits as a percentage of income are very high for the low-income aged, exceeding 20 percent, whereas the corresponding figure for the high-income aged is less than 6 percent on average. Consequently, many low-income aged find the out-of-pocket expenses a financial hardship, and 11 percent must rely on Medicaid. Furthermore, almost all of the aged (97 percent) pay the same Part B premium and therefore receive the same subsidy. (Starting in 2006 Part B premium subsidies for high-income aged will be slightly reduced.)

How equitable is the financing of Medicare? Medicare beneficiaries do not pay the full costs of the medical services they receive; the aged are subsidized by those who pay state and federal taxes and Medicare HI taxes. The subsidy to Medicaid recipients is acknowledged to be "welfare," as they receive benefits in excess of any taxes they may have paid. As a welfare program, Medicaid is appropriately financed through the income tax system, whereby those with higher incomes contribute more in both absolute and proportionate payments in relation to their income. This is the fairest way to finance a welfare program.

Thus, the second concern with Medicare's redistributive system is that Medicare enrollees currently receive a very large intergenerational transfer of wealth (subsidy) from those currently in the labor force, which is no different from a conventional form of welfare. Several studies have estimated the difference between the Medicare payroll tax contributions made by the aged and the average value of the benefits they received; the difference between these contributions and benefits is the size of the intergenerational subsidy. For example, those aged who became eligible when Medicare started in 1966 received a 100 percent welfare subsidy. In subsequent years, as more aged became eligible, they made some contributions into the Hospital Trust Fund. Vogel (1988) estimates that 95 percent of Part A expenditures in 1984 should be regarded as subsidies, and Iglehart (1992, p. 966) states that, "for those who retired in 1991, the current average value of a beneficiary's Medicare hospital benefit far exceeds his or her contribution: $5.09 of services has been paid for under Part A for every $1 contributed. The ratio of benefits to contributions is even greater for people who retired earlier."

To these Part A subsidies should be added the 75 percent federal subsidy for Part B (SMI) premiums, which exceeded $116 billion in 2005, and the 75 percent federal subsidy for Part D (prescription drugs), which is estimated to exceed $890 billion over the next decade. However, because both the Part B and Part C subsidies are financed from general income taxes, those with higher incomes provide the intergenerational subsidy to the aged. With regard to Part A, on the other hand, the subsidy to the aged is financed by a payroll tax on all employees. Thus, an inequitable situation arises. Lower-income employees are taxed to subsidize the medical expenses of higher-income Medicare beneficiaries.

Payroll taxes are not a desirable method of financing a welfare program. Although the employer and the employee each pay half of the Medicare HI tax, studies confirm that employees end up paying most of the employer's share of the payroll tax as well (Brittain 1971; Summers 1989). When an employer decides how many employees to hire and what wage to pay, it considers all of the costs of that employee. Any tax or regulatory cost imposed on the employer based on its number of employees is the same as requiring the employer to pay higher wages to those employees. Whether the cost of that employee is in the form of wages, fringe benefits, or taxes does not matter to the employer; these costs are each considered a cost of labor. An increase in the employer's HI tax increases the cost of labor.

When the cost of an employee is increased and exceeds her value to the employer, the employer will discharge the employee unless it can reduce the employee's wage so the cost does not exceed the employee's value. Typically, when payroll taxes are increased, wages are eventually renegotiated. Employees receive less than they would otherwise have received because of higher payroll taxes imposed on the employer. Thus, most of the employer's share of the tax is shifted to the employee in the form of lower wages.

A tax per employee imposed on the employer rarely stays with the employer. Although the employer pays the tax, the part of the tax not shifted back to the employee in the form of lower wages will be shifted forward in the form of higher prices for goods and services. For example, most industries are competitive and do not earn excessive profits; otherwise, firms would enter the industry and compete away those profits. When the HI tax is increased on both the employee and employer, employment contracts cannot be immediately renegotiated. Rather than being forced to reduce its profits and leave the industry, the employer will shift the tax forward to the consumer by raising prices.

Whether the tax is shifted back to the employee or forward to the consumer, the tax is regressive; those with low incomes pay a greater portion of their income in Social Security taxes than do higher-income people. Only recently has the HI payroll tax become proportional to wages; because interest and dividend income is excluded from the tax, only a portion of an employee's income is subject to that tax. When the tax is passed on to consumers, the higher prices are a greater proportionate burden on low-income consumers.

If the tax is shifted either forward or backward, why is half of the tax imposed on the employer? The reason is related more to a tax's visibility than to who ends up paying it. Politicians would prefer to make employees believe their share of the tax is much smaller than it actually is.

If society makes the value judgment that it wants to help those with low incomes by providing them with a welfare benefit, the most equitable way to do so would be to provide the majority of benefits to those with low incomes and finance those benefits by taxing those with higher incomes. The burden of financing Medicare Part A, however, has fallen more heavily on those with lower incomes. Many aged who receive Part A benefits have higher incomes and assets than those who are providing the subsidies. An income tax, which takes proportionately more from those with higher incomes, would be a more equitable way to finance benefits to those with low incomes. Although the investment and retirement incomes of high-income aged are not subject to payroll taxes, they are subject to income taxes.

Efficiency Incentives in Medicare

Traditional Medicare was designed to provide limited efficiency incentives for either beneficiaries or providers of medical services. The elderly had no incentives to choose less-costly hospitals, as the deductible was the same and there were no copayments for inpatient admissions or lengths of stay. Hospitals were initially paid according to whatever their costs were for caring for an aged patient. In 1984, Medicare changed hospital payment to a fixed price per admission, but neither hospitals nor physicians have a financial incentive to manage the overall costs of an episode of care for an aged patient or provide preventive services that lead to lower acute medical costs. Only Medicare Advantage plans, such as HMOs, paid on a capitation basis have such incentives.

Medicare can best be thought of as a state-of-the-art 1960s health insurance plan. Congress modeled Part A after BlueCross, which paid for hospitalization, and Part B after BlueShield, which covered physician services. Cost-containment and utilization management methods used extensively in the private insurance market are virtually nonexistent in Medicare.

The lack of financial incentives for providers to be concerned with appropriate coordinated care and minimizing the cost of that care led to rapid increases in the cost of Medicare over time. In 2005, Medicare spent $342 billion, compared with $1.8 billion in 1966. As Medicare expenditures have exceeded government projections, every administration, regardless of political party, has increased the HI payroll tax and reduced the rate of increase in hospital payments for treating Medicare patients.

As shown in Figure 8.4, when the Medicare hospital DRG pricing system was introduced in the mid-1980s and an annual limit was placed on increases in the DRG price, the rate of increase in Medicare hospital expenditures declined. However, since the late 1980s, expenditures for skilled nursing homes, and particularly home health care, which were included in Part A, have increased very rapidly, causing total Part A expenditures to sharply increase.

In 1997, concerned by the rate of increase in Part A expenditures, Congress enacted several changes intended to keep the Medicare (Part A) HI Hospital Trust Fund solvent. Home health care expenditures, which were increasing very rapidly, were simply moved from Part A to Part B. This change shifted the financing of home health care from the payroll tax to the income tax. Congress also reduced payments to hospitals and to Medicare HMOs, which caused many HMOs to reduce their enrollment of Medicare beneficiaries. (Both of these changes resulted in a reduction in Medicare Part A expenditures, as shown in Figure 8.4.)

To limit the rise in Part B expenditures, in 1997 Congress also changed the method by which physicians' fees would be updated annually. Medicare physician fee increases were to be based in part according to the percentage increase in real GDP per capita, which is unrelated to the supply and demand for physician services by Medicare beneficiaries.

Figure 8.4: Growth in Real Medicare Expenditures per Enrollee, Parts A and B, 1966–2005

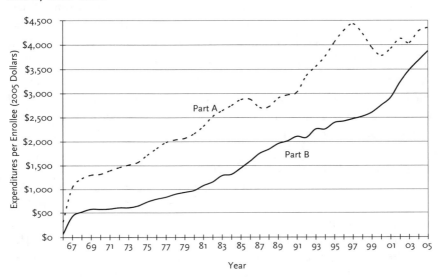

Note: Values adjusted for inflation using the consumer price index for all urban consumers. Part A and Part B expenditures exclude patient deductible. In 1997, home health care was moved from Part A to Part B. As a result, Part A expenditures per enrollee dropped.

Sources: Data from U.S. Department of Health and Human Services, Social Security Administration. 2000. *Social Security Bulletin, Annual Statistical Supplement.* Washington, DC: U.S. DHHS; 2000–2005 data from Centers for Medicare & Medicaid Services, Office of the Actuary. 2006. *2006 Annual Report of the Boards of Trustees of the Federal Hospital Insurance and Federal Supplementary Medical Insurance Trust Funds.* May 1. [Online information.] http://www.cms.hhs.gov/ ReportsTrustFunds/downloads/tr2006.pdf.

(This is referred to as the "sustainable growth rate," or SGR). The consequences of the SGR were not to be felt for several years.

At the same time Congress was limiting provider payment increases, the aged were provided with additional benefits by expanding Medicare coverage for preventive services such as mammograms, Pap smears, and prostate and colorectal screening tests.

Perhaps the clearest indication of Medicare's inefficient design is the wide variation that exists in Medicare expenditures per beneficiary with chronic illness across states, without any difference in life expectancy or in patient satisfaction.[1] For example, in 2005 Medicare spent, on average, $39,810 per beneficiary in New Jersey, compared with an average of $23,697 per beneficiary in other states. Patients with chronic illness in New Jersey had an average of 41.5 physician visits during the last six months of their lives, compared with an average of 17 visits for similar patients in Utah. Hospital days during the last six months of their lives varied from 32.1 per beneficiary at one medical center to 12.9 at another medical center. During the last two years, Medicare spent an average of $79,280 at one academic medical center, compared with $37,271 at another academic center. Medicare pays for quantity, not quality.

Medicare Modernization Act of 2003

The largest and most significant change to Medicare since its inception was the passage of the Medicare Modernization Act, which provided the aged with an outpatient prescription drug benefit. The initial cost of this drug benefit was estimated at $400 billion over ten years. This estimate has since been revised upward to almost $1 trillion over ten years. To receive the political support of hospitals and physician groups, Congress included in the legislation additional payments for hospitals and reversed the 4.5 percent decrease in Medicare physician fees that were to occur, based on the SGR. Instead, physicians were provided with a 1.5 percent increase.

IMPENDING BANKRUPTCY OF MEDICARE

The current Medicare program, without improvements, is ill suited to serve future generations of seniors and eligible disabled Americans.

---

1. The Dartmouth Atlas Project (2006) online report, *The Care of Patients with Severe Chronic Illness*, examined differences in the management of Medicare patients "with one or more of twelve chronic illnesses that accounts for more than 75% of all U.S. health care expenditures. Among people who died between 1999 and 2003, per capita spending varied by a factor of six between hospitals across the country. Spending was not correlated with rates of illness in different parts of the country; rather, it reflected how intensively certain resources—acute care hospital beds, specialist physician visits, tests and other services— were used in the management of people who were very ill but could not be cured. Since other research has demonstrated that, for these chronically ill Americans, receiving more services does not result in improved outcomes, and since most Americans say they prefer to avoid a very 'high-tech' death, the report concludes that Medicare spending for the care of the chronically ill could be reduced by as much as 30%—*while improving quality, patient satisfaction, and outcomes.*"

Medicare's future faces a series of challenges. The numbers of aged are increasing both in absolute and percentage terms. The aged are also living longer. Medical care costs continue to increase, and technology is driving medical costs still higher. To continue maintaining the solvency of Medicare Part A by imposing higher payroll taxes on the working population will be both politically infeasible as well as inequitable for those with low incomes. Medicare Part B and Part C expenditures, which are funded from general tax revenues, will eventually consume the entire federal budget and require politically unpopular income tax increases.

Medicare expenditures for Parts A, B, and D are expected to increase from 2.7 percent of GDP in 2005 to 5.4 percent by 2015. As a percentage of the federal budget, total Medicare expenditures are estimated to increase from 13.5 percent to 21.0 percent by 2015, based on the more likely pessimistic projections (U.S. Congressional Budget Office 2005).

In addition, the Medicare Supplementary Medical Insurance Trust Fund that pays for physician services and the new prescription drug benefit will require substantial increases over time in both general revenue financing and premium charges. As the reserves in HI are drawn down and SMI general revenue financing requirements continue to grow, the pressure on the federal budget will intensify.

The currently projected long-run growth rates of Medicare are not sustainable under current financing arrangements.

In coming years the aging of the population will place great pressures on the HI Trust Fund. The first of the 77 million baby boomers will retire in 2011. In 1960, just 9.2 percent of the population was older than 65 years. In 2005, 12.4 percent of the population was aged 65 or older. Under the demographic pressure of the baby boomers, the number of Medicare recipients will almost double by 2030 (from 37 million to 71 million), when the last of the baby boomers will have turned 65 (see Figure 8.5). At that time, almost one in five Americans (19.6 percent) will be older than 65.

People older than 65 years have four times the medical costs of younger Americans. Large numbers of retirees, combined with increased longevity and more expensive and advanced medical technology, will generate huge increases in Medicare spending. The magnitude of this projected shortfall is shown in Figure 8.6.

The pressure to reform Medicare will most likely occur as the Medicare Trust Fund approaches insolvency. The HI Trust Fund had negative cash flows in 2007, and annual cash flow deficits are expected to

Figure 8.5: Population Pyramid, United States, 1960, 2005, and 2030

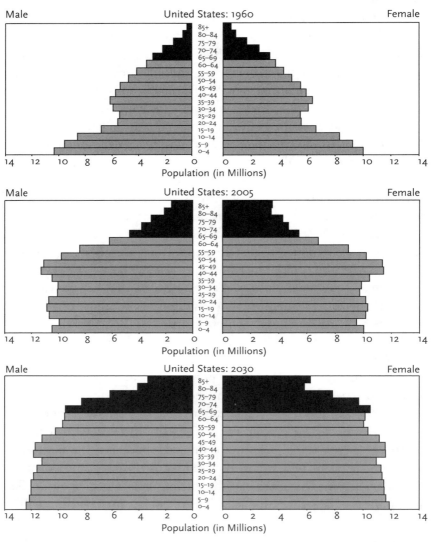

Source: Data from Department of Commerce, U.S. Census Bureau. 2006. *International Data Base.* [Online information.] http://www.census.gov/ipc/www/idbpyr.html.

continue and to grow rapidly after 2011 as baby boomers begin to retire. The growing deficits will exhaust the Trust Fund reserves in 2020.

At the same time Medicare expenditures are projected to sharply increase, the employee base supporting Medicare is eroding. Per aged

Figure 8.6: Net Cash Flow of the Medicare HI Trust Fund, 2002–2015

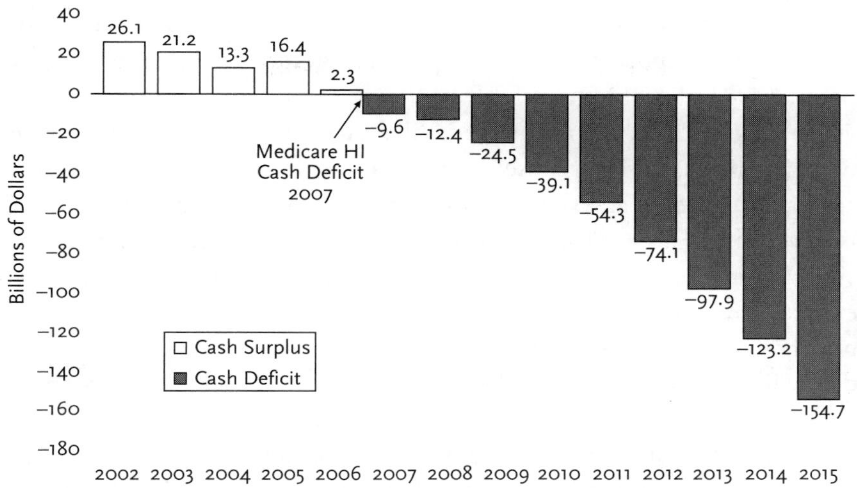

Source: Centers for Medicare & Medicaid Services, Office of the Actuary. 2006. *2006 Annual Report of the Board of Trustees of the Federal Hospital Insurance and Federal Supplementary Medical Insurance Trust Funds.* May 1, Tables III.B4., III.B5. [Online information.] http://www.cms.hhs.gov/ReportsTrustFunds/downloads/tr2006.pdf.

person, the number of workers paying taxes and financing the program has been steadily declining, increasing the tax burden on each employee. In 1960 there were 5.1 workers per beneficiary, in 1970 that ratio declined to 3.7:1, and currently it is 3.4:1. By 2030, when the last of the baby boomers retire, that ratio will fall to 2.2:1.

Intermediate projections indicate that the HI tax will have to be increased from 2.9 percent to 6.21 percent. However, as actual experience has been much closer to the pessimistic (high cost) assumptions, the HI tax rate will likely have to be increased to 10.86 percent by 2030.[2] These increased tax rates are only for Part A. The annual subsidy for Medicare

2. The rate of growth in real wages (because HI is a payroll tax) and life expectancy at retirement are important components of these projections. Pessimistic projections assume a rate of growth in real wages similar to the growth rate in the past 25 years, which is half as large as that used in the intermediate assumption. Advances in medicine, genetics, and biotechnology are also projected to result in a more rapid increase in life expectancy at retirement than the intermediate projections that assume the same rate as for the past 50 years.

Parts A, B, and D (in constant 2005 dollars) will rise from $299 billion (2005) to $701 billion by 2015 (total expenditures minus premium income).[3] Unless taxes are increased or Medicare benefits are reduced, these federal expenditures will require reductions in other politically popular federal programs.

Political support for Medicare is likely to decline as the costs to the nonaged increase, with a consequent increase in intergenerational political conflict. Our political system cannot wait until 2011 to resolve an issue that involves such a large redistribution of wealth among different groups in society. When the baby boomers start retiring in 2011, they will have certain expectations about what they will receive from Medicare. Politicians cannot change Medicare's benefits at the last moment. No presidential candidate will likely campaign on decreasing Medicare benefits. Any changes will have to be agreed upon in nonelection years and gradually phased in. Yet the longer Congress waits, the higher the payroll tax will be.

Enacting legislation to decrease Medicare benefits or eligibility in either a presidential election year or a congressional election year will be very difficult, as Medicare has such widespread political support among the elderly, the near elderly, and their children, who might be faced with an increased financial burden of paying their parents' medical expenses. Given that a new Medicare system must be phased in and there are few nonelection years in which to enact such controversial legislation, any changes must be enacted within the next few years.

PROPOSALS FOR MEDICARE REFORM

The financial problems of Medicare cannot be solved by using only past approaches—increasing the HI tax and reducing hospital and physician payments—because the funds required would be too great and the tax base too small. Employees will begin to oppose politicians who want to increase their payroll taxes, hospitals and physicians will reduce access to care for the aged, and quality of services will decline as costs exceed government payments. Instead, Medicare will have to be restructured. Furthermore, the financial burden will likely be spread over several constituencies—taxpayers, employees, health care providers, and the baby

---

3. In 2005, annual federal expenditures were $184 billion for Medicare Part A, $152 billion for Part B, and $1.2 billion for Part D—a total of $337 billion. Projected federal subsidies (expenditures minus premiums) in 2015 for each part of Medicare, in constant dollars, are $352 billion for Part A, $220 billion for Part B, and $129 billion for Part D—a total of $701 billion.

boomers. As in previous attempts to save the Trust Fund, the current aged are least likely to be adversely affected by these changes.

Proposals to restructure Medicare should be based on two criteria: equity and efficiency. To make Medicare an equitable redistribution system, the "entitlement" myth of Medicare must be recognized, and its large welfare component acknowledged. Medicare should either become similar to a pension system whereby people save for their own medical (and long-term-care) expenses, or government subsidies should be used to help the low-income aged. Health plans should also compete for beneficiaries based on price, quality, outcomes, and enrollee satisfaction. Health plans will then have incentives to be efficient and responsive to beneficiary preferences.

The following approaches have been proposed for reforming Medicare. A combination of proposals will likely be used to spread the financial burden.

Increase the Eligibility Age to 67

Similar to one of the solutions used to increase the solvency of the Social Security system, the age of eligibility would be increased by one month each year so that the eligibility age for Social Security and Medicare are the same at 67. With increased life expectancy, people could work longer and maintain their employment-based health insurance.

Reduce the Rate of Increase in Medicare Provider Payments

This approach has been used previously and is likely to be part of any long-term solution. However, decreasing provider payments will ultimately reduce provider participation and access to care by Medicare beneficiaries.

Increase the HI (Part A) Tax

This approach, which has also been used previously, is likely to be part of any proposed solution. An increase in the HI tax would increase the financial burden on low-wage workers.

Increase the Part B Premium

The elderly currently pay a premium that covers only 25 percent of Part B expenditures; a higher percentage will likely be phased in over time. A uniform premium increase for all of the aged places a greater financial burden on low-income aged.

Make the Part B Premium Income Related

As the Part B premium is increased, the percentage of the Part B premium paid by the aged could be related to their incomes, which would minimize the hardship on the low-income aged. The Medicare Modernization Act of 2003 was a start in this direction by making very high income aged (3 percent of the total) receive smaller federal subsidies (Pauly 2004). Equity would be improved if subsidies to higher-income aged were completely phased out.

Change Medicare from a Defined-Benefit to a Defined-Contribution Plan

Medicare currently pays for a defined (and continually expanding) set of benefits regardless of their costs, which is an open-ended government commitment. A defined contribution is a predetermined amount of money (including Parts A, B, C, and D), similar to a voucher, that the government would pay to a health plan on behalf of the aged. (This capitation payment should be risk adjusted based on age, health status, and geographic location to reflect the expected variation in a beneficiary's health costs.) Older and sicker beneficiaries would receive higher amounts to provide health plans with an incentive to enroll them. Health plans would compete for the defined contribution, and the aged would have an incentive to shop for the most cost-effective plan.

In addition to providing greater predictability to the government, the financial risk of caring for the aged is shifted to the health plan. Under a defined-contribution plan the government would pay the premium for the low-cost health plan (an HMO) in an area. The aged would be able to join other, more expensive plans by paying the additional cost of those plans. (This approach is similar to the Federal Employees Health Benefits Plan.)

Change Medicare to an Income-Related Program

Medicare benefits can be made income related by providing the aged with a voucher for a uniform set of benefits. The value of the voucher would equal the entire premium for low-income aged and would decline in value the higher the income of the aged. As a transition to this approach, all of the current aged could receive the full value of the voucher. The income-related voucher would be phased in for future aged.

In addition to improving equity, the income-related approach would also improve efficiency, unlike traditional fee-for-service Medicare, because managed care plans would compete for the vouchers. An income-related approach would reduce both the cost of the program and the huge intergenerational subsidies from low-income workers to high-income aged. Income-related benefits would also help the low-income aged, who are less able to afford the same deductibles, cost sharing, and Part B and C premiums than high-income aged.

Medical Individual Retirement Account

Medicare could be changed from a pay-as-you-go plan (in which the contributions from current employees pay the expenses of current retirees) to a true pension-type system in which the funds contributed by current employees are invested and available to pay their future retirement medical benefits. Under this scenario employees would be able to invest their 2.9 percent HI tax in a medical individual retirement account (medical IRA) to be used only when they retire. Obviously, such a plan would have to be phased in over a long transition period, as many workers have already contributed to Medicare. Additional government funds would be required under this approach because the government would lose the HI payroll tax revenues from those employees who choose the medical IRA option. Individuals would have greater control (and incentive) over how their health care funds are spent; they could be used to buy a high-eductible plan or join a health plan. These funds could also be used for long-term care.

POLITICS OF MEDICARE REFORM

The popularity of Medicare means that politicians who attempt to change it without the endorsement of both political parties are at great political risk. Previously, imposing financial burdens on providers by paying them less and increasing payroll taxes was easier than increasing the financial burden on the elderly.[4]

Unfortunately, the longer it takes to phase in a system that is more equitable, the greater will be the political problems. Current workers will have to pay higher payroll taxes, intergenerational transfers from

---

4. The Medicare Catastrophic Act of 1989 provides an illustration of how much difficulty Congress will face in enacting equitable Medicare reform. High-income aged were required to increase their Part B contributions to finance greater benefits to low-income aged. Protests by the high-income aged were so great that Congress repealed the legislation the following year, and this attempt to increase fairness failed.

low-income workers will increase, beneficiaries will have less access to providers as provider fees are reduced, and the financial hardship on low-income aged who cannot afford high out-of-pocket expenditures and rising Part B and C premiums will increase. The sooner the financial burden is shared among the different groups in a more equitable manner, the smaller future tax increases will be as more baby boomers retire.

SUMMARY

The potential cost of suggesting dramatic solutions is very high to any one political party. Whatever the combination of approaches selected, a vast redistribution of wealth will result. A bipartisan commission whose recommendations are adopted by Congress has in the past resolved such highly visible redistributive problems. Although the National Bipartisan Commission on the Future of Medicare (created by Congress as part of the 1997 Balanced Budget Act) was unable to reach agreement (by just one vote) on reforming Medicare in 1999, whether and when a commission approach will again be used for reforming Medicare remains to be seen.

DISCUSSION QUESTIONS

1. Which population groups are served by Medicare, what are the different parts of Medicare, and how is Medicare financed?

2. Discuss how Medicare's patient and provider incentives affect efficient use of services.

3. How equitable are the methods used to finance Medicare?

4. How does the Medicare Hospital Trust Fund differ from a pension fund?

5. Why is it necessary to reform Medicare?

6. Evaluate proposals to reform Medicare in terms of their equitability and effects on efficiency.

REFERENCES

Brittain, J. A. 1971. "The Incidence of Social Security Payroll Taxes." *American Economic Review* 61 (1): 110–25.

Dartmouth Atlas Project. 2006. *The Care of Patients with Severe Chronic Illness.* [Online publication; retrieved 11/15/06.] http://www.dartmouthatlas.org/press/ 2006_atlas_press_release.shtm.

Iglehart, J. K. 1992. "The American Health Care System—Introduction." *The New England Journal of Medicine* 326 (14): 962–67.

Pauly, M. 2004. "Means-Testing in Medicare." *Health Affairs* Web exclusive, December 8, W4-546–W4-557. [Online article; retrieved 11/15/06.] http://content. healthaffairs.org/cgi/reprint/hlthaff.w4.546v1.

Summers, L. 1989. "Some Simple Economics of Mandated Benefits." *American Economic Review* 79 (2): 177–83.

U.S. Congressional Budget Office. 2005. *The Budget and Economic Outlook: An Update.* [Online publication; retrieved 12/6/06.] http://www.cbo.gov/ftpdocs/66xx/ doc6609/08-15-OutlookUpdate.pdf.

Vogel, R. J. 1988. "An Analysis of the Welfare Component and Intergenerational Transfers Under the Medicare Program." In *Lessons from the First Twenty Years of Medicare*, edited by M. V. Pauly and W. L. Kissick, 73–114. Philadelphia: University of Pennsylvania Press.

Chapter 9

Medicaid

MEDICAID IS A means-tested welfare program for the poor, providing medical and long-term care to more than 16 percent of the population. In 1985, Medicaid covered 22 million people, the federal government spent $23 billion on the program, and it represented 2.4 percent of the federal budget. By 2005, Medicaid covered 57 million people, total federal expenditures reached $182 billion, and the program increased its share of the federal budget to 7.5 percent. Despite these rapidly increasing Medicaid expenditures, which represent a growing financial burden on federal and state budgets, many low-income persons do not qualify for Medicaid.

Medicaid is administered by each state, but policy is shared by the federal government, which pays between 50 percent and 76 percent matching funds based on each state's financial capacity (per capita income).[1] These federal dollars make Medicaid a less-expensive approach for the states to use in expanding access to medical care by those with

---

1. Many states have used various financing schemes, sometimes using intergovernmental transfers, to make large supplementary payments to government-owned or government-operated health care providers, such as nursing homes, to inappropriately increase federal Medicaid payments. These supplementary payments are in excess of the established Medicaid payment rate and create the illusion that these are valid payments for services delivered to Medicaid beneficiaries. The state payments above the usual payment rate allow states to obtain federal reimbursement, only to have the local government providers, under agreements with the states, transfer the excessive federal and state payments back to the state. Once the states receive the returned funds, they have increased their federal matching rate above the established federal law and can use those funds to substitute for their share of future Medicaid spending or even for non-Medicaid purposes.

low incomes, compared with other state programs such as General Assistance. Each state Medicaid program must cover certain federally mandated population groups to qualify for federal matching funds.

The first, and largest, of the federally mandated population groups are those receiving cash welfare assistance, which include single-parent families, who were previously eligible for Aid to Families with Dependent Children (AFDC), and low-income aged, blind, and disabled persons who qualify for Supplemental Security Income. The second mandatory eligibility group is low-income pregnant women and children who do not qualify for cash assistance. Third are those considered to be "medically needy," that is, persons who do not qualify for welfare programs but have high medical or long-term-care expenses. The fourth group consists of low-income Medicare beneficiaries who cannot afford the deductibles, cost sharing, premiums for Medicare Part B, or cost of services not covered by Medicare.

States may expand eligibility and enroll additional groups (and add services beyond those for groups mandated by the federal government). Thus, wide variations in coverage and eligibility exist among the states. Groups typically added at the state's option include medically needy individuals, children and pregnant women at a higher percentage in excess of the federal poverty level (e.g., 200 percent), and all uninsured persons with incomes below a certain level. However, the percentage of the Medicaid-covered population that is poor (less than 100 percent of the poverty level) varies greatly by state, between 33 percent and 65 percent. Just being poor is insufficient to qualify for Medicaid. *On average, only 40 percent of those classified as poor are enrolled in Medicaid.* The percentage of near-poor (100 percent to 199 percent of poverty) enrolled by states varies from 7 percent to 28 percent (average 16.5 percent).

In 1996, Temporary Assistance to Needy Families (TANF) was enacted to replace AFDC. TANF retains the same eligibility rules as AFDC. Before welfare reform many poor children qualified automatically for Medicaid because their families were receiving AFDC, the national cash benefits program for poor children. Welfare reform ended that link because it abolished AFDC. Because Congress did not want anyone to lose Medicaid eligibility as a result of welfare reform, it decreed that states should continue using their old AFDC rules for determining Medicaid eligibility, such as covering pregnant women, the medically needy, and children, if their parents would have qualified for AFDC under the old law. The children of women who leave welfare for work are still eligible for Medicaid because of low family income.

AN ILLUSTRATION OF MEDICAID ELIGIBILITY

Within federal guidelines, states may set their own income and asset eligibility criteria for Medicaid. Following is an illustration of how those who are medically needy qualify for Medi-Cal (Medicaid in California). A person cannot have more than $2,000 in assets ($3,000 for two people), excluding a house, car, and furniture. One's financial assets can be reduced in many legitimate ways to qualify for Medicaid. Money could be spent fixing up one's house, purchasing a new car, or taking a vacation, or it could be put in a special burial account. Selling one's house and giving the cash to one's children will make one ineligible for Medicaid for 29 months.

When a couple is involved, special spousal financial protections exist. If a husband enters a nursing home, the wife can remain in their home and is entitled to have about $2,000 a month in income and $95,100 in financial assets. If the wife's Social Security payments are below $2,000, the husband's Social Security can be used to bring her monthly income to $2,000.

Retirement accounts and other assets can be partially shielded from the government by counting the income from those retirement accounts toward the $2,000 monthly income. For example, if a person has $100,000 in an IRA and takes out $500 a month, the $500 counts toward his monthly income, but the $100,000 does not count as an asset. A number of states have begun to crack down on various schemes used by some wealthy aged to shield their assets to become Medicaid eligible, such as setting up annuities, trusts, and life contracts.[2] In general, however, many middle-class elderly become distraught when they find they must spend down their hard-earned assets for a spouse to become Medicaid eligible.

---

2. As part of deficit-reduction legislation in 2005, Congress included limits on the ability of people with homes and assets to get Medicaid to pay their nursing home costs. The legislation toughens rules that prevent individuals seeking to become Medicaid eligible from transferring assets, usually to their children. Examples of these changes include lengthening the time period states are to examine for inappropriate transfer of assets to five years and excluding from Medicaid coverage persons whose home equity is in excess of $500,000 (previously there was no limit on home equity).

STATE CHILDREN'S HEALTH INSURANCE PROGRAM (SCHIP)

A major expansion of Medicaid eligibility occurred in 1997. As part of the 1997 Balanced Budget Act, Congress enacted the State Children's Health Insurance Program (SCHIP). SCHIP was enacted to provide coverage for low-income children whose family incomes were not low enough to qualify for Medicaid. Politically, children are considered to be a vulnerable and more deserving group than other uninsured groups; consequently, this program expansion received bipartisan support. (Medical benefits for children are considered to be relatively inexpensive compared with benefits for uninsured adults.) Furthermore, providing coverage to older children was viewed as an expansion of existing Medicaid policies, which expanded Medicaid coverage to infants, younger children, and pregnant women in the late 1980s. This program provided the states with federal matching funds to initiate and expand health care assistance for uninsured low-income children, up to age 19, with family incomes as high as 200 percent of the federal poverty level. (Federal matching funds may be as high as 85 percent.)

The number of children eligible for public coverage increased dramatically, as did participation rates in SCHIP. The percentage of uninsured children whose family income was between 100 percent and 200 percent of the poverty level (as well as those whose family income was less than 100 percent of the federal poverty level) has declined since 1997 (Cunningham and Kirby 2004). In each of these groups, the percentage of children with public coverage has increased; the percentage of children with private insurance decreased over this same period. Not all of the increase in public coverage for poor and low-income children, however, was the result of uninsured children being enrolled in SCHIP. A significant increase in public coverage also resulted from a shift away from private insurance to free or lower-cost public coverage.

Bipartisan support for SCHIP was also achieved as a result of an ideologic compromise on how SCHIP services would be delivered to eligible children. States may either purchase health insurance coverage for eligible children in the private market or they may be included in the state's Medicaid program.

Although SCHIP is considered to be successful in having increased the number of low-income children with health insurance, states are undertaking additional marketing efforts to further increase the enrollment of eligible children in SCHIP (the "take-up" rate).

MEDICAID BENEFICIARIES AND MEDICAID EXPENDITURES

Broadened eligibility requirements for Medicaid have caused the number of recipients to sharply increase, from 22 million in 1975 to 57 million in 2005. Most of the enrollment growth resulted from federal and state expansions in coverage of low-income children and pregnant women. Currently (as of 2006), the major beneficiary groups consist of low-income children (47.6 percent); nondisabled low-income adults (pregnant women and adults in families with children receiving cash assistance, 26.3 percent); aged persons receiving Medicare who need Medicaid ("dual eligibles") to pay for their deductibles, cost sharing, premiums for Medicare Parts B and D, and other services not covered by Medicare (9.6 percent); and blind and disabled persons receiving acute medical and long-term care services (16.5 percent).

As shown in Figure 9.1, the distribution of Medicaid expenditures does not match the distribution of Medicaid enrollees. Although about 74 percent of Medicaid recipients are low-income parents and children, they account for only about 31 percent of Medicaid expenditures. By comparison, about 69 percent of Medicaid expenditures are for medical services and institutional care for the aged, disabled, and mentally retarded (26 percent of Medicaid recipients).

Although the number of Medicaid beneficiaries has increased over time, from 22 million in 1975 and 1985 to about 35 million in the 1990s, to almost 60 million in 2005, the distribution of beneficiary groups has stayed roughly constant over this period.

State and federal Medicaid expenditures have been rapidly increasing and are expected to continue to rise sharply over the next decade. *Medicaid represents the largest single item in state budgets,* exceeding elementary and secondary education expenditures. Total Medicaid expenditures were $55.1 billion in 1988, rose to an estimated $313 billion in 2005, and are expected to reach $450 billion by 2010. The federal share of Medicaid expenditures is expected to increase from $182 billion in 2005 to $259 billion by 2010. The remaining expenditures represent the state's financial burden. During this same period, the number of beneficiaries is expected to increase by 7 percent (see Figure 9.2).

Figure 9.3 shows the distribution of Medicaid expenditures by type of service. The largest share of Medicaid expenditures is for acute care (62 percent), which comprises fee-for-service payments (69 percent), managed care (28 percent), and Medicare premiums (3 percent). Long-term

Figure 9.1: Percentage Distribution of Medicaid Enrollees and Benefit Payments, by Eligibility Status, Fiscal Year 2006

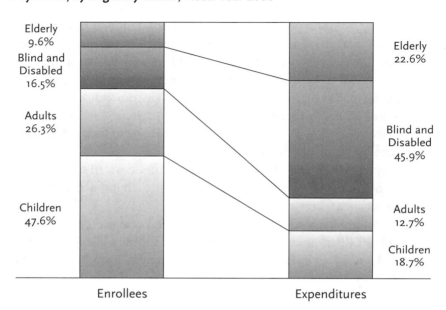

Elderly 9.6%
Blind and Disabled 16.5%
Adults 26.3%
Children 47.6%

Elderly 22.6%
Blind and Disabled 45.9%
Adults 12.7%
Children 18.7%

Enrollees   Expenditures

Source: Congressional Budget Office. 2006. *Medicaid Spending Growth and Options for Controlling Costs.* July 13. [Online information.] http://www.cbo.gov/ftpdocs/73xx/doc7387/07-13-Medicaid.pdf.

care (which includes nursing home care and home health care) represents the second-largest category (33 percent). Given the low rates Medicaid pays providers, payments to disproportionate-share hospitals (4.9 percent) compensate those hospitals that serve proportionately more Medicaid beneficiaries and low-income people.

MEDICAID POLICY ISSUES
Major Medicaid policy issues include:

- Providing Medicaid coverage for all those eligible for Medicaid;
- Providing full or partial coverage for those with low incomes who are not Medicaid eligible;
- Providing high-quality coordinated care to those receiving Medicaid services; and
- Reducing the rate of increase in Medicaid expenditures.

Figure 9.2: Number of Medicaid Beneficiaries and Total Medicaid Expenditures, Actual and Projected, 1975–2010

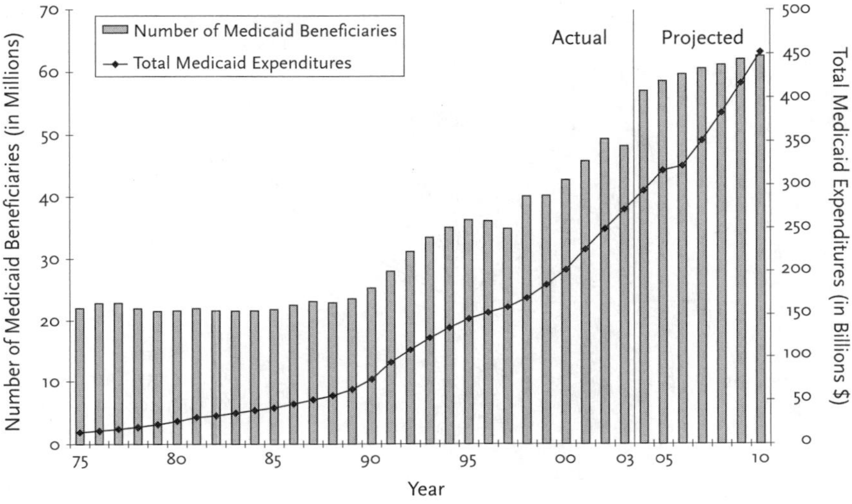

Sources: Data on the number of Medicaid beneficiaries from Centers for Medicare & Medicaid Services. 2006. [Online information.] http://www.cms.hhs.gov/Medicaid DataSourcesGenInfo/Downloads/MSISTables2003.pdf; Projected data from Congressional Budget Office. 2006. *Current Budget Projections.* March 3. [Online information.] http://www.cbo.gov/budget/factsheets/2006b/medicaid.pdf; Data on the total Medicaid expenditures from Centers for Medicare & Medicaid Services, Office of the Actuary, National Health Statistics Group. 2006. [Online information.] http://www.cms.hhs.gov/NationalHealthExpendData/downloads/tables.pdf.

These policy issues are not mutually exclusive; in fact, several of these goals are contradictory. To cover all those who are eligible, expand coverage to low-income persons who are not Medicaid eligible, and provide quality coordinated care cannot be achieved if federal and state policy at the same time emphasizes reducing the rate of increase in Medicaid expenditures. Rising Medicaid expenditures have become an increasing financial burden to the states and the federal government. At the federal level, the administration has attempted to limit its commitment to Medicaid by changing the program from a federal matching program into a program of block grants to each of the states. Federal Medicaid spending would therefore be "capped" and, in return, states would be granted greater flexibility in defining Medicaid eligibility and benefits. State governors have opposed the block grant approach, believing

Figure 9.3: Medicaid Expenditures, by Service, 2003

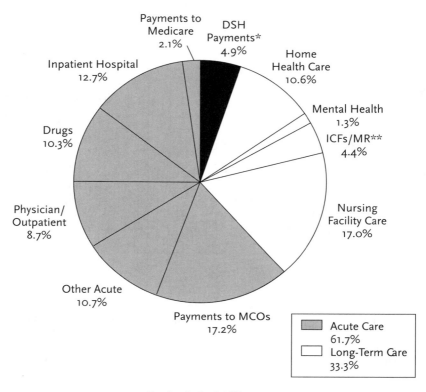

Total = $262.6 Billion

*DSH = disproportionate-share hospital payments.

**ICFs/MR = intermediate care facilities for the mentally retarded.

Source: Centers for Medicare & Medicaid Services. 2006. *2005 CMS Statistics.* [Online information.] http://www.cms.hhs.gov/MedicareMedicaidStatSupp/ downloads/ 2005_CMS_Statistics.pdf.

they will have to bear an even greater financial burden for the poor in their states.

States are limited in the amount of funds that can be spent on Medicaid. To continue spending an increasing portion of state budgets on Medicaid would require expenditures on politically popular programs, such as education and prisons, to be reduced or taxes increased. Each option is politically costly. Instead, many states have resorted to reducing Medicaid eligibility and setting low provider-payment rates, which reduce provider participation and reduce access to care by those on Medicaid.

Increasing the "take-up" rate, that is, increasing enrollment of those eligible, involves two benefit/cost trade-offs by those who are eligible but not participating in Medicaid. An eligible, but not participating, person must weigh the additional medical benefits she would receive if she participated in Medicaid versus the stigma "costs" of participating. Second, because income is one criterion for Medicaid eligibility, a person would lose his eligibility if his income increases above a certain level. Thus, another trade-off is between earning a higher income versus losing all Medicaid benefits. (This is referred to as the "notch" effect.) Medicaid eligibility would be increased if, as people's wages increased, they would lose only a portion of their Medicaid benefits. Graduating Medicaid benefits according to income would provide an incentive for those who want to keep their benefits to work more hours and to seek higher-paying jobs.

Expanding Medicaid coverage to a greater portion of those with low incomes involves addressing state funding issues as well as maintaining incentives for working low-income persons who have health insurance to maintain their private insurance. Working low-income people with insurance have an incentive to drop their private insurance and accept the free public insurance. (This phenomenon is referred to as "crowd out," that is, public insurance "crowds out" private insurance.) Although Medicaid is considered to be less valuable than private insurance (the stigma "cost" and access to physicians is more restricted because of low Medicaid reimbursement), as the cost of private insurance increases, Medicaid becomes a more desirable substitute. Expanded public coverage in some states has displaced existing private coverage with little additional overall gain in coverage. (Part of the private coverage replaced by public coverage may have had relatively limited benefits.)

To lessen the cost of expanding Medicaid eligibility to the working poor, incentives, such as partial Medicaid subsidies, should be developed to lessen employees' incentive for shifting from private coverage to Medicaid.

The remaining two Medicaid policy issues, providing high-quality coordinated care to Medicaid beneficiaries and reducing the rate of increase in Medicaid expenditures, are related. Medicaid has traditionally relied on fee-for-service provider payment. To reduce rising Medicaid expenditures Medicaid programs reduced the fees paid to health care providers. The consequence of both fee-for-service payment and reduced provider fees led to a lack of coordinated care and low provider participation rates in Medicaid. Physician fees affect not only access to care but also which physicians are willing to treat Medicaid patients and how much time physicians are willing to spend with their Medicaid patients (Gruber 2000).

Managed care offered Medicaid programs an approach to reduce rising Medicaid expenditures as well as provide coordinated care to its enrollees. By paying managed care plans, such as HMOs, a fixed fee per person per month (i.e., a "capitation" fee), states were able to shift their risk for higher expenditures to a managed care plan. In addition, states could monitor how well the managed care plan achieved specific goals, such as immunization rates, preventive care, reduced use of hospital emergency departments, and so on. Medicaid managed care has become an important approach for providing Medicaid services.

MEDICAID MANAGED CARE

The largest change in the distribution of Medicaid expenditures has been the growth in Medicaid managed care. Almost all states rely on some form of managed care for their Medicaid populations. About 60 percent of Medicaid beneficiaries are enrolled in some form of managed care program. The types of managed care plans used by states vary. Initially many states used primary care case management, whereby Medicaid beneficiaries are enrolled with a primary care "gatekeeper," who does not assume financial risk but receives a monthly fee of about $2 to $3 per enrollee per month and is responsible for coordinating the enrollee's care. Under the primary care case management concept providers are paid on a fee-for-service basis. In the mid-1990s, many states moved toward contracting with HMOs and paying them a capitated amount for each enrolled Medicaid beneficiary. Under full risk capitation the HMO provides a comprehensive range of required benefits that include both preventive and acute care services.

States contract with managed care plans for two reasons. The first is to reduce the rate of increase in Medicaid expenditures. Managed care produced substantial savings in the private sector. Similar savings have not occurred in fee-for-service Medicaid programs, where providers do not have similar incentives to reduce inpatient utilization, use less-costly outpatient settings, and reduce unnecessary use of the emergency department.

Second, contracting with managed care plans is expected to increase Medicaid enrollees' access to care. To save money Medicaid programs have reduced payments to hospitals and physicians (well below rates paid by other insurers) so that many health providers refuse to serve Medicaid patients. Medicaid enrollees have typically had to rely on emergency departments and on clinics that predominantly serve large numbers of Medicaid patients. By contracting with managed care plans, the states expect their Medicaid enrollees to have greater access to primary care providers, receive coordinated care, and spend fewer dollars than previously.

Until 1997, states had to seek federal waivers to mandate enrollment of their Medicaid beneficiaries in managed care plans. The 1997 Balanced Budget Act changed this requirement so that states no longer had to receive federal permission to enroll their Medicaid populations in managed care plans. The percentage of Medicaid beneficiaries enrolled in managed care plans increased rapidly, from 4.5 percent in 1991 to 63 percent in 2005. Eliminating federal waivers dramatically accelerated enrollment growth in managed care plans.

Initially, the Medicaid populations enrolled in Medicaid managed care programs were similar to those enrolled in private health plans, namely, children and working-age adult caregivers. Managed care plans have had a great deal of experience caring for these relatively young demographic groups in their commercial businesses. However, these population groups—nondisabled, low-income adults and children (who make up about 74 percent of Medicaid beneficiaries)—account for a relatively small share of Medicaid spending (about 31 percent of Medicaid expenditures). Managed care plans have had less experience in caring for chronically ill and disabled populations. Managing care for these groups is much more difficult but the potential savings of providing coordinated care to these populations is much greater. The aged, blind, and disabled and those in nursing homes (about 26 percent of beneficiaries) account for most Medicaid expenditures (about 69 percent). States have now begun to extend Medicaid managed care to these populations as well. Until managed care plans enroll and manage care for the chronically ill, AIDS patients, those with severe mental illness, and the institutionalized aged who require long-term care, managed care savings will not be very large.

It is very important for the states to provide managed care plans with appropriate financial incentives to enroll these more costly Medicaid beneficiaries. Capitation payments will have to reflect the costs of caring for different types of beneficiaries (risk-adjusted payments). If the payment rate is set too low, managed care plans will be unwilling to enroll these groups. To date, it has been very difficult to develop capitation rates that adequately reflect the costs of caring for elderly and chronically ill population groups.

It is essential for state Medicaid programs to monitor the care provided and the access to care by beneficiaries in any delivery system, managed care or traditional fee for service. Unfortunately, many states' performance in monitoring the quality of care received by their Medicaid populations has been notoriously inadequate. For budgetary reasons, some states are unwilling to monitor and punish low-performing providers. Nursing home scandals continue to surface, and many Medicaid programs are inadequate in terms of both the quality of care received and accessibility by Medicaid patients.

A challenge for many states will be to adequately monitor the care provided by managed care plans to the chronically ill and disabled, as well as to other Medicaid enrollees. In the past several years, a number of states have developed measurement tools to monitor the care received by their beneficiaries (Landon et al. 2004). In the private sector, insurers are beginning to use "pay for performance" to reward providers who practice high-quality care. It remains to be seen how well state agencies will use the quality information they receive to similarly reward and penalize different Medicaid providers.

REFORMING MEDICAID

Although Medicaid is the main program for providing medical services and long-term care to those with low incomes, it is generally perceived to be inadequate. Medicaid does not cover a large portion of those with low incomes; fewer than 50 percent of those who are considered poor and near-poor are covered. In addition, the percentage of low-income groups covered by Medicaid varies greatly among the states, from fewer than 40 percent to more than 60 percent. Only those with very low incomes are eligible; no more than 40 percent of people with incomes below the federal poverty level ($20,000 for a family of four, $13,200 for a couple, and $9,800 for a single person as of 2007, except in Hawaii and Alaska, where poverty levels are higher) are eligible.

Those on Medicaid lose their eligibility once their incomes rise above the Medicaid cut-off level, which could still be below the federal poverty level. The potential loss of their medical benefits is a disincentive for Medicaid recipients to accept low-paying jobs.

Medicaid should be reformed to include all those with low incomes through an income-related voucher, and the size of the subsidy would decline as income increases. An income-related voucher would include a uniform set of benefits for all persons with low incomes in a managed care plan. As incomes increased, the value of the voucher would decline. If those on Medicaid lost only a portion of their vouchers as their incomes rose, they would no longer have a disincentive to accept low-paying jobs. Furthermore, as a result of differences in states' financial capacity and willingness to broaden eligibility levels, large variations exist among the states in access to medical care by those with low incomes. An income-related voucher would eliminate these large differences in the percentage of low-income populations eligible for Medicaid.

This income-related approach, in addition to improving equity, would improve efficiency. An income-related voucher would reinforce the movement to Medicaid managed care, with its emphasis on coordinated care, increased access to primary care physicians, and incentives to provide care in less-costly settings.

To be effective in having health plans compete for Medicaid enrollees, the income-related voucher should be risk adjusted, namely, chronically ill enrollees should receive higher or more expensive vouchers than those who are younger and in better health. Risk-adjusted premiums will result in MCOs competing for chronically ill enrollees and developing disease management programs to better care for them.

When contracting with managed care plans, some states allow their Medicaid beneficiaries a choice of such plans. If they do not select an HMO, they are assigned to one. Managed care plans therefore have an incentive to compete for Medicaid patients. States, however, need to provide the Medicaid population with relevant information on their plan choices. To the extent that beneficiaries do not choose and are assigned to a managed care plan, the role of choice in disciplining plan performance is negated.

Several states, such as Florida, are trying innovative approaches for serving their Medicaid populations. Florida's Medicaid program covers more than 2 million people, and Medicaid expenditures have been increasing at about 13 percent per year over the past six years (as of 2005). In 2005, Medicaid consumed about 24 percent of the entire state budget and is estimated to increase to 60 percent of the state budget by 2015, unless Medicaid expenditures are better controlled. Previously, to control rising Medicaid expenditures, provider fees were reduced, medical benefits were limited, Medicaid eligibility was reduced, and access to prescription drugs was limited.

Florida hopes that using patient choice and health plan competition will improve patient care and reduce rapidly rising Medicaid expenditures. Each Medicaid enrollee will receive a defined contribution that will be based on her risk level and health status; a disabled enrollee, for example, will receive a larger amount than a healthy child. Medicaid enrollees then select among several competing, state-approved health plans, such as HMOs and PPOs, or they can use their defined contribution to join their employer's health plan. With risk-adjusted defined contributions, health plans have an incentive to enroll chronically ill enrollees, as they will receive higher premiums for doing so. Under this arrangement health plans have a financial incentive to develop disease management programs for patients with diabetes, heart disease, and other chronic conditions.

Previously, Medicaid programs relied on fee-for-service payment, which often resulted in poor care management for the chronically ill and led to fraud and abuse. The movement to having health plans compete for Medicaid enrollees, who can choose among several plans, and be paid premiums reflecting the care needs of the diverse Medicaid population, is likely to result in greater patient satisfaction and improved care outcomes.

To reduce Medicaid expenditures, attention must be focused on those groups consuming the largest portion of Medicaid expenditures, namely the chronically ill and disabled. (These groups will also be the fastest-growing segment of the Medicaid population.) States must be vigilant in monitoring the care these groups receive, whether in a fee-for-service or managed care setting. The challenge for the states in coming years is to include these vulnerable population groups in managed care, pay managed care plans and PPOs appropriately for their care, and vigorously monitor the care received.

Medicaid's movement to managed care has made survival difficult for many traditional "safety-net" providers, such as public and not-for-profit hospitals and community clinics who have traditionally served large Medicaid and uninsured populations. These traditional safety-net providers who rely on Medicaid and disproportionate-share hospital payments need Medicaid patients if they are to survive. As managed care firms seek less-expensive hospital settings and reduce inpatient use, these safety-net providers must become part of a provider network that competes for Medicaid capitation contracts. Unless they are able to do so, their financial stability is threatened. The loss of these safety-net providers would be unfortunate, as an income-related voucher will not likely be enacted in the near future. Until then, those without private insurance or Medicaid coverage will need access to medical care, which is likely to be provided primarily by safety-net providers.

SUMMARY

Medicaid is a means-tested program to provide medical services to those with low incomes. Although Medicaid programs are federally required to serve designated population groups, states have discretion to include additional medical services and population groups in their programs. Medicaid does not cover all those with low incomes or all of the uninsured. In contrast to Medicare, Medicaid recipients and their supporters are not able to provide legislators with political support. For these reasons the generosity of Medicaid programs (eligibility levels and included services) varies across states, and Congress does not mandate the level of funding as it does with Medicare. (Medicare is a defined-benefit program to specific population groups, which requires the federal government to fund those benefits.) In times of budget difficulties many states attempt to reduce their budget deficits by cutting Medicaid eligibility and benefits. Furthermore, Medicaid is permitted to enroll its recipients in managed care plans, whereas Medicare recipients make their own decisions as to whether they want to join such health plans.

It is widely recognized that Medicaid either needs to be reformed or replaced by a new program if all those with low incomes are to have similar access to medical services. One reform proposal is to provide an income-related voucher to those with low incomes for use in a managed care plan. Such a proposal would eliminate state variations in benefits and eligibility and provide recipients with incentives to choose a managed care plan.

An important challenge facing Medicaid reform, however, concerns the most costly Medicaid beneficiaries, disabled and long-term nursing home patients. The current Medicaid system has not performed adequately in this arena, and managed care plans have to demonstrate their ability to care for such patients.

DISCUSSION QUESTIONS

1. Describe the Medicaid program. What are the differences between Medicare and Medicaid?

2. How well does Medicaid achieve its objectives?

3. Why will it be difficult to enroll all of the Medicaid population in HMOs?

4. What are some approaches for reforming Medicaid?

5. What are the arguments for and against having one government program instead of both Medicare and Medicaid?

REFERENCES

Cunningham, P., and J. Kirby. 2004. "Children's Health Coverage: A Quarter-Century of Change." *Health Affairs* 23 (5): 27–38.

Gruber, J. 2000. *Medicaid.* Working Paper No. 7829. Cambridge, MA: National Bureau of Economic Research, 55, 1–101. [Online publication; retrieved 11/15/06.] http://www.nber.org/papers/w7829.

Landon, B., E. Schneider, C. Tobias, and A. Epstein. 2004. "The Evolution of Quality Management in Medicaid Managed Care." *Health Affairs* 23 (4): 245–54.

ADDITIONAL READINGS

Allen, K. G. 2005. "Medicaid: States' Efforts to Maximize Federal Reimbursements Highlight Need for Improved Federal Oversight." Testimony Before the Committee on Finance, U.S. Senate. June 28, 1–27. GAO-05-836T. [Online information; retrieved 12/28/06.] http://www.gao.gov/new.items/d05836t.pdf.

Cannon, M. 2005. *Medicaid's Unseen Costs.* Policy Analysis No. 548, 1–21. Washington, DC: Cato Institute.

Lueck, S. 2005. "Stiffer Rules for Nursing Home Coverage." *The Wall Street Journal* December 21, D1.

The September/October 2004 (volume 23) issue of *Health Affairs* contains several articles on children's health coverage and the State Children's Health Insurance Program.

Chapter 10

How Does Medicare Pay Physicians?

MEDICARE REPRESENTS, ON average, more than 20 percent of total physician revenues, although for many physicians and specialties it represents a sizable portion of revenues. As such, it is important to understand how Medicare pays physicians for care of Medicare patients. In 1992, a new payment system was instituted for physician services under Medicare. Why was it necessary to change the system? How does the new payment system compare to the previous one? What are the effects of this new payment system on access to care by Medicare patients, on physician fees paid by the nonaged working population, and on physicians' incomes?

PREVIOUS MEDICARE PHYSICIAN PAYMENT SYSTEM

When Medicare Part A, which pays for hospital care, was enacted in 1965, Part B, which pays for physician and out-of-hospital services, was included. (Part B is a voluntary benefit for which the aged pay a monthly premium that covers only 25 percent of the total cost of that program.) Physicians were paid on a fee-for-service basis for Medicare patients and given the choice to be a participating physician (or even participate for some medical claims but not others). When physicians participated, they agreed to accept the Medicare fee for that service, and the patient was responsible for only 20 percent of that fee after she paid the annual deductible.

If a physician was not a participating physician, the patient would have to pay the physician's entire charge, which was higher than the Medicare fee, and apply for reimbursement from Medicare. When the government reimbursed the patient, however, it would only pay the patient 80 percent of the Medicare-approved fee for that service. Thus, a patient who visited a nonparticipating physician would have to pay 20 percent of the physician's Medicare-approved fee plus the difference between the approved fee and the physician's actual charges. This difference is referred to as *balance billing*. Medicare patients who saw nonparticipating physicians were also burdened by the paperwork involved with sending their bills to Medicare for reimbursement.

As physicians' fees and Medicare expenditures rapidly increased, in 1972 the government placed a limit on physicians' Medicare fees, referred to as the Medicare Economic Index. Physicians' fees, however, continued to increase sharply in the private sector, and as the difference between private physician fees and the Medicare-approved fee became larger, fewer physicians chose to participate in Medicare. Consequently, more of the aged were balance billed for the difference between their physician's fee and the Medicare-approved fee.

Medicare fee-for-service payment also encouraged greater use of services. Limits on participating physicians' fees raised concerns that physicians would encourage more visits and engage in more testing to increase their Medicare billings ("induced demand"). Even with limits on physicians' fees, Medicare Part B expenditures continued to increase rapidly, as shown previously in Figure 8.4.

REASONS FOR ADOPTING THE NEW PAYMENT SYSTEM

The new Medicare physician payment system was adopted for three reasons. The most important was the federal government's desire to limit the rise in the federal budget deficit, an issue of great political concern in the early 1990s. In 1992, physicians received 75 percent of all Part B payments (this decreased to 38 percent as of 2005); the remaining expenditures were for other nonhospital services and had been increasing rapidly, at approximately 10 percent per year. Part B expenditures increased from $777 million in 1967 to more than $50 billion by 1992 and were expected to continue their rapid rise. (In 2005, Part B expenditures reached $152 billion; they are expected to be $295 billion by 2015.) As Medicare physician payments continued to increase, the government's portion, 75 percent of the total, contributed directly to the growing federal budget deficit. Both Republican and Democratic administrations believed that if the government was to reduce the size of the federal deficit, the growth in Part B expenditures had to be slowed.

The government, however, was constrained in the approaches it could use to limit Part B expenditures. Given the political power of the aged, the government was reluctant to ask them to pay higher Part B premiums or to increase their cost sharing. Furthermore, the government could not simply limit Medicare physician fees for fear that physicians would reduce their Medicare participation, which would adversely affect the aged.

Second, members of Congress were concerned that unless the aged had access to physicians, they would lose their political support at election time. As limits were placed on Medicare physician fee increases, fewer physicians were willing to participate (accept Medicare payment); more aged were either charged additional amounts by nonparticipating physicians (balanced billed) or, if they could not afford the additional payments, had decreased access to physician services. Congress wanted to increase physician participation in Medicare.

Third, many physicians and academicians believed the previous Medicare payment system was inequitable and inefficient. A newly graduated physician establishing a fee schedule with Medicare could receive higher fees than could an older physician whose fee increases were limited by the Medicare Economic Index. Physicians who performed procedures such as diagnostic testing and surgery were paid at a much higher rate per unit of physician time than were physicians who performed cognitive services, such as office examinations. Medicare fees for the same procedure varied greatly across geographic areas and were unrelated to differences in practice costs. The fee-for-service payment system encouraged inefficiency by rewarding physicians who performed more services. These inequities and inefficiencies caused differences in physician incomes and affected their choice of specialty and practice location.

COMPONENTS OF THE NEW PAYMENT SYSTEM

Reducing the federal deficit by limiting Part B expenditures, achieving greater Medicare fee equity among physicians, and limiting the aged's payments led to the three main parts of the physician payment reform package. The inefficiencies inherent in the fee-for-service system were not addressed by the new payment system.

Resource-Based Relative Value Scale Fee Schedule

The first, and most publicized, part of the physician payment reform package was the creation of a resource-based relative value scale (RBRVS) fee schedule. The RBRVS attempted to approximate the cost of performing each physician service. Its premise was that, in the long run, in a competitive market the price of a service will reflect the cost of producing that service. Thus, the payment for each physician service should reflect his resource costs. However, this cost-based approach to determining relative values was very complex, as it required a great deal of data, relied on interviews, was based on certain assumptions such as the time required to perform certain tasks, and would have to be continually updated because any of the elements of cost and time could change.

Three resource components were used to construct the fee for a particular service. The first, the work component, estimated the cost of providing a particular service, including the time, intensity, skill, and mental effort and stress involved in providing the service.[1] Second were the physician's practice expenses, such as salaries and rent. Third was malpractice insurance, because its cost varies across specialties. Each component was assigned a relative value that was summed to form the total relative value for the service; the greater the costs and time required for a service, the higher the relative value unit (RVU) was. A procedure with a value of 20 was believed to be twice as costly as one with a value of 10.

The actual fee was then determined by multiplying these RVUs by a politically determined conversion factor. For example, "transplantation of the heart" was assigned 44.13 work RVUs, 49.24 practice-expense RVUs, and 9.17 malpractice RVUs for a total of 102.54 RVUs. The 1992 conversion factor was $31, making the fee for this procedure $3,178 ($31 × 102.54). This fee was then adjusted for geographic location. (The initial conversion factor was set so that total payments under the new system would be the same as under the previous one, that is, the system was "budget neutral.") A separate conversion factor was used for surgical services, primary care, and other nonsurgical services. (In 1998, a single conversion factor was instituted for all services.) Table 10.1 illustrates how the RBRVS and the conversion factor are used to calculate the fee for an office visit.

---

1. Two methods were used to estimate the complexity of a task: personal interviews, and a modified Delphi technique in which each physician was able to compare her own estimate to the average of physicians within that specialty. Many assumptions were required; for example, in calculating opportunity cost, it was assumed that the years required for training in a specialty were the minimum necessary. Further assumptions were made regarding the lengths of working careers across specialties, residency salaries, hours worked per week, and an interest rate to discount future earnings.

Table 10.1: Calculations of Physician Payment Rate Under RBRVS Office Visits (Midlevel), New York City (Manhattan)

	Relative Value		Geographic Adjustment	Adjusted Relative Value
Physician work	0.67	×	1.09	0.73
Physician expense	0.69	×	1.35	0.93
Professional liability insurance	0.03	×	1.67	0.05
				1.71
		Conversion factor		× 36.20
		Payment rate		$61.90

RBRVS reduces the variation in fees both within specialties and across geographic regions. New physicians receive 80 percent of the Medicare fee schedule in their first year, and the percentage rises to 100 percent by the fifth year. Medicare fees can still vary geographically by 12 percent less and 18 percent more than the average, but this is greatly reduced from the previous geographic variation. As a result, fees were reduced for physicians in California, whereas fees in Mississippi increased by 11 percent.

The new payment system reflected the cost of performing 7,000 different physician services. When constructing the RBRVS fee structure, Harvard professor William Hsiao and colleagues (1988) found that physician fees were not closely related to the resource costs needed to produce those services. In general, cognitive services, such as patient evaluation, counseling, and management of services, were greatly undervalued compared with procedural services, such as surgery and testing. The RBRVS reduces the profitability of procedures while increasing payment for cognitive services. By changing the relative weights of different types of services, the RBRVS system caused substantial shifts in payments, and consequently incomes, among physicians. In large metropolitan areas, for example, surgeons' fees declined by 25 percent. The "winners" and "losers" among physician specialties after the new system was introduced are shown in Figure 10.1.

Medicare Expenditure Limit

The RBRVS approach is still fee-for-service payment and by itself does not control the volume, mix of services, nor total physician expenditures.

Figure 10.1: Medicare Physician Fee Schedule, Effect on Fees, by Specialty, 1992

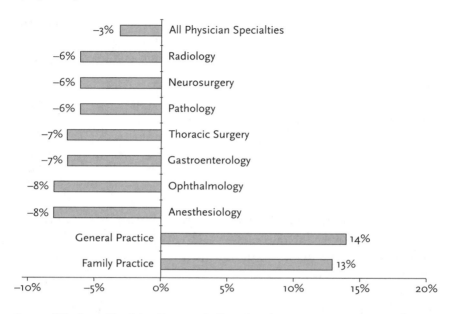

Source: "Medicare Physician Payment Reform Regulations." 1991. Hearing Before the U.S. Senate Subcommittee on Medicare and Long-Term Care of the Committee on Finance. July 19.

Because the government was concerned that physicians would induce demand to offset their lower Medicare fees, the second part of the new payment system limited overall physician Medicare expenditures. This limit was achieved by linking the annual update on physician fees (the conversion factor) to the growth in volume and mix of services. If volume increased more rapidly than a target rate based on increases in inflation, number of beneficiaries, newly covered services, and technological advances, Congress would reduce the annual fee update the following year. Too rapid an increase in services would result in a smaller fee update.

As it turned out, volume and mix of services increased less rapidly than expected for surgical services. Consequently, to maintain the target rate of Medicare payments for surgical services, the conversion factor increased more rapidly. These changes in fees were unrelated to any supply or demand changes for such services.

As part of the Balanced Budget Act of 1997, the annual update method was changed. An SGR in Medicare physician expenditures became the new government objective. The SGR was designed to reduce physician fee updates if physician spending growth exceeded a specified target. This new system holds Medicare spending growth for physician services to that of the general economy (GDP), adjusting for several factors. (Tying the SGR to GDP per capita represented an affordability criteria: how much the government could afford to subsidize physician Part B expenditures.) The SGR consists of four elements: the percentage increase in real GDP per capita, a medical inflation rate of physician fee increases, the annual percentage increase in Part B enrollees (other than Medicare Advantage enrollees), and the percentage change in spending for physicians' services resulting from changes in laws and regulations (e.g., expanded Medicare coverage for preventive services).

Under the SGR system, physician fee updates are adjusted up or down depending on whether actual spending has fallen below or has exceeded the target. Over time, fees tend to increase at least as fast as the cost of providing physician services as long as volume (number of services provided to each beneficiary) and intensity growth (complexity and costliness of those services) remain below a specified rate, about 2 percent per year. *If volume and intensity grow faster than the specified rate, the SGR lowers fee increases or causes fees to fall.*

During the late 1990s and early 2000s, physicians received generous fee increases from Medicare (5.4 percent in 2000 and 4.5 percent in 2001). However, physician organizations raised concerns about the SGR when fees dropped by 5.4 percent in 2002, a decline that was, in part, a correction for fees (overpayments) that had been set too high in prior years because of errors in forecasting. (The government revised upward its estimate of previous years' actual physician expenditures and lowered the spending target based on revised GDP data.) Responding to pressure from physicians, Congress repealed the scheduled fee reductions for 2002 and projected fee reductions for 2003 to 2005. Beginning in 2006, however, fees were projected to fall by about 5 percent per year until 2012, partly to recoup excess spending accumulated from averted cuts in previous years and partly because real spending per beneficiary (volume and intensity) on physician services is projected to grow faster than allowed under the SGR (Steinwald 2004).

Congress faces a dilemma. Recognizing that rapid expenditure growth in Medicare physician expenditures is not sustainable, Congress can maintain fiscal discipline by relying on an automatic mechanism, such as the SGR. By doing so, however, Congress risks having physicians limit their participation with Medicare, thereby dramatically reducing Medicare beneficiaries' access to physician services.

Tying Medicare physician fees to economic growth completely ignores changes in physician supply and demand; Medicare physician payment increases will be either too generous or too low.

Balance Billing Limit

The third part of the new payment system limits the amount physicians are able to balance bill Medicare patients. Physicians can no longer decide to participate in Medicare for some patients but not others; they must either participate for all of their patients or for none. Few physicians are able to forgo such a significant source of revenue. Physicians who decide not to participate in Medicare still cannot charge a Medicare patient more than 109 percent of the Medicare-approved fee. *Thus, even physicians who decide not to participate in Medicare are restricted in how much they can charge for treating a Medicare patient.*

EFFECTS OF MEDICARE'S PAYMENT SYSTEM
Initial Effects of the RBRVS System

To analyze the likely effects of Medicare's physician payment system, assume initially that physicians do not induce demand, that is, as specialist fees and incomes are reduced, physicians are not motivated to manipulate patients' demand. It is also important to keep in mind that physicians work in at least two markets; they serve Medicare patients and private or non-Medicare patients. (The private market could also be subdivided into HMO and non-HMO patients.)

RBRVS reduces fees for procedures and increases fees for cognitive services. With lower fees for surgery, for example, surgeons might be expected to perform fewer Medicare surgeries and reallocate their time to performing surgeries for private patients, whose fees were not reduced. However, if surgeons are not as busy as they would prefer, and the Medicare fee still exceeds the value of their time spent doing nonsurgical tasks, surgeons will not reduce their Medicare surgeries and will continue to perform the same number of procedures. The effect of lower fees for procedures with no change in the number of procedures will result in a decrease in Medicare procedure-type expenditures and lower specialists' incomes.

Would specialists increase their fees to their private patients to make up for lower Medicare fees? Specialists' fees for private patients are presumably already at their highest level, consistent with making as much profit as possible from those patients. If specialists do not charge as much as the market will bear, they forgo income they could have earned. If private fees are increased beyond what the market will bear, the loss in revenue from lower volume would exceed the gain in revenue from those higher fees. The specialist would be worse off. (See Chapter 17: Cost Shifting.) A specialist might be able to increase his volume from private-pay patients by *decreasing* his fees to MCOs to increase the number of private patients. Lowering the fee would be a more profitable strategy than raising it if the gain in revenue from increased volume more than offsets the loss in revenues from decreased fees.

Assume that before Medicare lowered specialist fees, specialists were allocating their time between private and Medicare patients so that the profit from each type of patient was the same. Once Medicare reduces its fees, the profit per hour of the specialist's time becomes greater when serving private patients. The specialist should serve fewer Medicare patients and more private patients. However, the only way the specialist can serve more private patients is to reduce her fees (to MCOs). Thus, the specialist would not likely want to or be able to "cost shift" to private patients.

If a specialist has excess capacity and does not attempt to induce demand, the aged would have the same access as before. Specialists would provide the same volume of services, but their incomes would be reduced and Medicare expenditures for specialist services would decline.

Physicians who are willing to "create" demand to offset declines in their incomes would first attempt to induce demand among their private patients. A greater volume of private patients would be more profitable because the private fee has not been reduced. Only after private fees were reduced would the specialist create demand among the Medicare patients, whose fees had already been reduced. If specialists are not busy enough, they have probably already tried to induce as much demand as possible and would be unable to induce much further demand. Instead, they might engage in such fraudulent practices as "code creep" as a way of increasing their Medicare fees.

Medicare expenditures and specialist incomes would still be expected to decline among physicians who are inclined to induce demand, assuming that these specialists previously had excess capacity. To the extent that demand inducers are able to engage in code creep they will be able to offset some of the decline in their incomes. If specialists were fully busy, the reductions in Medicare specialist fees would result in a reallocation of specialists' time to private patients (whose fees are higher) and, consequently, reduced access by Medicare patients.

Given the excess capacity that existed among specialists, when Medicare introduced the new RBRVS system and reduced Medicare fees to surgical specialties, the new, lower, fees likely reduced such specialists' incomes, reduced Medicare expenditures for such services, and did not reduce Medicare patients' access to these services.

Under RBRVS, Medicare fees for cognitive services increased. Because the higher fees increase the profitability of Medicare patients, primary care physicians were expected to serve more Medicare patients and fewer private patients. As physicians were expected to decrease their available time to private patients, and demand exceeded the available physician time for private patients, fees for private patients were expected to increase. Total Medicare expenditures for cognitive services, particularly for primary care physicians, increased.

Primary care physicians who may have been willing to induce demand to increase their incomes might have been less inclined to do so because their incomes increased as a result of their fee increases. Those still inclined to induce demand will have found that doing so for their Medicare patients, whose fees increased, was more profitable than for their private patients.

What was the RBRVS fee schedule's likely overall effect on expenditures? Assuming specialists were not busy enough, little additional demand inducement occurred, and (adjusting for the increased number of aged) Medicare Part B expenditures for specialists did not increase. Medicare expenditures for primary care physicians were expected to increase because their fees were increased; however, these increases were less than the decreases in specialist expenditures. Figure 8.4 (in Chapter 8) illustrates these changes in the trend in Part B expenditures after the new physician payment system was introduced in 1992. (Part B expenditures have increased slightly more rapidly in recent years as a result of Congress shifting home health care expenditures from Part A to Part B in 1997 to solve an impending bankruptcy in the Part A Trust Fund.)

The expenditure limit that was part of the RBRVS system was meant to control demand inducement. If specialists already had excess capacity, demand inducement of additional procedures was likely to be small.

Demand inducement, hence volume of surgical services, was less than the government anticipated.

The Present Period

The aged's demand for physicians is continuing to increase because of growth in the aged population, new technologies, and legislated new services. Unless Congress permits the SGR to reflect these pressures for higher expenditures, shortages will result. As demands for care by both Medicare and private patients increase, primary care physicians will attempt to increase their fees. To the extent that Medicare fee increases match fee increases to private patients, physicians would not find it profitable to change their allocation of time to each group of patients. If, however, Congress limits Medicare fee increases to save money, the relative profitability of Medicare patients would decline.

If Medicare fees fall relative to private fees, only by "raising" their Medicare fees—by such methods as reducing the time spent per Medicare visit or having the patient return more often—would it be profitable for primary care physicians to continue seeing the same number of Medicare patients.

Greater fee increases for private patients will cause physicians to reallocate their time to such patients. Medicare patients would then have less access to primary care physicians. However, if physicians were able to balance bill their Medicare patients, relative fees between Medicare and private patients would remain the same, and physicians would not reallocate their time away from Medicare patients. The inability of primary care physicians to balance bill may eventually result in shortages of physician services for Medicare patients; the demand for such services will exceed the amount physicians are willing to supply at Medicare's relatively lower fee.

To determine whether Medicare's physician fees are too low, the Medicare Payment Advisory Commission (MedPAC) undertakes two types of studies. The first is a survey of physicians' willingness to serve Medicare patients; the second is a survey of Medicare patients' access to care.[2] As of 2005, these data indicate that access to care by Medicare patients was generally good and Medicare fees relative to private fees had not fallen.[3]

---

2. Results of telephone surveys on Medicare beneficiaries, access to physicians are included in MedPAC (2006).

Recent anecdotal information, however, indicates that an increasing percentage of primary care physicians are not accepting new Medicare patients. Because of the SGR formula, reductions in Medicare physician fees for 2006 (and the projected decrease in fees for the next several years under current law) will change Medicare patients' access to care.

Given the three-year delay in receiving information with which to evaluate the adequacy of Medicare physician fees, MedPAC will not likely be able to bring the demand and supply for physicians into equilibrium. No automatic mechanism, such as increases in balance billing, is in place to indicate a current shortage, hence access problems.

Limiting balance billing and establishing a uniform fee schedule among physicians within the same specialty have another unfortunate effect. Previously, differences in fees for the same service may have reflected differences in that service. For example, some physicians are of higher quality or spend more time listening to the patient's concerns. Although the service code may be nominally similar, the content of that service may differ. In the above examples, the costs of providing that service in terms of the physician's time differ. Patients are willing to pay more for certain physician attributes, such as their ability to relate to the patient. By having a uniform fee schedule with virtually no balance billing, the physician treating Medicare patients is unable to charge for these extra attributes. Busy primary care physicians could provide additional visits and earn a higher income instead of spending time cultivating these extra attributes, which are not rewarded.

SUMMARY

The RBRVS national fee schedule, with expenditure controls and limits on balance billing, attempted to limit federal expenditures for Medicare physician services, improve equity among different medical specialties, and limit out-of-pocket payments and Part B premiums by the aged, while

---

3. According to ongoing tracking studies by the Center for Studying Health System Change, the proportion of U.S. physicians accepting Medicare patients stabilized in 2004–2005, with nearly three-quarters saying their practices were open to all new Medicare patients. In 2004–2005, 72.9 percent of physicians reported accepting all new Medicare patients, statistically unchanged from 71.1 percent in 2000–2001. Only 3.4 percent of physicians reported that their practices were completely closed to new Medicare patients in 2004–2005, also statistically unchanged from 2000–2001 (Cunningham, Staiti, and Ginsburg 2006).

increasing the aged's access to care. Medicare expenditures, however, will continue to rise as the number of eligible aged increases along with inflation, legislated new Medicare benefits, and advances in technology.

Under the present Medicare formula for paying physicians, Congress will be continually faced with the trade-off of limiting Medicare physician expenditures or decreasing the aged's access to care.

Congress is unlikely to be able to accurately forecast the "right" rate of increase in Medicare expenditures (SGR) because it is more likely to be concerned with limiting the rise in Medicare expenditures than with properly adjusting for changes in the number of aged, inflation, and technology. The consequences to the aged of "too slow" an increase in Medicare expenditures will be a shortage of primary care services.

A uniform fee schedule cannot indicate that a shortage is developing in some geographic areas or among certain physician specialties, nor can uniform fees eliminate such shortages. Unless a national fee schedule is flexible and allows fees for some services, physicians, and geographic regions to increase more rapidly than others, shortages will arise and persist. Furthermore, using three-year-old data to determine whether the aged have physician access problems is unlikely to be accurate. Permitting physicians to balance bill their Medicare patients would be a market mechanism to indicate that an imbalance between demand and supply has occurred. The government could then raise fees in those areas and among those specialties where balance billing is increasing.

Fees provide information; they signal that changes have occurred in the costs of providing care, the demands for that care, or both. If the government does not want to overpay specialties and services that are in oversupply while underpaying those that are in short supply, a flexible mechanism such as balance billing is needed. Otherwise, the aged will find that they have reduced access to care, and the government will not be spending its money wisely.

DISCUSSION QUESTIONS

1. What were the reasons for developing a new Medicare physician payment system?

2. In what ways does the current physician payment system differ from the previous system?

3. What are the likely effects of Medicare's payment system on its patients' out-of-pocket expenses, Part B premiums, and access to physicians (primary care versus specialists)?

4. What, if any, are the likely effects of Medicare's payment system on patients in the non-Medicare (private) sector?

5. What are the likely effects of Medicare's physician payment system on physicians (by specialty)?

REFERENCES

Cunningham, P., A. Staiti, and P. Ginsburg. 2006. *Physician Acceptance of New Medicare Patients Stabilizes in 2004–05*. Tracking Report, 1–4. Washington, DC: Center for Studying Health System Change.

Hsiao, W. C., P. Braun, D. Yntema, and E. R. Becker. 1988. "Estimating Physicians' Work for a Resource-Based Relative Value Scale." *The New England Journal of Medicine* 319 (13): 835–41.

Medicare Payment Advisory Commission (MedPAC). 2006. *Report to the Congress: Medicare Payment Policy.* [Online publication; retrieved 11/15/06.] http://www.medpac.gov/publications/congressional_reports/Mar06_EntireReport.pdf.

Steinwald, B. 2004. "Medicare Physician Payments: Information on Spending Trends and Targets." Testimony Before the Subcommittee on Health, Committee on Energy and Commerce, House of Representatives. Washington, DC: U.S. General Accounting Office, May 5. GAO-04-751T.

ADDITIONAL READINGS

Centers for Medicare & Medicaid Services. 2005. *2005 Annual Report of the Boards of Trustees of the Federal Hospital Insurance and Federal Supplementary Medical Insurance Trust Funds.* [Online publication; retrieved 11/15/06.] http://www.cms.hhs.gov/ReportsTrustFunds/downloads/tr2005.pdf.

Frech, H. E., III., ed. 1991. *Regulating Doctors' Fees: Competition, Benefits and Controls Under Medicare.* Washington, DC: AEI Press.

Pauly, M. V., H. Erder, R. Feldman, J. Eisenberg, and J. Schwartz. 1992. *Paying Physicians: Options for Controlling Cost, Volume, and Intensity of Services.* Chicago: Health Administration Press.

Chapter 11

Is There an Impending
Shortage of Physicians?

ABOUT EVERY 10 to 20 years, there is concern that the United States is either producing too many or too few physicians. The Council on Graduate Medical Education (COGME), which advises the government on the size of the physician workforce and its training, recently issued a report warning that there is likely to be a shortfall of 85,000 to 95,000 physicians by 2020 (COGME 2005).

Yet as late as 1992, COGME was warning that by 2000 the surplus of specialists would be as high as 15 percent to 30 percent of all physicians and that there would be a shortage of primary care physicians (COGME 1992).

Evidence for the prior belief in a large physician surplus was the rapid growth in the number of active physicians, which increased from 311,000 in 1970 to 435,000 in 1980, 560,000 in 1990, and 792,000 in 2004. When adjusted for population, the number of active physicians per 100,000 population (the physician–population ratio) increased from 156 in 1970 to 195 in 1980, 229 in 1990, and 275 in 2004. (See Figure 4.1 in Chapter 4.) Some researchers, assuming that a large portion of the U.S. population would be enrolled in HMOs, compared the relatively low physician ratio within HMOs to the national physician ratio and claimed that an overall surplus of 165,000 physicians, or 30 percent of the total number of patient care physicians, would be seen by 2000. A 30 percent surplus in the number of specialists was also projected.

The projected physician surplus was expected to have adverse effects on physician incomes, especially specialist incomes, for many years. To forestall such surpluses the COGME and physician organizations recommended to the administration and the Congress reducing medical school enrollments, reducing the number of specialists and expanding the number of primary care physicians (from 30 percent to 50 percent of all physicians), and limiting the number of foreign medical school graduates entering the United States.

The projected huge surplus of physicians did not materialize.

The COGME's current recommendations are the *opposite* of their prior policy recommendations of fewer than 15 years ago. More physicians are needed, and medical students should be encouraged to become specialists and not primary care physicians.

What is the basis for these projections of physician surpluses and shortages? Should public policy attempt to manipulate the supply of physicians based on such supply projections? What is an economic definition of a physician surplus or shortage? And what are the consequences and self-correcting mechanisms of a shortage or surplus?

DEFINITIONS OF A PHYSICIAN SHORTAGE OR SURPLUS

Physician–Population Ratio

Different approaches have been used to determine whether a surplus (or shortage) exists in a profession. One approach often used in the health field is a physician–population ratio. This type of definition often relies on a value judgment about how much care people should receive or on a professional determination of how many physician services are appropriate for the population.

This method generally uses the existing physician–population ratio and compares it with the physician–population ratio that is likely to occur in some future period. First, the likely physician–population *supply ratio* is estimated by projecting the future population and then calculating the likely number of medical graduates that will be added to the stock of physicians, less the expected number of deaths and retirements. Second, *physician requirements* are projected by estimating the extent of disease in the population (usually based on survey data), the physician services necessary to provide care for each illness, and the number of physician hours required to provide preventive and therapeutic services. (Some studies attempt to modify the requirements ratio by basing it on utilization rates of population subgroups, such as age, sex, location, and insurance coverage, and multiplying these utilization rates by the future population in each category.) Third, assuming a 40-hour workweek per physician, the number of hours is translated into number of physicians and into a physician–population ratio. The same approach is used to determine the number of physicians in each specialty. The difference between the supply ratio and the requirements ratio is the anticipated shortage or surplus.

The Graduate Medical Education Advisory Committee to the government (the predecessor organization to COGME) also used a physician–population ratio methodology somewhat similar to one first used in the 1930s to determine the appropriate number of physicians.

The ratio technique has served as the basis for much of the health manpower legislation in this country and has resulted in many billions of dollars of subsidies by both federal and state governments. Nonphysician health professional associations, such as those for registered nurses, have also used this approach in their quest for government subsidies.

Using a physician–population ratio for judging whether a shortage (or surplus) exists has serious shortcomings. First, the use of a ratio, either one based on need for services or one that currently exists, does not consider changes that are occurring in *demand* for physicians. For example, if demand is increasing faster than the supply of physicians because of an aging population, because of new medical advances that increase the public's use of medical care, or because patients' insurance coverage has changed, maintaining a particular ratio is likely to result in too few physicians. Second, the ratio method does not include *productivity* changes that are likely to occur or possible to attain. It is possible to achieve an increase in physician services without increasing the number of physicians. Technology, such as health information systems, and personnel with less training can be used to relieve physicians of many tasks; delegation of some tasks would permit an increase in the number of physician visits. A smaller physician–population ratio would be needed if productivity increases were considered. Conversely, if the percentage of female physicians (who work fewer hours on average than male physicians [Cooper et al. 2002]) increases or if physicians prefer an easier lifestyle, will a greater number of physicians be needed?

Third, the ratio technique does not indicate *how important a surplus or shortage is*, if in fact one exists. Is a shortage or surplus of 10,000 physicians significant, or does it have to reach 200,000 before the numbers are of concern? What are the consequences in terms of physician fees, incomes, and patients' access to care of shortages or surpluses of varying numbers of physicians?

Projections of shortages and surpluses using the ratio technique have been notoriously inaccurate over time. Many assumptions are used in calculating future ratios, and public policies based on inaccurate projections will take many years to correct, thereby exacerbating future shortages or surpluses.

Rate of Return

Economists prefer a different approach to determining whether a surplus or shortage exists. The economic approach relies on the concept of a *rate of return*. Medical education is viewed as an investment similar to other types of investments. The rate of return is calculated by estimating the costs of that investment and the expected higher financial returns achievable as a result of that investment.

If a person decides to enter medical (or any graduate) school, he is in effect making an investment in an education that offers a higher future income. The cost of that investment includes tuition, books, and the income forgone by going to school. (The largest part of this investment is often the income that could have been earned had a job been taken; this is known as the "opportunity cost" of a graduate education.)

The return earned on this educational investment is the higher income received. Because this income is earned in the future, and future income is valued less than current income, it must be discounted to the present. Does the discounted rate of return on a medical education exceed what the student could have earned had she invested the money in a savings or bond account? If the rate of return is higher than what could have been earned by investing an equivalent sum of money, there is a "shortage." If the return on a medical education is lower than alternative investments or an investment in education for other professions, a "surplus" exists.[1]

The rate-of-return approach does not imply that every prospective student makes a rate-of-return calculation before deciding on a medical or other graduate education. Many students would become physicians even if future income prospects were very low, simply because they believe medicine is a worthwhile profession. However, some students are "at the margin"; they may be equally excited about a career in medicine, business, or computer science. Changes in rates of return affect

---

1. If physician incomes do not increase as fast as other professions, the rate of return on becoming a physician decreases because the opportunity cost to prospective physicians has increased—their forgone income has increased.

these students. High rates of return in medicine shift more students to medicine (eventually lowering the rate of return), whereas low rates of return shift them into other professions, eventually eliminating the physician surplus.

The rate-of-return approach incorporates into its calculations all of the relevant economic factors, such as likely income lost if the person does not become a physician (opportunity cost), the longer time to become a specialist (greater opportunity costs), likely physician incomes by specialty, and educational costs such as tuition. Changes in any of these factors will cause changes in the rate of return on a medical education.

CONSEQUENCES OF AN IMBALANCE IN THE SUPPLY AND DEMAND FOR PHYSICIANS

What is likely to occur if demand for physicians exceeds supply (or, under a surplus scenario, supply exceeds demand)? Each scenario has a short- and a long-term consequence. And these effects will vary depending on whether the patient is a private-pay patient or publicly funded patient for whom the government regulates the physician's fee.

Private Market for Physician Services
Short-Term Effects of a Physician Shortage

An increase in the number of patients seeking physician services will initially mean patients will find it more difficult to schedule an appointment with a physician. Waiting times will increase. Physicians will be unlikely to immediately realize that they are experiencing a permanent increase in demand for their services. Physicians' bargaining position with insurers will improve, and they will eventually increase their fees. They will likely add staff to increase their productivity so they can see more patients. And physician incomes will increase.

Equilibrium will be reestablished, similar to what existed before the increase in demand occurred; however, physician fees and incomes will be higher, patients will pay higher copayments each time they go to the physician, and some patients will not see the physician as often as they did previously.

Long-Term Effects of a Physician Shortage

Over time, as physician incomes increase, the demand for a medical education will increase, as will demand for those residency positions in specialties experiencing the largest increases in demand for services. An important issue is whether medical schools will accommodate the higher demand for a medical education. If medical schools expand and new medical schools start, the supply of U.S.-trained physicians will slowly increase. If not, more students desiring a medical education will seek such an education overseas and return to the United States for their residencies.

The resulting greater supply of physicians, generated by the higher rate of return on a medical education, will moderate physician fee increases, and physicians' incomes will no longer increase more rapidly than those of other professions. The specialties in which demand has increased fastest will have a greater number of physicians.

The response by patients, physicians, college graduates, and medical schools will result in the elimination of a shortage. The response by these different parties will not be immediate, as it takes time for patients and physicians to realize there is an increase in demand, for some college graduates to decide to enter medicine, and then for these students to graduate, complete their residencies, and enter practice.

Short-Term Effects of a Physician Surplus
A surplus is characterized by patients not having to wait to see a physician, physicians not being as busy as they would like and more willing to participate with insurers to receive a greater volume of patients, a greater willingness among physicians to discount their fees, and physician incomes not keeping up with inflation. The rate of return on a medical education will decline as incomes fail to rise as rapidly as those for other professions.

Long-Term Effects of a Physician Surplus
Under the physician surplus scenario, a medical profession becomes less desirable. Physicians may decide to retire early, less use will be made of staff to increase physician productivity, and the applicant-to-acceptance ratio for medical schools will decline. Although medicine will always be a desirable profession, some students who might have chosen a career in medicine will choose another profession. The supply of physicians will increase more slowly than if the rate of return on a medical education were higher. Over time, as demand for physician services increases more rapidly than physician supply, the surplus situation will disappear. Physicians will become busier, their fees and incomes will increase, and

the rate of return on a medical education will increase to become comparable to the rate of return for other professions.

Public Market for Physician Services
Short-Term Effects of a Physician Shortage
The main difference between the private and public (Medicare and Medicaid) markets is that in public markets the government regulates the price of physician services. Governments are rarely able to accurately determine the price for physician services and for each specialty so that it equilibrates supply and demand for physician services for Medicare and Medicaid patients. Often budget considerations influence how much should be spent on physician services.

If a shortage situation occurs in the private market for physicians, physicians will serve fewer Medicare and Medicaid patients unless the government also increases physician fees. They will shift their time to higher-paying private patients. This has previously occurred with Medicare patients and is a continual problem for Medicaid patients. A growing shortage in the private market will exacerbate the shortage of physician services for Medicare and Medicaid patients unless the government increases Medicare and Medicaid fees.

Long-Term Effects of a Physician Shortage
Unlike the private market, a shortage may continue indefinitely in the public market if government fees are not sufficiently increased to match those in the private market. Low out-of-pocket payments by Medicare and Medicaid patients result in a high demand by publicly paid patients, which will continue to exceed the supply of services physicians are willing to devote to these patients. Waiting times will increase, and fewer physicians will be willing to serve new public patients. To increase their access to physician services, more publicly funded patients will join an MCO. Physicians will be able to receive a higher rate of pay from these organizations by providing preventive and disease management services to publicly funded patients, which reduces costly hospital care.

Short-Term Effects of a Physician Surplus
Physicians will serve more Medicare and Medicaid patients when they are not as busy as they would prefer. As physicians accept lower fees from

private insurers, government fees may become more attractive, and they will be willing to shift more of their time to publicly funded patients.[2]

Long-Term Effects of a Physician Surplus

As the physician surplus is resolved in the private market, and fees by privately insured patients begin increasing, publicly funded patients may experience some access problems, depending on whether government fees are increased in line with privately determined fees.

The public and private markets are interrelated. Physicians will allocate their time to each market depending on the relative profitability of serving patients in each market. (This is not meant to imply that all physicians behave similarly, but that a sufficient number of physicians are willing to shift their services based on the profitability of serving Medicare, Medicaid, and private patients [Rice et al. 1999].) Consequently, the effects on patients of a physician shortage or surplus depend on the flexibility of fees in each market. Markets that permit greater flexibility in fees and entry of new physicians are more likely to resolve a shortage situation than markets that rely on government-regulated fees, which are slow to recognize and adjust to changes in demand and supply.

A crucial assumption regarding long-term shortages in the private market is whether the supply of medical schools and spaces responds to student demands for a medical education.

ECONOMIC EVIDENCE ON TRENDS IN PHYSICIAN DEMAND AND SUPPLY

Data on rates of return on a career in medicine are only available up to 1985. What do they indicate? Throughout the post–World War II period, rates of return on a medical career were sufficiently high to suggest that a shortage existed. In 1962, the rate of return was estimated to be 16.6 percent. By 1970, it had risen to 22 percent. The rate of return declined slightly between 1975 and 1985, when it was estimated to be 16 percent, which still indicates a shortage, not a surplus (Feldstein 2005).

Rates of return varied greatly among physician specialties. In 1985, some specialties, such as anesthesiology and surgical subspecialties, earned 40 percent and 35 percent returns, whereas pediatrics earned only 1.3

---

2. Medicare payment as a percentage of private insurer payments has increased substantially in the past ten years, from about 71 percent on average in 1996 to 81 percent in 2003 (Cunningham, Staiti, and Ginsburg 2006, 7).

percent (indicative of a surplus). Rates of return were typically higher for hospital-based specialties than for those in primary care. (During this period, the rate of return on a physician education was more than 100 percent greater than the rate of return for a college professor.)

As recent rate-of-return data are unavailable, other data must be used to indicate whether this country is facing a physician shortage. Demand increasing faster than supply, rising physician fees and incomes (adjusted for inflation), and an increasing applicant-to-acceptance ratio for medical schools would be indicative of a trend toward a shortage. If, however, these data were trending in the opposite direction, it would be more indicative of a trend toward a surplus.

Trends in Physician Fees

In the late 1980s, physician fees rose much more rapidly than inflation and more rapidly than in the 1990s, when managed care began having an effect. Physician fee increases shown in Figure 11.1 are probably overstated. Previously, the Bureau of Labor Statistics, the federal agency that collects data on medical prices, collected data on physicians' "list" prices rather than the prices they actually received. As managed care discounting increased, the difference between a physician's list price and actual price became greater. Thus, it appears that in recent years physician fee increases have barely exceeded inflation.

Trends in Physician Incomes

Median physician incomes (i.e., the 50th percentile) fell in the latter part of the 1990s.[3] At the beginning of the 1980s a severe recession caused median physician incomes to decline, but they rose during the second half of the decade. Although physician incomes suffered a sharp drop in 1994, they recovered, but after peaking in 1995, they declined for the next three years. In 1997 and 1998, physician incomes not only increased less rapidly than inflation, but they actually fell in absolute dollars!

Throughout the 1980s and 1990s, physician incomes showed a great deal of variability. Several times in past years—in 1985, 1989 and 1990, and 1994—physician incomes, adjusted for inflation, fell. In subsequent

---

3. Physician incomes are highly skewed; that is, the physician income distribution contains large values at the high end of the income distribution. Therefore, using the average income per physician is a less accurate measure of the "typical" physician's income. For this reason, the middle of the income distribution, the median, is used in Figure 11.2.

Figure 11.1: Annual Percentage Changes in the Consumer Price Index and in Physicians' Fees, 1965–2005

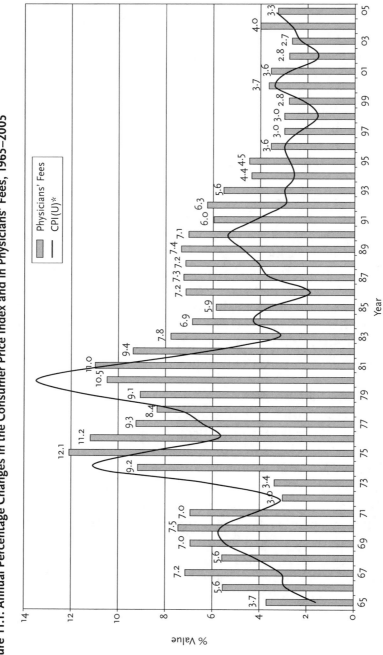

*CPI(U) = consumer price index for all urban consumers.

Source: U.S. Census Bureau. 2006. [Online information.] http://stats.bls.gov/cpihome.htm.

years physician incomes rose sharply. Using a longer time period, the 1980s, median physician incomes increased on average 2.4 percent per year (adjusted for inflation). However, from 1991 to 1998 median physician incomes (adjusted for inflation) fell on average 0.075 percent per year. The 1990s appear to be different from the 1980s, indicating a downward trend in physician incomes (Figure 11.2).

Managed care and the increased supply of physicians began to negatively affect physician fees and incomes by the mid-1990s. Furthermore, these data indicate that the ability of physicians to increase the demand for their services ("supplier-induced demand") appears to be limited; otherwise, physician incomes would not have fallen as much as they have.

Physician income data are not adjusted for changes in the number of hours worked. To the extent that in more recent years there are a greater number of female physicians (who, as mentioned earlier in this chapter, work fewer hours on average than male physicians [Cooper et al. 2002]) and more male physicians also decide to work fewer hours, physician incomes will not rise as rapidly. This change in physicians' lifestyle may have contributed to the downward trend in physician incomes.

The data presented in Figure 11.2 are based on all physicians. An examination of changes in physician incomes by specialty allows better observation of the effect of managed care. Between 1985 and 1990, physicians in surgical specialties, hospital-based physicians (anesthesiologists and radiologists), obstetric/gynecologic physicians, and those in internal medicine received the largest annual increases in incomes compared with those in general practice (Figure 11.3). Physician specialties better able to benefit from the development of new diagnostic and surgical techniques during the 1980s received greater increases in income. In the 1990s physicians in general practice (in greater demand by managed care plans) received the greatest increases in their incomes. Other physician specialties actually experienced decreases in their real (adjusted for inflation) incomes; obstetric/gynecologic physicians suffered the largest decline.

Unfortunately, the American Medical Association no longer conducts its annual survey of physician incomes. More recent data on physician incomes are, however, available from the Center for Studying Health System Change, which found that from 1999 to 2003, average physician incomes, adjusted for inflation, continued to decline, but less rapidly than from 1995 to 1999. The largest declines in real incomes occurred for primary care physicians. Tu and Ginsburg (2006) claim that specialists, whose average incomes were 86 percent higher than primary care physicians,

Figure 11.2: Annual Percentage Changes in Median Physician Net Income, After Expenses and Before Taxes, 1982–1998

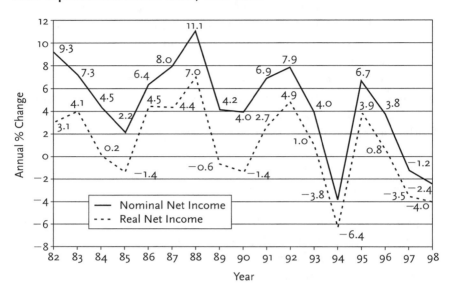

Source: Data from American Medical Association, Center for Health Policy Studies. 2001. *The Profile of Medical Practice, Socioeconomic Characteristics of Medical Practice,* and *Physician Socioeconomic Statistics,* various editions. Chicago: AMA.

have been able to perform procedures associated with advanced technology, thereby performing more procedures per day, whereas primary care physicians, relying on cognitive-based services, are unable to substantially increase their productivity.

Despite the decline in real physician incomes, Tu and Ginsburg conclude that "medicine overall remains one of the most well-paid professions in the United States" (2006, 1).

Applicant-to-Acceptance Ratio in Medical Schools

Another indicator of trends in rates of return on a medical education, in addition to physician fees and incomes, is the demand for a medical education. The applicant-to-acceptance ratio has always been greater than one. (See Figure 23.1 in Chapter 23.) After reaching a high of almost 3:1 in the mid-1970s, the ratio fell to a low of 1.56:1 in 1988 to 1989; it increased to 2.7:1 in 1996 to 1997 but has been declining since, falling to 2.1:1 in 2005 to 2006. An excess demand for a medical education still exists.

Figure 11.3: Average Annual Percentage Change in Net Income from Medical Practice, by Specialty, 1985–2000

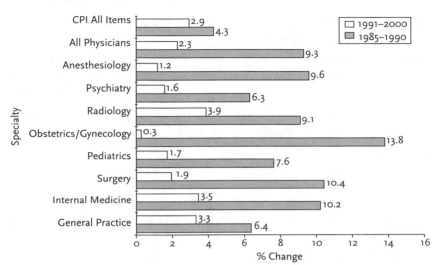

Source: Data from American Medical Association. 2003. *Socioeconomic Characteristics of Medical Practice* and *Physician Socioeconomic Statistics,* various editions. Chicago: AMA.

What can one conclude from the above data on physician fees, incomes, and the applicant-to-acceptance ratio? The 1990s were not as financially rewarding as the late 1980s. According to the most recent available data (2005 to 2006), the applicant-to-acceptance ratio appears to lag changes in physician incomes by several years, falling in the late 1980s after physician incomes fell in the early 1980s, rising again in the early 1990s after the rise in physician incomes in the late 1980s, and then falling in the late 1990s with the decline in incomes in the early 1990s. The demand for a medical education is still high; more qualified students seek admission to medical school than are accepted.

Given the variability in annual percentage changes in physician incomes, additional years of data are needed before more definitive statements can be made regarding whether a downward trend in physician incomes will continue. A medical career is not as attractive as it was previously. Even with the annual percentage decline in physician incomes, however, the level of physicians' incomes is still sufficiently high to offer a higher return on a medical career relative to other careers available to prospective medical students. Also indicative of a shortage is the continual excess demand for a medical education.

LONGER-TERM OUTLOOK FOR PHYSICIANS
Trends in Physician Supply

One study examining the adequacy of physician supply estimates that the supply of physicians will increase from 270 per 100,000 population in 2000 to a peak of 283 per 100,000 by 2010, and will then decline to 280 per 100,000 by 2020 (primarily because the population will increase faster than supply) (Cooper et al. 2002). In addition, physician supply will effectively be reduced as a result of decreased work effort (aging of the physician supply, increasing number of female physicians, and younger physicians placing a greater emphasis on lifestyle).[4] However, offsetting this reduced work effort is the growth in nurse practitioners, physician assistants, and nurse midwives, who all perform some physician-type (mostly primary care) services. The net effect of these offsetting factors is an estimated increase in physician supply of about 8 percent by 2020, or equivalent to about 300 per 100,000 population.

Factors Affecting Demand for Physician Services

Many factors affect the demand for physician services. The population has been growing by a rate of about 1 percent per year since the 1960s. In addition, the population is aging; the first of the baby boomers are expected to become eligible for Medicare in 2011. The aged have much higher visit rates than the non-aged, and these use rates have been increasing over time. Per capita incomes are also increasing, and use of physicians, especially specialists, is highly correlated with higher incomes. In addition, technology is being improved and there is greater use of existing technology, which results in greater complexity of a physician visit. Laboratory tests and diagnostic imaging services are also being used to a greater extent.

Most of the aged purchase private supplementary health insurance (Medigap) policies. This coverage pays for their Medicare deductibles and copayments, reducing the price they must pay for physician services and decreasing their price sensitivity to physician fees. With virtually

---

4. The age distribution of physicians in 2004 was as follows: under 35 years, 16 percent; 35 to 44 years, 23 percent; 45 to 54 years, 24 percent; 55 to 64 years, 17 percent; 65 years and older, 18 percent. Sixty-one percent of physicians are 45 years and older.

Figure 11.4: Percentage Distribution of Physician Expenditures, by Source of Funds, Selected Years 1965–2005

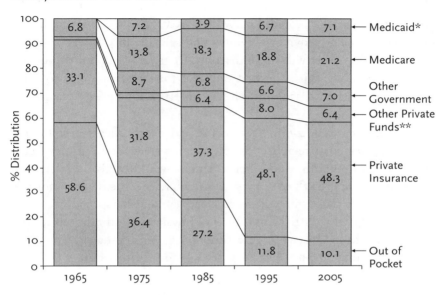

*Total Medicaid (excluding Medicaid expansion).

**Includes industrial inplant and other private revenues (including philanthropy). Other Private Funds in 1965 and 1975 were 1.5% and 2.1%, respectively.

Source: Centers for Medicare & Medicaid Services, Office of the Actuary, National Health Statistics Group. 2007. [Online information.] http://www.cms.hhs.gov/NationalHealthExpendData/downloads/tables.pdf.

complete coverage for physician services, a larger number of aged are likely to further increase their demand for physician services.

The growth in private insurance has reduced the out-of-pocket price of physician services paid by private patients. As shown in Figure 11.4, consumers' out-of-pocket payments for physician services have declined, reaching 10 percent by 2005. As patients' out-of-pocket payments declined, they became less price sensitive to physicians' fees and their demand increased. Previously, managed care plans were able to limit their enrollees' use of physician services and pay discounted fees to physicians who had excess capacity.

The growth of managed care had two main effects on physicians. Patients enrolled in managed care plans were required to use providers who were part of their plan's provider network; otherwise, the patient had to pay the full price charged by a nonnetwork provider. For physicians to have access to an insurer's enrollees, the physician had to be part of the insurer's provider network. MCOs limited the number of physicians in their provider networks and selected physicians based on how much they were willing to discount their fees (and not overutilize medical services). Thus, the first effect of managed care was to force physicians to deeply discount their fees in return for a greater volume of the plan's enrollees.

Managed care's second effect was to reduce enrollee access to specialists. Managed care relied on physician gatekeepers, primary care physicians, to determine whether a patient would receive a referral to a specialist. The growth of managed care increased the demand for primary care physicians while decreasing the demand for specialists.

Managed care's restrictions on use of physicians and referrals to specialists have been loosened. Unless more stringent managed care plans return, demand for physician services in the private sector is likely to expand.

A very important factor increasing use of medical services is new medical technology, such as new diagnostic and surgical procedures. Technological advances are likely to continue, further expanding demand for physicians, particularly specialists. (More expensive diagnostic and surgical procedures have raised average fees, resulting in procedure-oriented specialists receiving much higher profit margins per hour than physicians in primary care, who perform few procedures.)

To sum up the factors affecting demand for physicians, demographic trends, the aging of the population, increased incomes, and the decline of managed care's use of gatekeepers and limits on specialist referrals, together with advances in medical technology, are likely to greatly increase the demand for physician services. The first of the baby boomers will become eligible for Medicare in 2011, and those physicians likely to be in greatest demand are specialists, such as cardiologists and gerontologists, who care for the aged.

Comparing the projected increases in physician supply and likely increases in physician demand results in a shortfall of 50,000 physicians by 2010 (about 6 percent less than projected demand) and a much larger shortfall of 200,000 physicians by 2020 (about 20 percent of projected demand). Most of the shortfall is estimated to be for specialists rather than primary care physicians (Cooper et al. 2002). The COGME also forecasts a physician shortage in 2020, but by a lesser amount, 85,000 physicians. (A medical career will become more attractive than it is currently.)

The key to eliminating a long-term shortage is a large expansion in the number of new medical schools. To increase the number of medical school graduates, from the 16,000 graduating currently to the 26,000 a year needed to reduce the estimated 200,000 physician shortfall in 2020, will require 90 new medical schools. Whether the expansion of new medical schools will occur, how many will open, and how rapidly are serious concerns. Medical schools are nonprofit, and the accrediting commission places strict requirements on curriculum and sources of funding. Unless the nonprofit medical education sector is able to respond, more medical education will occur overseas and osteopathic medical schools will expand, as will training of physician assistants and nurse practitioners.

An increase in the projected demand for physicians so much greater than projected increases in supply will lead to large increases in physician fees and incomes (as well as higher health insurance premiums). Shortages in the private sector are resolved through higher prices, thereby reducing demand. If these shortage projections are approximately accurate, access to physician services will become a greater problem for many patients. Unless Medicare and Medicaid increase the fees paid to physicians during this period when demand is increasing faster than supply, those with low incomes (Medicaid) and the aged (Medicare) will suffer significant reductions in access to physician services.

SUMMARY

Forecasting physician shortages or surpluses is subject to a great deal of error. The COGME has proven itself to be a faulty prognosticator of future trends in the demand and supply for physicians. Public policy based on COGME's recommendations has adversely affected the career paths of many students. Projecting the future supply of physicians is less uncertain than demand projections.

Shortages and surpluses are resolved over time through the adjustment of rising or falling fees. Market imbalances are not resolved quickly, as it takes many years to train additional physicians (in a shortage situation) and many years before physicians retire (in a surplus case). Given the uncertainties regarding the future, information on future trends is important to prospective medical students; they will be able to make a more informed decision on the attractiveness of a medical career. Students who have to bear the cost of their decisions would prefer to have the freedom to choose their professions, rather than have their choices limited by expert panels (that are often wrong) deciding on the need for different types of physicians.

A particular problem with medical education is that it is highly regulated by the medical profession. It is difficult for entrepreneurs to develop new medical schools with innovative curricula, have their students graduate in a shorter time period, and achieve the same outcome measures as graduates from more traditional medical schools. As long as these restrictions continue, along with an excess demand for a medical education, medical schools will be unresponsive to increased demands for a medical education and to curriculum innovations.

Whether a shortage or surplus is beneficial often depends on whether one is a patient or a physician. A smaller physician supply increases physician incomes, whereas greater competition among physicians benefits patients by increasing their access to care.

DISCUSSION QUESTIONS

1. Evaluate the use of the physician–population ratio as a means of determining a surplus or a shortage of physicians.

2. Describe and evaluate how a rate of return on a medical education would determine the existence of a physician surplus or shortage.

3. What demand and supply trends in the physician services market will affect the incomes of surgical specialists and primary care physicians?

4. Prices change in a competitive market for two basic reasons, increased operating costs and changes in physician demand. In what ways are these reasons applicable for explaining physician fee increases?

5. Based on the evidence presented on physician incomes, physician fees, physician–population ratio, and applicant-to-acceptance ratio in medical schools, would you conclude that a physician shortage currently exists?

REFERENCES

Cooper, R., T. Getzen, H. McKee, and P. Laud. 2002. "Economic and Demographic Trends Signal an Impending Physician Shortage." *Health Affairs* 21 (1): 140–54.

Council on Graduate Medical Education (COGME). 1992. *Improving Access to Health Care Through Physician Workforce Reform: Directions for the 21st Century.* Third Report. [Online publication; retrieved 11/15/06.] http://www.cogme.gov/rpt3.htm.

———. 2005. *Physician Workforce Policy Guidelines for the United States, 2000–2020.* Sixteenth Report. [Online publication; retrieved 11/15/06.] http://www.cogme.gov/report16.htm.

Cunningham, P., A. Staiti, and P. Ginsburg. 2006. *Physician Acceptance of New Medicare Patients Stabilizes in 2004–05*. Tracking Report No. 12, Center for Studying Health System Change. [Online publication; retrieved 11/15/06.] http://www.hschange .org/CONTENT/811.

Feldstein, P. J. 2005. "Health Manpower Shortages and Surpluses." In *Health Care Economics*, 6th ed., 328–54. Albany, NY: Delmar Publishers.

Rice, T., S. C. Stearns, D. E. Pathman, S. DesHarnais, M. Brasure, and M. Tai-Seale. 1999. "A Tale of Two Bounties: The Impact of Competing Fees on Physician Behavior." *Journal of Health Politics, Policy and Law* 24 (6): 1307–30.

Tu, H., and P. Ginsburg. 2006. *Losing Ground: Physician Income, 1995–2003*. Tracking Report No. 15, Center for Studying Health System Change, 1–5. [Online publication; retrieved 11/15/06.] http://www.hschange.com/CONTENT/851/.

Chapter 12

The Changing Practice of Medicine

THE PRACTICE OF medicine has changed dramatically since the mid-1980s. For many years the predominant form of medical practice was solo practice with fee-for-service reimbursement. With the increase in medical knowledge and technological advancements, however, more physicians became specialists. Insurer payment and federal education subsidies also encouraged the growth of specialization. The development of managed care changed the practice of medicine; more physicians joined together in increasingly large medical groups.

What are the reasons for this shift away from solo and small group practice toward larger medical groups? Is the consolidation of medical practices into larger groups likely to continue?

TYPES OF MEDICAL GROUPS
Different types of medical groups have developed to serve the differing needs and preferences of practicing physicians. Following is a description of the two basic types of medical groups.

Single- or Multispecialty Groups
Physicians in this type of group share facilities, equipment, medical records, and support staff. Physicians may be paid according to one or more methods: salary plus a share in remaining net revenues, discounted fee for service with a share in remaining net revenues, or capitation. Leaving a group practice is difficult for physicians, as they cannot take their patients with them. Any contracts the group has with a health plan belong to the group and include the patients covered by those contracts.

Independent Practice Associations

Physicians who want to be associated with other physicians (on a nonexclusive basis) for the purposes of joint contracting with a health plan will form a very loose organization, such as an independent practice association (IPA). These physicians continue to practice in their own offices, see their own patients, hire and pay their own staff, and do their own billing.

When the IPA contracts with a health plan, the IPA physicians are paid on a discounted fee-for-service basis. If an IPA receives a capitation contract from a health plan, the physicians may be paid a discounted fee for service with the possibility of receiving additional amounts if total physician billings are less than the total capitation amount at the end of the year. The IPA may also subcapitate some specialists. As IPAs competed for capitated contracts and assumed financial risk, they began to exercise more oversight of their physicians' practice patterns.

CHANGES IN THE SIZE OF MEDICAL GROUPS

An indication of physicians' changing practice settings is provided in Table 12.1, which shows the changing distribution of office-based physicians according to group affiliation and size of group over time. The percentage of physicians in individual practice has declined from 78 percent in 1969 to about 54 percent in 1996. Although the largest percentage of group-practice physicians are in multispecialty groups, the growth in single-specialty groups has been more rapid, rising from 7 percent of all physicians in 1969 to 20 percent by 1996.[1]

Multispecialty group practices have on average the largest number of physicians per group. The average size of single-specialty and family practice groups is about the same.

Table 12.2 shows the increasing size of groups over time. The largest groups (50 or more physicians), which had about 15 percent of all group physicians in 1969, now account for almost 40 percent of all group-practice physicians. This growth occurred at the expense of the smallest groups. In some regions of the country, multispecialty groups have in excess of 200 physicians.

In a highly competitive managed care market, physicians in individual and small group practices were at a disadvantage. Therein lies an important explanation for the formation of large medical groups.

---

1. The latest publicly available data on the distribution of office-based physicians by group affiliation are from 1996.

Table 12.1: Number, Average Size, and Distribution of Office-Based Physicians, by Group Affiliation, 1969, 1980, and 1996

Type of Practice	Distribution of Physicians According to Type of Practice			Number of Group Practices			Average Size of Physician Group		
	1969	1980	1996	1969	1980	1996	1969	1980	1996
Total office-based physicians (nonfederal)*	100.0	100.0	100.0	—	—	—	—	—	—
Individual practice**	78.3	67.2	53.8	—	—	—	—	—	—
Group practice	21.7	32.8	46.2†	6,371	10,762	19,658‡	6.2	8.2	9.3
Single-specialty group practice	7.1	10.9	19.6	3,169	6,156	13,934	4.1	4.8	6.4
Multispecialty group practice	13.2	20.1	24.9	2,418	3,552	4,396	10.1	15.2	23.4
Family or general group practice	1.5	1.8	1.7	784	1,054	1,328	3.5	4.5	5.4

*Includes all patient care physicians except residents, interns, and full-time hospital staff. In 1996 there were 445,765 office-based physicians.

**The AMA defines a "group" as three or more physicians. Therefore, Individual Practice includes offices with a single physician and offices with two physicians.

†Excludes 477 physician positions in groups with unknown specialty composition.

‡Excludes 162 groups whose specialty composition was unknown.

Sources: National Center for Health Statistics. 1986. Health, United States. U.S. DHHS Publication (PHS) 87-1232, Public Health Service, 163. Washington, DC: U.S. Government Printing Office; Hung, J. N., and G. A. Roeback. 1970. Distribution of Physicians, Hospitals, and Hospital Beds in the United States, 1969, vol. 2. Metropolitan Areas Center for Health Services Research and Development. Chicago: American Medical Association; Havlicek, P. L. 1999. Medical Group Practices in the U.S.: A Survey of Practice Characteristics, 1999 ed., 44–46. Chicago: American Medical Association; The number of nonfederal office-based physicians in 1996 comes from Havlicek, P. L., of the American Medical Association. 1999. Personal correspondence. December 10.

Table 12.2: Distribution of Groups and Group Physicians, by Group Size, 1969, 1980, 1996, and 2005

Group Size	Distribution of Groups				Distribution of Physicians			
	1969	1980	1996*	2005	1969	1980	1996**	2005
Total number	6,371	10,762	19,468	19,913	40,093	88,290	206,557	240,773
				% Distribution				
3–4	65.0%	55.3%	45.9%	39.9%	34.6%	22.7%	15.0%	11.4%
5–15	30.3	37.5	44.2	48.2	34.2	32.9	30.7	30.3
16–25	2.4	3.6	4.8	5.6	7.6	8.7	8.9	9.0
26–49	1.5	2.2	2.7	3.5	8.2	9.1	9.1	9.9
50+	0.8	1.4	2.3	2.8	15.4	26.6	36.2	39.5
Total	100.0	100.0	99.9†	100.0	100.0	100.0	99.9	100.1

*Excludes 352 groups with unknown size.

**These figures represent physician positions. These figures were obtained by asking groups to report the number of physicians in their groups. Because physicians may practice in more than one group, some physicians may be counted more than once. Thus, these figures may overestimate the number of group physicians.

†Percentages do not sum to 100 because of rounding.

Note: In 1980, 100+ group size totaled 18,899 (21.4%) physicians; in 1996, 100+ group size numbered 59,179 (28.7%) physicians; in 2005, 100+ group size numbered 75,486 (31.4%) physicians.

Sources: Vahovich, S. G. 1973. *Profile of Medical Practice*, 1973 ed., Table 11. Chicago: American Medical Association; Henderson, S. R. 1980. *Medical Groups in the U.S.*, Table 3-2. Chicago: American Medical Association; Havlicek, P. L. 1999. *Medical Group Practices in the U.S.: A Survey of Practice Characteristics*, 1999 ed., Table 3-1. Chicago: American Medical Association; Smart, D. M. 2006. *Medical Group Practices in the U.S.*, 2006 ed., Table 1. Chicago: American Medical Association.

Medical Groups as a Competitive Response

Before managed care became dominant in the insurance marketplace, physicians were less concerned with being included in an insurer's provider panel or competing for insurance contracts. Patients had access to all physicians, who were paid according to their established fee schedules. Patients had similar insurance (indemnity) and limited, if any, information on physician qualifications or the fees they charged.

Price competition among managed care plans for an employer's enrollees changed all that. To be price competitive insurers had to reduce the price they paid for their inputs (physician and hospital services) and reduce the quantity of services used.

The physician services market in the 1980s consisted of a rising supply of physicians, particularly specialists, and a high proportion of them were in solo or small group practices. In the managed care environment, physicians were eager to contract with these new health plans. Insurers and HMOs were able to form limited provider networks by selecting physicians according to whether they were willing to sharply discount their fees in return for a greater volume of patients. Physicians excluded from such networks lost patients.

The growth of medical groups was a competitive response to the greater bargaining power of insurers and HMOs. Being part of a medical group, particularly a large group, provided physicians in that group with a competitive advantage over physicians who were not similarly organized. Medical groups also gained increased bargaining power over hospitals that desired their referrals and with managed care plans in negotiating physician contracts.

Negotiating and contracting with one large medical group is less costly (both administratively and in terms of performance evaluation) for health plans than contracting with an equivalent number of independent physicians. Tasks performed by the insurer, such as utilization management, can be delegated to the medical group.

HMOs were also able to shift their insurance risk to a large medical group by paying that group on a capitation basis instead of a fee-for-service basis. Similarly, a large medical group can spread financial risk over a large number of capitated enrollees and physicians.

Capitation also provided medical groups with financial incentives to be innovative in the delivery of medical services and the practice of medicine, because by saving part of the capitation payment they could increase their profits. These incentives do not exist in small group practices that are paid on a fee-for-service basis. As a consequence, several large medical groups developed expertise in managing care and in developing "best-practice" guidelines.

In the 1990s, medical groups in California, more so than medical groups in other states, sought greater financial risk and rewards by accepting a greater percentage of the HMO premium. These medical groups believed that by being responsible for all of the patient's medical services they could better manage care; furthermore, by reducing hospital admissions, lengths of stay, and payments to hospitals they could make greater profits. (Unfortunately, many of these medical groups were inexperienced in managing the financial risk associated with capitation and suffered financially. Most medical groups no longer accept capitation payments.)

Increased Market Power

Large medical groups were able to bid for HMO contracts and serve as PPOs for employers and insurers. The size of these groups enabled a health plan to negotiate with one physician organization rather than carry out separate, time-consuming negotiations with a large number of individual physicians. Thus, large medical groups were better able than individual physicians and smaller medical groups to compete for patients.

An employer or health plan contracting with a large medical group has less reason to be concerned with physician quality. Large medical groups have more formalized quality control and monitoring mechanisms than do large numbers of independently practicing physicians. Within a large group, physicians refer to their own specialists; thus, specialists who are not part of a group are less likely to have access to patients. These contracting, quality review, and referral mechanisms provide physicians in large medical groups with a competitive advantage over physicians who are unaffiliated with such groups.

The advantages of large groups enabled them to have greater bargaining power over health plans compared with independent and small physician practices. As a result, large groups were more likely to be able to negotiate higher payments from health plans as well as increased market share (receiving a greater portion of the health plan's total number of enrollees).

Large medical groups also have greater leverage over hospitals. Because such groups control large numbers of enrollees, the group can determine to which hospitals it will refer its patients. Hospitals in turn were willing to share some of their capitated revenues with these groups. (When hospitals were capitated, a "risk-sharing pool" was formed from part of the hospital's capitation payments whereby the savings from reduced hospitalization were shared between the hospital and the medical group.) These risk-sharing pools enabled physicians in medical groups to increase their incomes compared with what they would have earned in independent or small group practices.

Economies of Scale in Group Practice

An obvious reason for moving toward larger medical groups in a price-competitive environment is to take advantage of economies of scale. Larger groups have lower per unit costs than do smaller groups. Larger groups are also better able to spread certain fixed costs over a larger number of physicians. The administrative costs of running an office (including making appointments; billing patients, government, and insurance companies for services rendered; maintaining computerized information systems to keep track of patients; and staffing aides to assist the physician) do not increase proportionately as the number of physicians increases. Larger group practices are also able to receive volume discounts on supplies and negotiate lower rates on their leases than the same number of physicians practicing separately or in smaller groups.

The greater the number of physicians in a group, the lower will be their administrative and practice costs per physician. Group practice is a more efficient form of organization (Romano 2004, 2005).

"Informational" economies of scale also provide large groups with a competitive advantage over small or independent practices. A distinguishing characteristic of the physician services market is the lack of patient information on physicians, including their quality, fees, accessibility, and how they relate to their patients. Physicians are better able than patients to evaluate other physicians. Evaluating and monitoring member physicians is less costly for the medical group than for patients. Being a member of a medical group conveys information regarding quality to patients, giving physicians in that group the equivalent to a "brand name."

A new physician entering a market is at a disadvantage compared with established physicians, in that developing a reputation among patients and building a practice takes time. Joining a medical group immediately transfers the group's reputation to the new physician. The reputation of the group is more important to the patient for those specialist services that are less frequently used and more difficult for the patient to evaluate.

Multispecialty groups offer greater informational economies of scale than do groups comprising family practitioners.

REVERSAL OF FORTUNES OF LARGE MULTISPECIALTY GROUPS

The promise of large multispecialty medical groups in managing patient care and being rewarded for accepting greater capitation risk foundered in the late 1990s, particularly in California.

Changing Market Environment

The prosperity created by the economic expansion in the United States in the late 1990s led employees to demand broader provider networks and freer access to specialists from their HMOs. Large medical groups had been using primary care gatekeepers to control specialist referrals and utilization management to control the growth in medical costs. The market had changed; it was no longer willing to reward large capitated medical groups for strict cost-control measures.

During this time, competition among HMOs led to very low premium increases, leaving large capitated groups with low capitation rates. Medical groups found themselves in financial difficulty as their costs increased and state and federal governments enacted "patient protection" measures. These included 48-hour hospital stays for normal deliveries, requiring HMOs to allow obstetricians/gynecologists to serve as primary care physicians, and prohibiting limited lengths of stay after a mastectomy, all of which further increased the medical groups' costs.

HMOs were wary of being sued for withholding appropriate treatment even when the HMO had delegated such treatment decisions to its large medical groups. As HMOs began undertaking those decisions themselves, some advantages of capitation payment to large groups faded.

Difficulty of Developing a Group "Culture"

A well-functioning medical group cannot be formed overnight; the group may not coalesce even after years. An important difference between group and nongroup physicians is the willingness of group physicians to give up some of their autonomy and abide by group decisions. Physicians may not share values or accept the same assumptions regarding their external environment, mission, and relationships with one another. This "cultural difference" often determines whether physicians will remain in a group. Many physicians are very independent and do not want other physicians prescribing their behavior, whether it relates to contracting with certain HMOs, reviewing their practice patterns, or determining their compensation.

A large multispecialty group must have various committees, one of which determines physician compensation. Disputes among physicians over their compensation are an important reason why such groups have dissolved. For example, when a multispecialty group is capitated for a large number of enrollees, the group must decide how the primary care physicians and each specialist will share in those capitation dollars. Because the primary care physicians control the specialist referrals, some groups pay them more than they would earn under a discounted fee-for-service environment. These funds must come from paying specialists less.

Another issue in medical group compensation is how much of each physician's income should be tied to productivity. Productivity incentives decline when a physician's payment is not directly related to his clinical work. More productive physicians may decide to leave if there are large differences between productivity and compensation.

When physicians in a large group share the use of inputs, that is, personnel and supplies, they are less concerned with those costs than if they were in independent or small group practice, where their costs are more directly related to their earnings. This lack of efficiency incentives offsets some savings from economies of scale.

Lack of Management Expertise

As medical groups increased in size and number, many had inadequate management expertise to handle the clinical and financial responsibilities of the group. The groups did not have adequate information systems for tracking expenses and revenues; they lacked actuarial expertise for underwriting risk when they were receiving capitation payments; and they did not have sufficient management specializing in marketing, finance, and contracting. Unfortunately, many medical groups expanded more rapidly than their management ability to handle the increased risk and volume of patients.

As a substitute for developing such management expertise themselves, many groups joined for-profit (publicly traded) physician practice management (PPM) companies. These PPM companies promised a number of benefits to a participating medical group, such as including it in a larger contracting network with health plans, handling its administration, and improving its efficiency. In return for providing these services, the PPM company received a percentage of the group's revenues, for example, 15 percent. However, several publicly traded PPM companies were themselves poorly managed and declared bankruptcy. A further disappointment with PPM companies was that the cost savings they were able to achieve in the medical group and the additional contracting revenue they were able to bring to the group were lower than the 15 percent management fee they charged.

Lack of Capital

Medical groups typically pay out all of their net revenues to their member physicians. Thus, no funds are available to reinvest in expanding the group, such as by establishing new clinics, purchasing expensive diagnostic services, or buying costly hardware and software for information technology. Their lack of capital is an important reason why expanding medical groups seek partners.

Hospitals have generally been willing to provide the capital for medical groups to expand and to develop their infrastructures. In return for such investments, hospitals hope to secure the medical group's inpatient referrals and be able to negotiate joint contracting arrangements with a health plan. The hospital may also manage or become a part owner in a joint management company that contracts with the medical group for medical services.

The main concerns groups have with hospitals as capital partners are that the hospital will somehow control the group and that the hospital may not be the most advantageous facility to which the group could refer its patients. Many hospitals have lost a great deal of money investing in their physician partners because the hoped-for returns have been lower than anticipated, particularly when hospitals purchased physician practices and physician productivity, once separated from physician compensation, declined.

OUTLOOK FOR MEDICAL GROUP PRACTICES

Large multispecialty medical groups have matured. The advantages to physicians of participating in a large medical group have continued to increase. Large medical groups are more likely than physicians in solo or small group practices to invest in management and clinical information systems, such as electronic medical records. The growing emphasis by insurers, employers, and Medicare on monitoring systems to measure patient outcomes and satisfaction, and the growing interest in "pay for performance" provide large medical groups with a competitive advantage in competing for patients and receiving bonuses for achieving certain quality benchmarks. Pay-for-performance revenue is likely to become a larger share of physician incomes; thus, medical groups that invest in information technology and are able to demonstrate improved patient performance will receive a greater share of physician revenues.

Medical groups are also likely to use more recommended care management processes for patients with chronic illnesses. (In a 2003 study comparing California medical groups with those in the rest of the country, Gillies et al. found that California medical groups used 35 percent to 50 percent more care management processes, such as use of hospitalists, case management, diabetes, asthma, and depression care management, than physician organizations in other parts of the country.)

Medical groups have also become more entrepreneurial as they attempt to increase physician revenues. Concerned that growth in physician revenues from providing physician services to Medicare and Medicaid patients is limited, medical groups have become more aggressive in expanding the services they offer. Based on a large-scale interview survey, Pham et al. (2004) found that physicians' health care investments in new services have increased. Medical groups were more likely than physicians in solo practice to invest in equipment to provide ancillary services, such as imaging and laboratory testing, within their existing practices. Patients' use of such services has sharply increased. Some survey respondents stated that if it were not for the ancillary services, some groups would not be making any money.

An important trend is the growth in large single-specialty medical groups. During the managed care era, with its emphasis on multispecialty medical groups that used primary care physicians to coordinate and control patient care, expectations were that a surplus of specialists would occur. These predictions proved to be inaccurate.

Tightly managed care, with its use of primary care physicians as gatekeepers and preauthorization for referrals that limited the use of specialist services, declined and had to change to permit direct access to specialists; consequently, the demand for specialist services increased. Rather than being considered a cost center when medical groups were paid a capitation rate, specialist services became profit centers under the fee-for-service system.

The emergence of new imaging and surgical technologies has made it possible to provide outpatient imaging and surgical services. In addition to the advances in medical technology that made it possible to perform these services on an outpatient basis, these new technologies were very profitable to perform, as they were reimbursed by Medicare and health plans at very favorable rates. Specialists had an incentive to move these services out of the hospital and into their own facilities. Physicians with specialties in cardiology and orthopedics have invested in free-standing specialty hospitals and ambulatory surgical centers that compete with their own community hospitals. By investing in these facilities, specialists are able to receive the facility fees for such services and thereby increase their incomes.[2] Physicians have claimed that such "focused factories" are more convenient for patients and improve patient care.

The profit potential of performing services with a high markup over cost in their own outpatient facilities provided specialists with an incentive to form large single-specialty groups. Specialists are able to generate more profit than primary care physicians. Specialty groups that own their own expensive imaging equipment, magnetic resonance imaging (MRI) equipment, and facilities, such as ambulatory surgery centers, are more profitable when paid on a fee-for-service basis than are primary care physicians providing cognitive services. In contrast to a multispecialty group, single-specialty groups would not have to share revenues or governance with primary care physicians.

Additional reasons for the growth of large single-specialty (as well as multispecialty) groups include the increased leverage such groups have in bargaining with health plans and community hospitals when they combine with similar specialists. Health plans are reluctant to lose a large network of specialists. Physicians in solo practice and small groups are at a competitive disadvantage in dealing with health plans.

Large groups are able to hire professional management to deal with an increasingly burdensome regulatory environment and achieve operational efficiencies by taking advantage of economies of scale. Further, larger groups, particularly large single-specialty groups, have been able to secure private investment capital (Casalino, Pham, and Bazzoli 2004) for investing in costly imaging equipment, surgical services, and information technology, which are usually beyond the means of smaller groups.

---

2. To forestall such competition from specialists, the American Hospital Association was successful in having Congress, as part of the Medicare Modernization Act of 2003, place a moratorium on physician-owned single-specialty hospitals.

SUMMARY

The growth of large medical groups is likely to continue. In addition to being able to hire professional management, achieve economies of scale, and have greater bargaining leverage with health plans and hospitals, large medical groups, particularly large single-specialty medical groups, are able to increase their revenues by taking more services that were previously provided in the hospital to their own outpatient settings.

As budget pressures from both federal (Medicare) and state (Medicaid) governments limit physician fee increases, finding new sources of revenue will increase in importance for physicians. The trend by multi-specialty and single-specialty medical groups to invest in technologically advanced services that can be provided in an outpatient setting will continue. Hospitals, to prevent the loss in revenues, will likely participate with medical groups in joint ventures.

Medical groups face a number of challenges in coming years. Employers, insurers, and Medicare are increasing emphasis on monitoring patient outcomes and satisfaction. As payers become more sophisticated and quality is rewarded, medical groups should have an advantage because quality and outcome measures are more accurate for medical groups than for individual physicians. Medical groups will also have to become more proficient in managing chronic illness for an increasingly aged population while demonstrating improved medical outcomes and patient satisfaction. Large medical groups, however, will be better able than smaller medical groups to invest in the necessary information technology to evaluate practice patterns and patient outcomes.

As pay for performance among insurers and Medicare becomes a more important source of revenue for physicians, well-managed medical groups, using information technology, will be better able to compete for pay-for-performance bonuses.

Large medical groups have the potential to play an increasing role in the delivery of medical services. It is uncertain whether medical groups will achieve their promise in innovating in new treatment methods that decrease medical costs while demonstrating improved patient outcomes. If medical groups are unable to do so, insurers will take the initiative in developing the information systems and databases for analyzing physicians' practice patterns, disseminating practice guidelines to physicians, and monitoring the quality of care provided by physicians.

The types of health plans consumers demand will affect which types of medical groups will expand more rapidly. If tightly managed care were to return, with its emphasis on coordinated care, multispecialty groups will grow at the expense of single-specialty groups. Conversely, fee-for-service payment and fewer restrictions on access to specialist services are likely to promote the formation of large single-specialty medical groups.

DISCUSSION QUESTIONS

1. Why has the size of multispecialty medical groups increased?

2. Why do large medical groups have market power?

3. Why do medical groups occasionally break up?

4. Describe how an IPA functions.

5. Who are the different types of capital partners available to medical groups? What do they expect in return for providing capital?

REFERENCES

Casalino, L., H. Pham, and G. Bazzoli. 2004. "Growth of Single-Specialty Medical Groups." *Health Affairs* 23 (2): 82–90.

Gillies, R., S. Shortell, L. Casalino, J. Robinson, and T. Rundall. 2003. "How Different Is California? A Comparison of U.S. Physician Organizations." *Health Affairs* Web exclusive, October 15, W3-492–W3-502. [Online publication; retrieved 11/15/06.] http://content.healthaffairs.org/cgi/reprint/hlthaff.w3.492v1.

Pham, H., K. Devers, J. May, and R. Berenson. 2004. "Financial Pressures Spur Physician Entrepreneurialism." *Health Affairs* 23 (2): 70–81.

Romano, M. 2004. "More Docs Say: Super-Size it." *Modern Healthcare* 34 (40): 24–26.

———. 2005. "A Bigger Brood." *Modern Healthcare* 35 (43): 28–30.

Chapter 13

The Malpractice Crisis

FOR THE THIRD time in 30 years, another malpractice "crisis" began in 2002. The median increase in malpractice premiums was between 15 percent and 30 percent in most states, and some states experienced rate increases as high as 73 percent (Figure 13.1). The first malpractice crisis occurred in the early 1970s when physicians' malpractice premiums rose more than 50 percent between 1974 and 1976; for some specialties, such as obstetrics/gynecology and surgery, the increases were even greater. During this first malpractice crisis, some insurers completely withdrew from the malpractice insurance market, whereas others increased their premiums by as much as 300 percent. Physicians threatened to strike if state legislatures did not intervene. To ensure access to malpractice insurance at the lowest possible rates, some medical societies formed their own insurance companies.

By the late 1970s and early 1980s, malpractice premiums had stabilized somewhat, but they rose sharply again in the mid-1980s, precipitating a second malpractice crisis. Again, physicians demanded that state legislators take action to alleviate the burden of high premiums. In the late 1980s, malpractice premiums and awards started to decline and then stabilized through the mid-1990s.

In 2002, malpractice premiums started to rise sharply once again (U.S. Government Accounting Office 2003). The annual percentage change in malpractice premiums appears to be cyclical. After a number of years of falling malpractice premiums, premiums are rising rapidly again, and premiums for some medical specialties are rising sharply (Figure 13.2). With the rapid rise in premiums, medical societies are once again pressuring the federal and state legislatures for malpractice

Figure 13.1: Medical Professional Liability Insurance Premiums for Self-Employed Physicians, 1974–1998

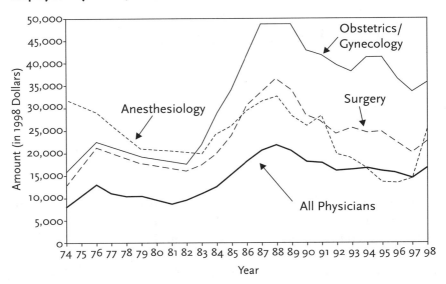

Note: Values adjusted for inflation using CPI(U).

Sources: Data from American Medical Association. 2002. *The Profile of Medical Practice, Socioeconomic Characteristics of Medical Practice,* and *Physician Socioeconomic Statistics,* various editions. Chicago: AMA.

"reform," that is, tort changes that would limit both malpractice awards and claims filed.

EXPLANATIONS FOR THE RISE IN MALPRACTICE PREMIUMS

Malpractice premiums consist of three components. The first is referred to as "economic" costs, which include current and future medical expenses and lost wages. Second are the costs of "pain and suffering"; this is the component damage caps seek to limit. And third are factors affecting the malpractice insurer's profitability, including its operating loss ratio, investment returns, and legal defense costs. To understand the cyclical rise in malpractice premiums, it is important to understand how each of these components has been changing.

Insurers' malpractice payments per physician are based on economic costs and the costs of pain and suffering. These payments consist of two

Figure 13.2: Annual Percentage Changes in Medical Professional Liability Insurance Premiums for Self-Employed Physicians, 1975–1998

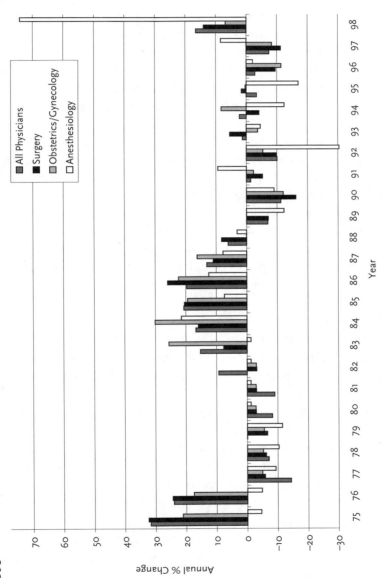

Note: Values adjusted for inflation using CPI(U).

Source: Data from American Medical Association. 2002. *The Profile of Medical Practice, Socioeconomic Characteristics of Medical Practice, and Physician Socioeconomic Statistics,* various editions. Chicago: AMA.

parts: the number of claims filed and the size of jury awards and out-of-court settlements per claim.

Claims Filed

The number of claims per physician has increased over the past 50 years. Two reasons account for the increase in malpractice cases over time. First, physicians are performing more procedures using complex new technologies, which carry greater risks of injury. Second, liberalized applications of tort law have created uncertainty among insurers concerning awards for "pain and suffering" and have placed some defendants (those with "deep pockets," such as insurers and hospitals) at greater financial risk, although their contributions to injuries may be minor. (Add to this the fact that the United States is a litigious society.)

The number of claims per 100 physicians has risen at various times and then declined. Since 1990, the number of claims per 100 physicians has been *declining* (U.S. Government Accounting Office 2003), as shown in Figure 13.3. Claims against obstetricians, typically the group with the highest number of claims filed, have declined sharply since the early 1990s.

Based on data showing a decline in the number of claims filed per 100 physicians, the number of claims filed does not appear to be the explanation for the latest increase in malpractice premiums.

Claims Payment

The second component of malpractice payments is the average payment per claim. Most claims are resolved by settlement with the insurer (about 14,000 per year), whereas successful jury awards to the injured party number only about 400 per year.

An interesting aspect of the rising costs for malpractice insurance is the difference between the average (mean) jury award and the median jury award, which represents the midpoint of all of the awards (half the awards are above and half are below the median award). Although a slight rise in median jury awards has been seen over time, the average jury award has increased sharply since the late 1990s and then has leveled out (Figure 13.4). The average jury award in any year is generally two to five times greater than the median award ($1.2 million in 2003), meaning that juries make many small awards and a few large ones, although the latter receive the greatest publicity. Trial judgments, which account for only 4 percent of all malpractice payments (settlements account for the remaining 96 percent of payments), are, on average, about twice the size

Figure 13.3: Average Incidence of Medical Professional Liability Claims, by Specialty, 1985–1997

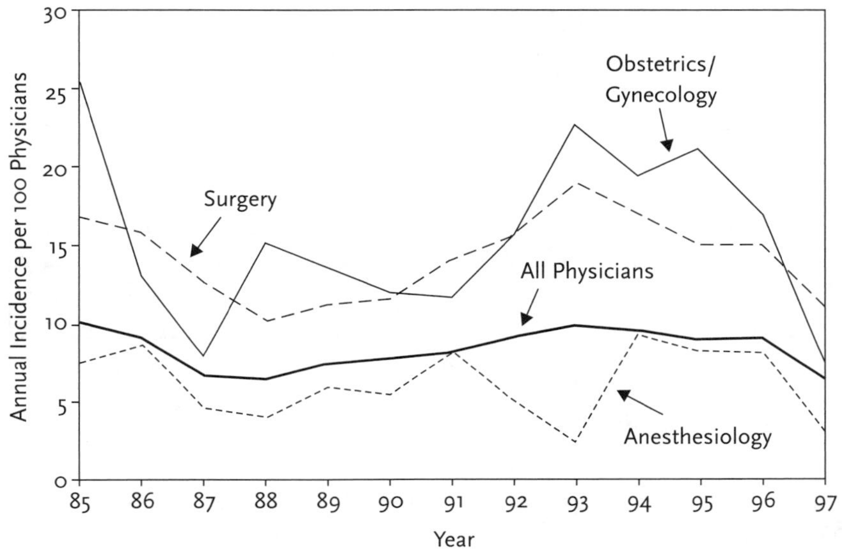

Source: Data from American Medical Association, Center for Health Policy Research. 2002. *Physician Marketplace Report,* Table 1. Chicago: AMA.

of settlements. (The median settlement award increased from $400,000 in 1997 to $700,000 in 2003.)

Large damage awards and financial settlements for patients, however, do not appear to be the driving force responsible for the "explosive" increase in physicians' malpractice insurance premiums. A recent study, based on data from the National Practitioner Data Bank, found that payments to patients between 1991 and 2003 increased by 4 percent annually, a figure that is similar to increases in overall medical costs over that same period (Chandra, Nundy, and Seabury 2005). Malpractice premium increases, however, increased much more rapidly.

Insurer Profitability
The third possible explanation for the recurrent crisis is based on the changing financial condition and market structure of malpractice insurers. Profitability of insurers is determined by both their loss ratio (jury awards, settlements, and defense costs as a percent of premiums) and

Figure 13.4: Jury Awards for Medical Malpractice Cases, 1974–2003

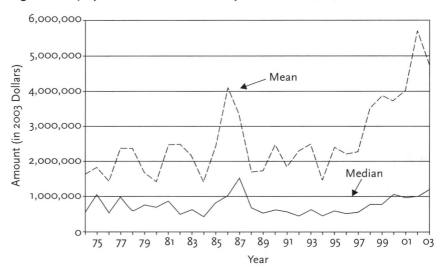

Sources: 1974–1990 data from American College of Surgeons. *Socioeconomic Factbook,* various editions. Chicago: ACS; 1991–1992 data from *Trends in Health Care Provider Liability*; 1993–2003 data from Jury Verdict Research. *Current Award Trends in Personal Injury,* various editions. Horsham, PA: LRP Publications.

their investment returns, which are often used to offset high loss ratios. If the loss ratio is high, the investment returns may still enable the insurer to be profitable.

As the frequency and size of physicians' malpractice claims rose in the early 1980s, several large insurers sharply increased their rates. The frequency and size of claims leveled off by the late 1980s, leaving insurers with large reserves that had been set aside for expected continued increases in malpractice payouts. During the early and mid-1990s, these insurers had substantial reserves against possible losses, so by "releasing" these reserves insurers greatly increased their income. Also during this period, insurers' loss ratios were favorable, about 92 percent, and investment returns were high; insurers were profitable and malpractice premiums were generally stable.

Seemingly unaware that insurers' high income was based on prior years' reserves (when insurance actuaries were predicting that previous claims trends would continue increasing) and believing large profits could be had in malpractice insurance, new insurers entered the business.

Table 13.1: Malpractice Insurers' Financial Ratios, 1995–2003

Year	Broad Combined Ratio*	Loss Ratio**	Investment Insurance Ratio†	Net Income†
1995	112%	97%	46%	23%
1996	109	92	43	19
1997	111	92	43	20
1998	114	92	42	16
1999	113	91	33	13
2000	120	98	32	6
2001	134	113	30	−7
2002	129	111	18	−11
2003	122	105	21	−2

*Awards, settlements, and defense costs plus dividends, administrative costs, and corporate income taxes as a percentage of premium.

**Awards, settlements, and defense costs as a percentage of premium.

†As a percentage of premiums.

Source: Hurley, J. D. 2004. "Medical Malpractice Update." Towers Perrin, CASE 2004 Fall Meeting, September 23. [Online information.] http://www.casact.org/affiliates/case/0904/hurley.ppt.

To attract business, these new insurers offered lower premiums; existing insurers responded by cutting their premiums. Intense price competition among insurers led to premiums that were inadequate to cover malpractice payouts (Zimmerman and Oster 2002). As a result, the loss ratio began to greatly exceed premium income, reaching 113 percent by 2001 (Table 13.1). Further, reserves were diminished, and investment returns fell sharply as bond yields and equities declined.[1] To improve their loss ratios and to compensate for their lower investment returns, insurers increased their premiums to return to profitability.

Two additional factors reinforced insurers' rate increases. Reinsurers, who cover larger insurance payments, began to increase their reserves, and consequently their rates to malpractice insurers, as the percentage of million-dollar jury awards increased. Second, the structure of the malpractice insurance industry changed. By 2001 many insurers were losing

---

1. A decline in investment returns of 1 percent is estimated to lead to a 2 percent to 4 percent increase in malpractice premiums (Thorpe 2004, W4-23).

money, became insolvent, and either exited the business or withdrew from markets in which they had been losing money. These temporary disruptions in availability of coverage in several markets led to much higher rates by the remaining insurers.[2]

The latest financial results of malpractice insurers indicate that insurer profitability is increasing and that the latest crisis of rapidly rising malpractice premiums is moderating.

OBJECTIVES OF THE MALPRACTICE SYSTEM

Tort law is the basis for medical malpractice. It entitles an injured person to compensation as a result of someone's negligence. Damages include economic losses (lost wages and medical bills) and pain and suffering. Thus, physicians should have a financial incentive to provide good treatment and perform only those procedures for which they are competent. *The purposes of tort law are compensation to the victim for negligence and deterrence of future negligence.*

How well does the malpractice system fulfill these two objectives? Can legislative reforms achieve these objectives at a lower cost than the current system? Physician advocates maintain that too many claims have little to do with negligence (so the insurer will settle to avoid legal expense) and that juries award large sums unrelated to actual damages. Furthermore, "defensive" medicine—additional tests prescribed by physicians to protect themselves against malpractice claims—adds billions of dollars to the nation's health expenditures.

Patient advocates claim that physician negligence is more extensive than is reflected by the number of claims filed, large jury awards are infrequent, incompetent physicians must be discouraged from practicing because physicians do not adequately monitor themselves, and defensive medicine is caused by an insurance system that eliminates patients' incentives to be concerned about the cost of care.

Compensation of Victims

Which arguments are correct? A 1990 Harvard University study found that too few of those injured by negligence are compensated under the

---

2. Rising malpractice premiums are not the result of collusion among insurers. Collusion would be difficult given the large number of insurers, including physician-owned insurance companies (although there are fewer companies from whom these insurance companies purchase reinsurance), and the high level of competition among them.

malpractice system (Localio et al. 1991). The authors examined hospital records in 51 New York hospitals and determined that almost 4 percent of all patients suffered an injury while in the hospital and that one-quarter of those injuries were the result of negligence. Thus, about 1 percent of all patients discharged from New York hospitals in 1984 experienced some type of negligence. Examples of injuries occurring in hospitals are errors in diagnosis, falls, hospital-caused infections, and surgical complications.

Surprisingly, fewer than 2 percent of the patients identified as victims of negligence filed a malpractice claim. Six percent of injured patients who had not been victims of negligence also filed claims. (Even though there may have been no negligence on the part of the surgeon, not all surgical procedures are successful, and the patient could be left with a disability or even die.) According to the Harvard researchers, only half of patient claims filed eventually receive some compensation. Most patients settle within two years without receiving any compensation, and the rest may wait years for compensation. Few victims of negligence ever receive compensation. *About 1 percent of victims of malpractice receive some compensation.* Of those patients injured through negligence who do not file claims (98 percent of negligence victims), 20 percent have serious injuries—disabilities that last six months or more—and this figure includes fatalities.

Several reasons account for the low percentage of negligence claims filed. A patient may not know that negligence caused an injury. Some claims may be difficult to prove. Recoverable damages may be less than the litigation costs, particularly when the injured patient earns low wages, which explains the low incidence of claims for minor injuries.

The cost of administering the compensation system is very high, and only a small portion of malpractice premiums, 28 percent to 40 percent, is returned to those injured through negligence. Overhead, including legal fees, consumes the major portion of premiums. Health insurance, on the other hand, returns 85 percent to 90 percent of the premium for medical expenses.

If the sole purpose of malpractice insurance is to compensate those who are negligently injured, more efficient means at lower administrative costs exist. A different approach could compensate a greater number of victims and return a greater portion of premiums to those injured.

Deterrence of Negligence
Justification of the current malpractice system must depend, therefore, on how well it performs its second, more important role, preventing

negligence. Compensation tries not only to make whole the injuries suffered by victims of negligence, but also to force negligent health care providers to pay that compensation so they will exercise greater caution in future caregiving situations. Concerns exist, however, that not enough injuries are prevented (the deterrence effect) by the current system to justify the high costs of practicing defensive medicine to prevent claims, determining fault, and prosecuting malpractice claims.

The standard of care used in determining negligence is what one would expect from a reasonably competent person who is knowledgeable about advances in medicine and exercises care. Some cases of malpractice, such as amputating the wrong leg or leaving surgical supplies in a patient's abdomen, are easily established. With other forms of physician behavior, however, uncertainties exist in both diagnosis and outcome of medical treatment. Many medical procedures are inherently risky. Even with correct diagnosis and treatment a patient may die because of poor health conditions, or a baby may be born with a birth defect through no fault of the obstetrician. Physicians do differ in the quality of care they provide and in their success rates, but it is difficult, hence costly, to determine whether a specific outcome is a result of physician negligence, poor communication of the risks involved, or the patient's underlying health condition.

The potential for malpractice suits increases the cost of negligent behavior to the physician. Physicians therefore would be expected to change their behavior and restrict their practices to forestall such costs, no longer performing procedures and tasks for which they lack competence. The deterrence effect should cause physicians to exercise proper care to minimize errors. Prevention costs time and resources; therefore, physicians should invest in prevention (their time, training, and medical testing) up to the point at which the additional cost of prevention equals the additional value of injuries avoided (forgone malpractice costs). "Too much" prevention could occur if a great deal of time and resources (the additional costs) are used to prevent occasional minor injuries. A requirement that the injury rate be zero would be too costly for society and would discourage skilled specialists from performing procedures that involve an element of risk of injury but could benefit the patient.

How well does the malpractice system deter negligence? More precisely, is the value (to patients) of the negligence prevented greater than the costs (defensive medicine, determining liability, and litigation) of the malpractice system? Experts differ on this issue.

First, critics of the current system claim that physicians are not penalized by negligence, as only 2 percent of negligence victims file claims (Localio et al. 1991). Second, because less than half of malpractice insurance premiums—approximately $6 billion, or one-third of one percent of total health care spending—are returned to victims of negligence and the remainder is spent on overhead and legal fees, the malpractice system is too costly. Third, because most malpractice insurance does not "experience rate" physicians within their specialties, incompetent physicians are not penalized by higher premiums; their behavior merely increases premiums for all physicians in that specialty. Fourth, not all physicians who are sued are incompetent. Although incompetent physicians may be sued more often, competent physicians may also be sued because of occasional errors or because they are specialists who treat more difficult cases; for example, board-certified physicians are sued more often than other physicians. Fifth, the current system results in high costs for tests and services that are not medically justified but are performed to protect physicians from malpractice claims. Physicians will engage in "defensive" medicine, resulting in medically unnecessary expenditures. Physicians overuse tests because the costs of such defensive medicine are borne by patients and insurers, whereas an injury claim could result in physician liability. Thus, physicians are able to shift the costs of their greater caution to others.

Defenders of the malpractice system claim that the incentive to avoid malpractice suits changes physicians behavior and makes them act more carefully. Physicians have limited their scope of practice, they are more conscientious in documenting their records, and they take the time to discuss the risks involved in a procedure with their patients. Although physician premiums are not experience rated, lawsuits are a costly deterrent in terms of time spent defending against them and in potential damage to the physician's reputation.

The costs of defensive medicine are probably overstated because, under a fee-for-service system, excessive testing would remain even if the threat of malpractice was eliminated. Physicians order too many tests because insured patients pay only a small portion of the price for physician-ordered tests. Although the patient benefits of the tests are less than the costs of performing those tests, it is rational for patients to want those tests because the benefit to them may be greater than their share of the costs. Physicians reimbursed on a fee-for-service basis also benefit by prescribing extra tests. Physicians in HMOs have less of an incentive to perform excessive testing. Thus, physicians' use of excessive testing results in part from traditional insurance payment systems and a lack of policing of such tests by insurers, not necessarily from malpractice.

However, one study that estimated the cost of defensive medicine using Medicare data concluded that the additional cost of defensive medicine is about 4 percent of total Medicare hospital expenditures (Kessler and McClellan 2002). Using the estimate of 4 percent and applying it to total hospital (public and private) expenditures of $616 billion suggests that about $30 billion was spent on defensive medicine in hospitals in 2005—not an insignificant amount. A recent survey of physicians in Pennsylvania found that 93 percent of physicians said they sometimes or often practiced defensive medicine (Studdert et al. 2005). Diagnostic tests were ordered more than was medically necessary as were referrals to other physicians.

Furthermore, removing the threat of malpractice leaves few alternatives for monitoring and disciplining physicians. The emphasis on quality control in organized medicine has always been on the "process" of becoming a physician, that is, the number of years of education, graduation from an approved medical school, and passing national examinations. However, once a physician is licensed, she is never reexamined for relicensure. State medical licensing boards do not adequately monitor physician quality or discipline incompetent physicians. Finally, patients have little or no access to information on physicians' procedure outcomes. Until recently the medical profession actively discouraged public access to such information. What recourse, other than filing a malpractice claim, would a patient have after being injured by an incompetent physician?

Few would disagree that victims of negligence are not adequately compensated. The controversial issues are whether malpractice actually deters negligence and whether alternatives are available for monitoring and disciplining incompetent physician behavior.

PROPOSED CHANGES TO THE MALPRACTICE SYSTEM

Many changes have been proposed to correct perceived inadequacies of the malpractice system. Generally, proposals seek to lower malpractice premiums by limiting the size of jury awards for "pain and suffering" (economic costs for medical expenses and lost wages are not subject to a cap) and reduce the number of claims filed. Both changes would reduce lawyers' incentives to accept malpractice cases.

Damage Caps

Proposals to limit the potential recovery of damages decrease the value of malpractice claims and thereby reduce the number of malpractice claims filed. One study found that malpractice premiums in states with damage caps are 17 percent lower than in states without damage caps (Thorpe 2004).[3] The current Bush Administration has proposed a damages cap similar to California's. In 1975, California enacted a $250,000 damages cap on pain and suffering, which has not been updated for inflation. (If adjusted for inflation, the cap would be almost $1 million.) Jury awards for pain and suffering (quality of life), such as occurs when an injured party has brain damage or paralysis, are reduced to the statutory cap. Caps such as California's reduce the amount of malpractice awards that can be used to pay legal fees, as the remainder of the award is for lost wages and medical expenses.

Collateral Offset Rule

An injured party, under the collateral offset rule, will have the amount of his award or settlement reduced by amounts paid by other sources. Proponents of this rule believe payments from other sources, in addition to the jury award or insurer's settlement, will provide an injured person with much more than they are entitled to. Opponents believe that unless the injured party collects the full amount of her award, even though she has already been paid by other sources, a negligent defendant benefits by having his liability reduced. Proposals to reduce awards by amounts already paid to the victim by other sources, such as health insurance and worker's compensation, would have the same effect as reducing damage

---

3. Physicians claim that the financial burden of high malpractice premiums has led some physicians to retire early, others to stop performing high-risk procedures, and still others to move to states with lower malpractice premiums—all of which affect patients' access to medical care.

States that capped noneconomic damages in malpractice cases experienced a relatively modest 3.3 percent increase in physician supply compared with states without such caps. Although all states experienced an increase in physicians over the period studied (1985–2001), states with damage caps experienced a higher-than-average increase than states without such tort changes (Kessler, Sage, and Becker 2005).

Rural counties in states with noneconomic damage caps had 3.2 percent more physicians per capita than rural counties in states without caps. Obstetricians and surgeons, who are considered more vulnerable to lawsuits, were most influenced by the presence or absence of caps (Encinosa and Hellinger 2005).

caps. Lawyers would have a reduced incentive to bring suits on behalf of patients.

Limits on Attorney's Fees

Fewer malpractice cases would be brought if a limit were placed on lawyers' contingency fees (currently these can be as high as one-third to one-half of the award). Lawyers accept malpractice cases based on the probability of winning and the size of the likely award. Lawyers have less financial incentive to invest their resources in cases whose awards would be smaller. Lawyers are in a competitive market and may represent either plaintiffs or defendants in malpractice cases. Lawyers for defendants are paid hourly rates. Fewer lawyers would choose to represent plaintiffs if contingency fees were reduced.

Joint and Several Liability

When a case is brought against multiple defendants, an injured person is able to collect the entire award from any of the defendants, regardless of the defendant's degree of fault. This rule creates an incentive for the injured party to sue as many defendants as possible to make sure the damages can be paid. Some states have limited a defendant's liability to the individual degree of fault. Limiting a defendant's liability decreases the potential size of the award and might lessen the defendant's (e.g., a hospital's) oversight of its staff physicians.

Local Versus National Standards

Proposals that make proving a malpractice claim more difficult, such as using local rather than national standards and excluding testimony from out-of-state experts, reduce the number of cases to which lawyers would be willing to devote their own time and resources.

Proposals that lessen the size of an award or that make it more difficult to bring claims *are addressing the wrong problem*. These "remedies" are directed at decreasing the number of claims, but the real problem appears to be that too few negligence claims are brought.[4] Malpractice

---

4. A recent federal proposal is to link damage caps to physician participation in reporting medical errors. Proponents of this approach believe the medical malpractice system, which is based on penalizing negligent providers, is a barrier to recognizing medical errors. Thus, providing an incentive (damage caps) for providers to report medical errors will, it is believed, lead to systems for preventing human errors.

reforms should be evaluated in terms of whether they deter negligent behavior and improve victim compensation.

NO-FAULT MALPRACTICE

One proposed reform, a "no-fault" system, would compensate an injured patient whether or not negligence was involved. In return patients would forfeit their right to sue. Two main advantages are seen with a no-fault system. First, litigation costs would be lower because it would not be necessary to prove who was at fault for the injury, and these savings could be used to increase victim compensation. Second, all injured patients, most of whom could not win malpractice suits because their claims were either too small to attract a lawyer's interest or no one was at fault in causing their injury, would receive some compensation. A no-fault system could have a schedule of payments according to types of injuries to compensate the injured for loss of income and for medical expenses. The schedule could include payment for pain and suffering in cases of severe injury.

A no-fault system, however, has two important problems. First, such a system has no deterrence mechanism to weed out incompetent providers or encourage physicians to exercise greater caution. Second, because all injuries would be subject to compensation, no clear line is drawn between injuries that result from negligence, injuries that are not the result of negligence, unfavorable treatment outcomes because of the patient's health condition and lifestyle, and outcomes of risky procedures that are never 100 percent favorable, such as transplants and delivery of low-birth-weight infants. Compensating patients for all injuries and unfavorable outcomes could be very expensive given the large number of injuries for which no claims are filed.[5] Who should bear these costs?

Problems with methods for deterring physician negligence continue to be difficult to resolve. Regulatory approaches, such as state licensing boards for monitoring and disciplining physicians, have performed poorly. Until other deterrent mechanisms are in place, eliminating the malpractice system would be premature.

---

5. The Institute of Medicine and others have issued reports documenting high rates of medical error in causing serious harm or death in the United States. Not all of these injuries to patients, however, are believed to be the result of provider negligence. Instead, appropriate systems are lacking to prevent human error (Kohn, Corrigan, and Donaldson 1999).

ENTERPRISE LIABILITY

One approach that seeks to improve on the malpractice system for deterring negligence is referred to as "enterprise liability." Changing the liability laws so that liability is shifted away from the physician (he can no longer be sued) to a larger entity of which the physician would be required to be a part, such as a hospital, medical group, or managed care plan, would place the incentive for monitoring and enforcing medical quality with that larger organization. These organizations would balance the increased costs of prevention and risk-reducing behavior against the potential for a malpractice claim.

The shift to enterprise liability is already occurring because of market trends and court rulings. The growth of MCOs and the fact that they are liable for physicians they employ or contract with have increased such organizations' monitoring of physician behavior. Furthermore, the concept of "joint and several" liability, wherein the physician is the primary defendant but the hospital or managed care plan is also named as a defendant with potentially 100 percent liability for damages (although it may have been only 10 percent at fault), provides hospitals and HMOs with an incentive to increase their quality assurance and risk management programs.

Many physicians, however, perform surgery only in outpatient settings or do not practice within a hospital. Others may have multiple hospital staff appointments, and still others do not belong to large health plans. These physicians would be most affected by such a shift in liability laws because they would lose some of their autonomy as they become subject to greater supervision by larger entities.

Placing liability for malpractice on a larger organization would enable insurers to experience rate the organization. As more health care organizations become experience rated, they will devote more resources to monitoring their quality of care and disciplining physicians for poor performance. Many organizations, such as HMOs, PPOs, and large medical groups, have information systems in place to profile the practice patterns of their physicians. Competition among health care organizations on price and quality provides them with an incentive to develop quality-control mechanisms. These organizations, rather than regulatory bodies, have both the incentives and the ability to evaluate and control physicians.

SUMMARY

Experts do not agree on malpractice reform (see, for example, the proposals of Newhouse and Weiler 1991, and Danzon 2000). Victim compensation could be improved under a no-fault system, but incentives for deterring negligence would be lacking. Proposals for change often reflect the interests of those who might benefit. Medical societies are often pitted against the trial lawyers' association, for example. The battle for changes in the malpractice system is occurring in almost every state, and federal legislation has been proposed in recent sessions of Congress. All proposals for reform, by whatever interest group, should be judged by how well they achieve the two goals of the malpractice system: compensating victims injured by negligence and deterring future negligence.

DISCUSSION QUESTIONS

1. How well does the malpractice system compensate victims of negligence?

2. How effective is the deterrence function of the malpractice system?

3. Discuss the advantages and disadvantages of no-fault insurance.

4. Do you think the costs of defensive medicine would be reduced under a no-fault system?

5. Evaluate the effects of the following on deterrence and victim compensation:

   a. Limiting lawyers' contingency fees

   b. Excluding testimony from out-of-state experts

   c. Limiting the size of malpractice awards

   d. Placing the liability for malpractice on the health care organization to which the physician belongs

REFERENCES

Chandra, A., S. Nundy, and S. Seabury. 2005. "The Growth of Physician Medical Malpractice Payments: Evidence from the National Practitioner Data Bank." *Health Affairs* Web exclusive, May 31, W5-240–W-249. [Online publication; retrieved 11/15/06.] http://content.healthaffairs.org/cgi/content/abstract/hlthaff.w5.240v1.

Danzon, P. 2000. "Liability for Medical Malpractice." In *Handbook of Health Economics*, vol. 1b, edited by A. J. Culyer and J. P. Newhouse, 1341–1404. New York: North-Holland Press.

Division of Practitioner Data Banks, Bureau of Health Professions, Health Resources and Services Administration. *National Practitioner Data Bank Public Use Data File.* Washington, DC: U.S. DHHS. The National Practitioner Data Bank (NPDB) is a national database maintained by the federal Department of Health and Human Services, which has been collecting data since 1991 on medical malpractice payments made on behalf of physicians.

Encinosa, W., and F. Hellinger. 2005. "Have State Caps on Malpractice Awards Increased the Supply of Physicians?" *Health Affairs* Web exclusive, May 31, W5-250–W5-258. [Online publication; retrieved 11/15/06.] http://content.healthaffairs.org/cgi/content/abstract/hlthaff.w5.250v1.

Kessler, D., and M. McClellan. 2002. "How Liability Law Affects Medical Productivity." *Journal of Health Economics* 21 (6): 931–55.

Kessler, D., W. Sage, and D. Becker. 2005. "Impact of Malpractice Reforms on the Supply of Physicians." *Journal of the American Medical Association* 293 (21): 2618–25.

Kohn, L., J. Corrigan, and M. Donaldson, eds. 1999. *To Err Is Human.* Washington, DC, National Academies Press.

Localio, A. R., A. Lawthers, T. Brennan, N. Laird, L. Hebert, L. Peterson, J. Newhouse, P. Weiler, and H. Hiatt. 1991. "Relation Between Malpractice Claims and Adverse Events Due to Negligence." *The New England Journal of Medicine* 325 (4): 245–51.

Newhouse, J. P., and P. C. Weiler. 1991. "Reforming Medical Malpractice and Insurance." *Regulation* 14 (4): 78–84.

Studdert, D., M. M. Mello, W. M. Sage, C. M. DesRoches, J. Peugh, K. Zapert, T. A. Brennan. 2005. "Defensive Medicine Among High-Risk Specialist Physicians in a Volatile Malpractice Environment." *Journal of the American Medical Association* 293 (21): 2609–17.

Thorpe, K. 2004. "The Medical Malpractice 'Crisis': Recent Trends and the Impact of State Tort Reforms." *Health Affairs* Web exclusive, January 21, W4-20–W4-30. [Online publication; retrieved 11/15/06.] http://content.healthaffairs.org/cgi/reprint/hlthaff.w4.20v1.

U.S. Government Accounting Office. 2003. "Medical Malpractice Insurance: Multiple Factors Have Contributed to Increased Premium Rates." [Online publication; accessed 12/7/06.] http://www.gao.gov/new.items/d03702.pdf.

Zimmerman, R., and C. Oster. 2002. "Assigning Liability: Insurers' Missteps Helped Provoke Malpractice 'Crisis.'" *The Wall Street Journal* June 24, A1 and A8.

ADDITIONAL READING

Budetti, P., and T. Waters. 2005. *Medical Malpractice Law in the United States.* Publication No. 7328. Washington, DC: The Henry J. Kaiser Family Foundation. [Online publication; retrieved 11/15/06.] http://www.kff.org/insurance/upload/Medical-Malpractice-Law-in-the-United-States-Report.pdf.

Chapter 14

Do Nonprofit Hospitals Behave
Differently than For-Profit Hospitals?

HOSPITALS INITIALLY CARED for the poor, the mentally ill, and those with contagious diseases such as tuberculosis. Many hospitals were started by religious organizations and local communities. They were charitable institutions; more affluent patients were treated in their own homes. Ether was developed in the mid-1800s, which allowed operations to be conducted under anesthesia. Surgery patients suffered a high rate of mortality from infection until the antiseptic procedures adopted by the late 1800s began to increase their chances of surviving surgery. Furthermore, the introduction of the x-ray machine around the beginning of the 20th century enabled surgeons to become more effective; the surgeon was better able to determine the location for the surgery and some exploratory surgery was eliminated.

As a result of these improvements, the role of hospitals changed; hospitals became the physician's workshop. Similarly, the type of patients served by the hospital changed. Hospitals were no longer a place to die or be incarcerated but rather places where paying patients could be treated and returned to society. The development of drugs and improved living conditions reduced the demand for mental and tuberculosis hospitals, and the demand for short-term general hospitals increased.

The control of private nonprofit hospitals also changed. As more of the hospital's income came from paying patients, reliance on trustees to raise philanthropic funds declined, and physicians, who admitted and treated patients, became more important to the hospital. As physicians were responsible for generating the hospital's revenue, their importance to and control over the hospital increased.

Most hospitals in the United States are nonprofit, either nongovernmental institutions or controlled by religious organizations. Together these are referred to as *private nonprofit hospitals*. The ownership of a majority of hospitals (2,958 of the 4,956 hospitals in 2005) is "voluntary," meaning private nonprofit. Next in ownership are state and local governmental (1,110) and federal hospitals (226). Investor-owned (for-profit) institutions account for 868 of the total hospitals. Together, private nonprofit and for-profit hospitals admit 83 percent of patients (70 percent and 13 percent, respectively) (Table 14.1).

Most physicians practice in the private nonprofit and for-profit hospitals. These hospitals have also been subject to much governmental policy and have been involved in managed care competition.

The main legal distinctions between nonprofit and for-profit hospitals are that nonprofits cannot distribute profits to shareholders and their earnings and property are exempt from federal and state taxes; they also have the ability to receive donations. Nonprofit hospitals are the beneficiaries of this differential treatment because they have a different mission from for-profit hospitals.

Since the mid-1980s, when managed care competition started, debate has ensued concerning whether nonprofit hospitals are really different from for-profit hospitals. In most industries the competing firms are for-profit. Why is the hospital industry different? The issues surrounding this debate concern the following questions. Do nonprofits charge lower prices than for-profits? Do nonprofits provide a higher level of quality? Do nonprofits provide more charity care than for-profits? Or, as some critics of nonprofits maintain, does no difference exist between the two other than the tax-exempt status of nonprofits' "surpluses"?

If the latter position is correct, is continuing nonprofit hospitals' tax advantages and government subsidies justified? Alternatively, if nonprofits provide more charity care and a higher quality of service as well as charge lower prices, will eliminating for-profit hospitals enable nonprofits to better serve their communities?

WHY ARE HOSPITALS PREDOMINANTLY NONPROFIT?

Several hypotheses have been offered to explain the existence of nonprofit hospitals. The most obvious is that when hospitals were used predominantly as institutions to serve the poor, they were dependent on donations for their funds. Although donations may have been an original motivation for the development of nonprofit hospitals to care for the

Table 14.1: Selected Hospital Data, 2005

Type of Hospital	Number of Hospitals	% Change, by Year			Beds	Admissions	% Distribution of Admissions	Occupancy Rate*
		75–85	85–95	95–05				
Short term								
General**	4,956	–3.3%	–9.8%	–5.1%	804,080	35,264,919	97.9%	67.4%
State and local government	1,110	–10.4	–16.5	–17.8	127,695	4,739,756	95.3	66.7
Not-for-profit	2,958	0.3	–8.1	–4.3	561,106	25,880,516	12.8	69.1
Investor owned	868	3.9	–6.6	15.4	113,510	4,618,401	69.9	59.6
Federal	226	–10.2	–12.8	–24.4	45,837	951,806	12.5	66.0
Long term†	574	-6.3	4.0	–25.6	97,080	789,302	2.6	86.9
							2.1	

*Ratio of average daily census to every 100 beds.

**Short-term general includes community hospitals and hospital units of institutions. The community hospitals group consists of state and local government, nongovernment not-for-profit, and investor-owned hospitals.

†Includes general, psychiatric, tuberculosis and other respiratory diseases, and all others.

Source: American Hospital Association. *Hospital Statistics,* various editions: 1986 ed., Table 2, 1995–96 ed., Table 3A, and 2007 ed., Table 2. Chicago: AHA.

poor, the reliance on donations does not explain why the majority of hospitals continue to be nonprofit. Donations account for a very small percentage of hospital revenue. As hospitals' revenue sources changed (public and private health insurance became the dominant sources of hospital revenue), the potential for profit increased, as did the number of for-profit hospitals.

Although both public and private insurance have increased, large numbers of people are still uninsured. Thus, some believe only nonprofit hospitals would provide uncompensated care to those who are unable to pay. Nonprofit hospitals would presumably be willing to use their surplus funds to subsidize both the poor and money-losing services.

Another related explanation is the issue of trust. A relationship based on trust is needed in markets in which information is lacking. Patients are not sure what services they need. They are dependent on the provider for their diagnoses and treatment recommendations, and they do not know the skill of the surgeon. The quality of medical and surgical treatments is difficult for patients to judge, and they cannot tell whether the hospital failed to provide care to save costs. In such situations patients are more likely to rely on nonprofit providers, believing that because they are not interested in profit, they will not take advantage of a patient who lacks information and is seriously ill.[1]

Another explanation for nonprofit status is that the hospital's managers and board of directors want to be part of a nonprofit hospital, where their activities would be subject to limited community oversight. The managers and board would have greater flexibility in pursuing policies according to their own preferences, such as offering prestigious but money-losing services, although these services are provided by other hospitals in the community.

Still another explanation is that hospitals are nonprofit because it is in physicians' financial interest. Being associated with nonprofit organizations allows physicians to exercise greater control over the hospital's policies, services offered, and investments in facilities and equipment. In a for-profit hospital, physicians would have less money available for facilities and equipment of their choosing because the surplus would

---

1. The trust relationship between the patient and provider, however, applies more strongly to the patient–physician relationship. The physician diagnoses the illness, recommends treatment, refers the patient to specialists, and monitors the care the patient receives from different providers. Yet physicians are not nonprofit.

have to be divided with shareholders and the government by paying dividends and taxes. The hospital's physicians would also benefit from the hospital's ability to receive donations and from the trust the community would have in a nonprofit hospital.

None of these explanations are mutually exclusive. However, the importance of trust, the provision of community benefits, and the financial interests of physicians appear to have been key reasons for the nonprofit status of hospitals.[2]

PERFORMANCE OF NONPROFIT AND FOR-PROFIT HOSPITALS

For-profit hospitals have a more precise organizational goal, namely profit, than nonprofit hospitals. A concern of any organization is monitoring its managers in achieving the firm's goal. In a for-profit firm the objective is straightforward, and the shareholders have an incentive to monitor the performance of its managers and replace them if their performance is lacking.

A nonprofit firm has multiple objectives, making it more difficult to monitor its managers. The various stakeholders of the nonprofit hospital—medical staff, board members, managers, employees, and the community—have different and conflicting objectives as to how the hospital's surplus should be distributed. Should the "profits" go to subsidizing the poor, increasing compensation for managers, increasing wages for employees, establishing prestige facilities, or providing benefits (e.g., low office rent and resources) to medical staff?

Less incentive exists to monitor a nonprofit hospital, as the board of directors has no financial interest in the hospital's performance and must depend on the managers for information on achieving the hospital's multiple goals. Furthermore, if the nonprofit hospital is not performing efficiently, it can still survive on community donations.

---

2. An additional explanation that has been offered for the existence of nonprofit status is that the stochastic nature of the demand for medical services requires hospitals to maintain excess capacity for certain services. It can be very "costly" to patients if they cannot have access to hospital care when needed. For-profit hospitals, some believe, would be unwilling to bear the cost of idle hospital capacity. Furthermore, certain hospital services (e.g., emergency departments, trauma centers, NICUs, teaching, and research, including care for certain groups such as AIDS patients and drug addicts, all of which benefit the community) are generally money-losing services and would otherwise not be provided.

Given these differing goals and incentive-monitoring mechanisms between for-profit and nonprofit hospitals, examining how the behavior of nonprofit hospitals differs from for-profit hospitals is important.

Pricing

For-profit hospitals are expected to set prices to maximize their profits.[3] Do nonprofit hospitals set lower prices than a for-profit hospital would? Three aspects of hospital pricing have been investigated to shed light on how nonprofit hospitals set prices. The first is the *cost-shifting* argument, namely that nonprofit hospitals price to earn sufficient revenues to cover their costs. The nonprofits set prices to private insurers below their profit-maximizing price and increase those prices when the government reduces the price it pays for Medicare or Medicaid patients. For cost shifting to occur, a hospital must (1) have market power (i.e., be able to profitably raise its price) and (2) decide not to exploit that market power before the government reduces its price. The extent to which cost shifting occurs is an indication that hospitals do not set profit-maximizing prices to private payers. (Chapter 17 provides a more complete discussion of cost shifting.)

Evidence on cost shifting is based on data prior to the mid-1980s, before managed care competition. With the start of intense price competition among hospitals, insurers became more sensitive to the prices charged by hospitals. Thus, hospitals' market power declined because insurers were willing to shift their volume to those hospitals offering lower prices. Since the mid-1980s, any ability nonprofit hospitals may have had to cost shift disappeared with hospital competition for managed care contracts. Instead, as the government reduced the prices it paid for Medicare and Medicaid patients, hospitals were under greater pressure to lower rather than raise their prices to be included in an insurer's provider network.

Second, the pricing practices of nonprofit hospitals to uninsured patients have received a great deal of media publicity recently. Large

---

3. In addition to its pricing strategy, the type of services a hospital chooses to offer will also affect its profitability. Horwitz (2005) examined more than 30 services that were categorized as relatively profitable, unprofitable, or variable. Over the period studied (1988–2000), for-profits were more likely to offer relatively profitable medical services, government hospitals were more likely to offer relatively unprofitable services, and nonprofits were often in the middle. For-profits were also more responsive to changes in service profitability than the other two types.

purchasers of hospital services, such as health insurers, Medicare, and Medicaid, receive large discounts from a hospital's billed charges—often as high as 50 percent. Patients who are uninsured have been asked to pay 100 percent of the hospital's billed charges. Newspaper stories have described the hardship faced by many of these patients who do not have the resources to pay their hospital bills (Lagnado 2004). Several lawsuits have been filed on behalf of the uninsured against nonprofit hospitals based on their differential pricing of charging those least able to pay the highest prices and hounding patients for unpaid debts (Davies 2004). These lawsuits (several of which have been settled by hospitals) claim that nonprofit hospitals have violated their charitable mission by overcharging the uninsured and seek to have their tax-exempt status revoked. The pricing practices of nonprofit hospitals with regard to the uninsured appear to be no different than those of for-profit hospitals.

The third indication of whether nonprofit hospitals set lower prices is how they determine prices once they achieve increased market power as a result of a merger between nonprofit hospitals. The number of hospital mergers has increased in recent years, resulting in fewer hospitals competing with one another within a market. Consolidation of for-profit firms or hospitals in a market raises concern that competition will be reduced when there are fewer competitors, enabling the hospitals to increase their prices. Consumers would thereby be harmed because higher hospital prices would be passed on in the form of increased health insurance premiums. Would a merger of nonprofit hospitals similarly result in higher hospital prices, or are nonprofit hospitals different?

In previous court cases in which the merger of nonprofit hospitals was contested by federal antitrust agencies, the presiding judge ruled that nonprofit hospital mergers are different from mergers of for-profits. The judges believed that merging nonprofit hospitals were unlikely to raise their prices, even if they acquired monopoly power, because the boards of directors are themselves local citizens and would not take advantage of their neighbors by raising prices.

Empirical studies, however (Melnick, Keeler, and Zwanziger 1999), contradict the judges' reliance on nonprofit ownership for limiting price increases after a merger. Researchers found that even nonprofit hospitals in more concentrated markets (in which there is greater market power) charge significantly higher prices than nonprofits in more competitive markets. These results suggest that some nonprofit hospitals merge simply as a means to increase their market power and be able to negotiate higher prices with managed care plans. This type of behavior is no different from what one would expect from for-profit hospitals.

In October 2005, the Federal Trade Commission (FTC) won an antitrust suit against nonprofit Northwestern Healthcare for a previously consummated hospital merger. The FTC claimed that a hospital merger that occurred in 2000 violated federal antitrust law because the newly created three-hospital system was able to sufficiently increase its market power to illegally control hospital prices in its market (Taylor 2005). The FTC claimed that, as a result of the merger, the nonprofit hospital system used its postmerger market power to impose huge price increases—of 40 percent to 60 percent, and in one case, 190 percent—on insurers and employers. If upheld on appeal, Northwestern will have to divest itself of one hospital. Mergers of nonprofit hospital are no longer likely to be viewed as being different from mergers of for-profit hospitals.

Quality of Care
Sloan (2000) reviewed several large-scale empirical studies of quality of care received by Medicare beneficiaries in nonprofit and for-profit hospitals. Various measures of quality were examined, such as the overall care process and the extent to which medical charts showed that specific diagnostic and therapeutic procedures were performed competently. Different hospital admissions were examined, such as hip fracture, stroke, coronary heart disease, and congestive heart failure, and different outcome measures were examined, such as survival, functional status, cognitive status, and probability of living in a nursing home. These studies found that although patients admitted to major teaching hospitals did better, no statistically significant differences were found between nonteaching private nonprofit hospitals and for-profit hospitals.

In an extensive study, McClellan and Staiger (2000) compared patient outcomes of all elderly Medicare beneficiaries hospitalized with heart disease (more than 350,000 per year) in for-profit and nonprofit hospitals between 1984 and 1994. They found that:

> On average, for-profit hospitals have higher mortality among elderly patients with heart disease, and . . . this difference has grown over the last decade. However, much of the difference appears to be associated with the location of for-profit hospitals. Within specific markets, for-profit ownership appears if anything to be associated with better quality care. Moreover, the small average difference in

mortality between for-profit and not-for-profit hospitals masks an enormous amount of variation in mortality within each of these ownership types. Overall, these results suggest that factors other than for-profit status per se may be the main determinants of quality of care in hospitals (p. 4).

Charity Care

Nonprofit hospitals have a long tradition of caring for the medically indigent. They were given tax-exempt status and community donations in the belief that they would provide charity care. However, the advent of price competition in the mid-1980s has changed the ability of nonprofit hospitals to provide the level of charity care some believe is necessary to maintain their tax-exempt status.

The extent of charity care provided by nonprofit hospitals has been examined with respect to (1) hospital conversions (a nonprofit becomes a for-profit hospital) and (2) the effect of increased competitive pressures resulting from managed care.

Concern has arisen that once a hospital converts to for-profit status its charity care will decline as the profit motive becomes dominant. Various studies, however, have found no difference in provision of uncompensated care once a hospital converts from nonprofit to for-profit status. Norton and Staiger (1994) found that for-profit hospitals are more often located in areas with a high degree of health insurance (Medicare, Medicaid, and private insurance). However, once differences in hospital location are accounted for, such as by examining nonprofit and for-profit hospitals in the same market, no difference was found in the volume of uninsured patients cared for by the two types of hospitals.

Price competition is expected to negatively affect a nonprofit hospital's ability to provide charity care by decreasing the "profits" or surplus available for such care. As competition reduces prices charged to privately insured patients, "profits" are reduced and less is available for charity care. Gruber (1994) found that increased competition among hospitals in California during the period from 1984 to 1988 led to a decrease in their revenues from private payers, as well as a decrease in their net income, and consequently a reduction in the hospitals' provision of uncompensated care.

The comptroller general, David Walker (2005), stated that in four of the five states studied in 2003, state and locally owned hospitals provided an average of twice as much uncompensated care as either not-for-profit or for-profit hospitals. In Florida, Georgia, Indiana, and Texas, not-for-profit hospitals provided more uncompensated care than for-profit hospitals. The difference, however, was small. In California, for-profit hospitals provided more uncompensated care than not-for-profit hospitals, according to the study. In another study of uncompensated care in five states, the U.S. Congressional Budget Office (2006, 2) found that the cost of uncompensated care as a percentage of hospital operating expenses was much larger in government hospitals (13 percent) than in nonprofit hospitals (4.7 percent) or for-profit hospitals (4.2 percent). Individual nonprofit and for-profit hospitals, however, varied widely in the amount of uncompensated care provided: "The distribution of uncompensated-care shares among these two types of hospitals overlap to a large extent."

Overall, competitive pressures result in less income being available for charity care in both nonprofit and for-profit hospitals, and public hospitals are finding themselves with increased uncompensated care costs.

THE QUESTION OF TAX-EXEMPT STATUS

Nonprofit hospitals have received tax advantages that obligate them to serve the uninsured. Nonprofits, however, vary greatly in the amount of care they provide to the uninsured. In a number of cases, the value of the hospital's tax exemption exceeds the value of charity care it provides. Consequently, it has been proposed that in return for their tax-exempt status nonprofit hospitals be required to provide a minimum amount of charity care.

If the tax exemption is to be tied to the value of charity care/community benefits, the measure to be used and the amount of care the hospital should provide must be defined. Following are different possible measures that have been proposed.

- *Pure charity care:* care for which payment is not expected and patients are not billed
- *Bad debt:* value of care delivered and billed to patients believed to be able to pay but from whom the hospital is unable to collect
- *Uncompensated care:* the sum of bad debt and charity care
- *Medicaid and Medicare shortfalls:* the difference between hospital charges and the amount Medicare and Medicaid reimburse the hospital

- *Community benefits:* include the previous items and the amount of patient education, prevention programs, medical research, and provision of money-losing services, for example, burn units and trauma centers

Deciding which definition should be used, and what percentage of a nonprofit hospital's revenue should be devoted to that measure, is an important public policy issue being debated by state and federal governments. For example, if the charity care definition is used, is the amount of free care provided measured using the hospital's full charges (which few payers actually pay), or the lower prices an HMO would pay? Furthermore, using the broadest definition, community benefits, may result in a hospital providing no charity care and relying instead on Medicare and Medicaid shortfalls as well as some community prevention programs, which may also be viewed as a marketing effort by the hospital. If such a broad definition were used, little difference would be found between many nonprofit and for-profit hospitals.

To date, many states have engaged in limited monitoring of the uncompensated care provided by nonprofit hospitals. Explicit rules should be specified for a hospital to maintain its tax-exempt status.

SUMMARY

In examining whether the behavior of nonprofit hospitals is different from that of for-profit hospitals, one must keep in mind that wide variations in behavior exist within both types of hospitals. Although little difference is found between ownership type in pricing behavior, quality of care delivered, or even the amount of uncompensated care provided, these comparisons are based on averages. For example, teaching hospitals often provide greater levels of charity care than other nonprofit hospitals.

As price competition among hospitals increases, ownership differences become less important in determining a hospital's behavior with regard to pricing, quality of care, and even charity care. In a price-competitive environment, both nonprofits and for-profits must have similar behavior to survive; nonprofits will have less of a surplus to pursue other goals.

Ideally, the poor and uninsured should not have to rely on nonprofit hospitals for charity care. Expanding health insurance to the uninsured, either through private insurance vouchers or Medicaid, will more directly solve the problem of providing care for the medically indigent. Unfortunately, providing coverage for all of the uninsured is unlikely to occur in the foreseeable future. Thus, hospitals will have to continue providing free care to the uninsured.

DISCUSSION QUESTIONS

1. Discuss the differences and similarities between the different theories about why hospitals are nonprofit.

2. Do you agree with the ruling by a federal judge that merging nonprofit hospitals should not be subject to the same antitrust laws as merging for-profit hospitals?

3. How has price competition affected the ability of nonprofit hospitals to achieve their nonprofit mission?

4. What conditions should be imposed on nonprofit hospitals for them to retain their tax-exempt status?

5. In what ways, if any, are nonprofit hospitals different from for-profit hospitals?

REFERENCES

Davies, P. 2004. "Hospital Chains Sued over Billing: Alabama Lawyer Claims Companies Inflated Profit by Overcharging Uninsured." *The Wall Street Journal* August 6, B2.

Gruber, J. 1994. "The Effect of Competitive Pressure on Charity: Hospital Responses to Price Shopping in California." *Journal of Health Economics* 13 (2): 183–212.

Horwitz, J. 2005. "Making Profits and Providing Care: Comparing Nonprofit, For-Profit, and Governmental Hospitals." *Health Affairs* 24 (3): 790–801.

Lagnado, L. 2004. "HHS Chief Scolds Hospitals for Their Treatment of Uninsured." *The Wall Street Journal* February 20, A1.

McClellan, M., and D. Staiger. 2000. "Comparing Hospital Quality at For-Profit and Not-for-Profit Hospitals." In *The Changing Hospital Industry: Comparing Not-for-Profit and For-Profit Institutions*, edited by D. Cutler, 93–112. Chicago: The University of Chicago Press.

Melnick, G., E. Keeler, and J. Zwanziger. 1999. "Market Power and Hospital Pricing: Are Nonprofits Different?" *Health Affairs* 18 (3): 167–73.

Norton, E., and D. Staiger. 1994. "How Hospital Ownership Affects Access to Care for the Uninsured." *RAND Journal of Economics* 25 (1): 171–85.

Sloan, F. 2000. "Not-for-Profit Ownership and Hospital Behavior." In *Handbook of Health Economics*, vol. 1B, edited by A. J. Culyer and J. P. Newhouse, 1141–73. New York: North-Holland Press.

Taylor, M. 2005. "Changing the Balance." *Modern Healthcare* 35 (43): 6, 7, and 16.

U.S. Congressional Budget Office. 2006. "Nonprofit Hospitals and the Provision of Community Benefit." [Online publication; accessed 1/4/07.] http://www.cbo.gov/ftpdocs/76xx/doc7695/12-06-Nonprofit.pdf.

Walker, D. M. 2005. "Nonprofit, For-Profit and Government Hospital Uncompensated Care and Other Community Benefits." Testimony before the Committee on Ways and Means, House of Representatives, GAO-05-743T. [Online information; retrieved 11/15/06.] http://www.gao.gov/new.items/d05743t.pdf.

ADDITIONAL READINGS

Rosenberg, C. 1987. *The Care of Strangers: The Rise of America's Hospital System.* New York: Basic Books.

Shen, Y., K. Eggleston, J. Lau, and C. Schmid. 2005. *Hospital Ownership and Financial Performance: A Quantitative Research Review.* NBER Working Paper No. 11662. Cambridge, MA: National Bureau of Economic Research. [Online publication; retrieved 11/15/06.] http://www.nber.org/papers/w11662.

Chapter 15

Competition Among Hospitals: Does it Raise or Lower Costs?

CURRENT FEDERAL POLICY (the antitrust laws) encourages competition among hospitals. Hospitals proposing a merger are scrutinized by the FTC to determine whether the merger will lessen hospital competition in that market, in which case the FTC will oppose the merger. Critics of this policy believe hospitals should be permitted, in fact encouraged, to consolidate and co-operate the facilities and services they provide. They claim that the result will be greater efficiency, less duplication of costly services, and higher quality of care. Who is correct, and what is appropriate public policy for hospitals—competition or cooperation?

Important to understanding hospital performance are (1) the methods used to pay hospitals (different payment methods provide hospitals with different incentives) and (2) the consequences of having different numbers of hospitals compete with one another.

ORIGINS OF NONPRICE COMPETITION

After the introduction of Medicare and Medicaid in 1966, hospitals were paid their costs for the services they rendered to the aged and poor. Private insurance, which was widespread among the remainder of the population, also reimbursed hospitals generously according to either their costs or charges. The extensive coverage of hospital services by both private and public payers removed patients' incentives to be concerned with the costs of hospital care. Patients pay less out-of-pocket costs for hospital care (3 percent) than for any other medical service.

Third-party payers (government and private insurance) and patients had virtually no incentives to be concerned with hospital efficiency and duplication of facilities and services. Furthermore, most hospitals are organized as not-for-profit (nongovernment) organizations that are either affiliated with a religious organization or controlled by boards of trustees selected from the community. With the introduction of extensive public and private hospital insurance after the mid-1960s, the use of nonprofit hospitals increased. Lacking a profit motive and being assured of survival by the generous payment methods, nonprofit hospitals also had no incentive to be concerned with efficiency. The lack of efficiency incentives caused the costs of caring for patients to rise rapidly.

Figure 15.1 illustrates the dramatic rise in hospital expenditures from the 1960s to the present. After Medicare and Medicaid were enacted in 1965, hospital expenditures increased by more than 16 percent per year. These large increases were primarily attributable to sharp increases in hospital prices, as shown in Figure 15.2. Hospital price increases moderated during the early 1970s when wage and price controls were imposed but then increased sharply once they were removed in mid-1974. Hospital expenditure increases were less rapid in the mid- to late 1980s as Medicare changed its hospital payment system and price competition increased.

The rate of increase in both hospital expenditures and hospital prices continued to fall during the 1990s.[1] These decreases, as will be discussed, are indicative of the changes that have occurred in the market for hospital services.

In the late 1960s, the private sector also did not encourage efficiency. Although services such as diagnostic workups could be provided less expensively in an outpatient setting, BlueCross paid for such services only if they were provided as part of a hospital admission. Small hospitals attempted to emulate medical centers by having the latest in technology, although those services were infrequently used. It did not matter whether larger organizations had lower costs per unit and higher-quality outcomes than smaller facilities, because cost was of little concern to patients or purchasers of the service.

The greater the number of hospitals in a community, the more intense was the competition among the nonprofit hospitals to become the

---

1. Starting in the mid-1980s, hospital price increases, as calculated in the CPI, have been greatly overstated because the CPI measured "list" prices rather than actual prices charged. The difference between the two has become greater with the increase in hospital discounting (Dranove, Shanley, and White 1991). To correct this discrepancy the Bureau of Labor Statistics, in constructing the CPI, began to use data on actual hospital prices in the early 1990s.

Figure 15.1: Trends in Hospital Expenditures, 1966–2005

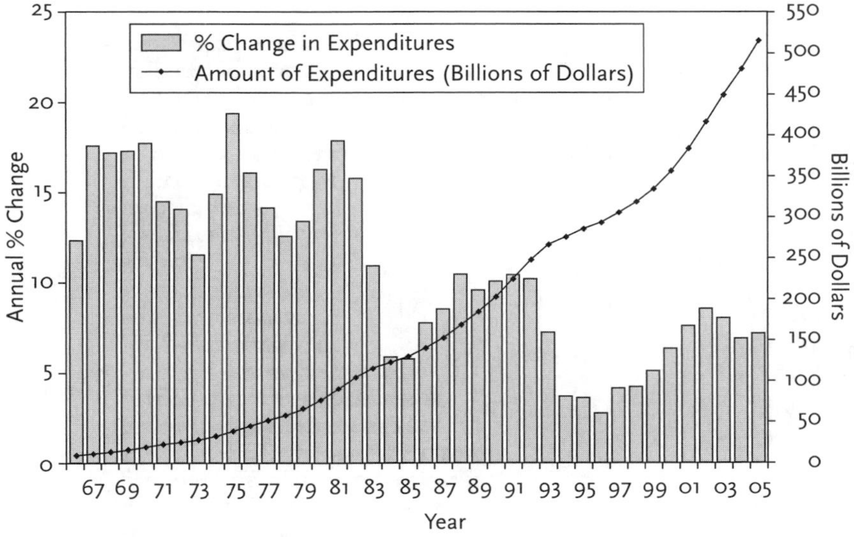

Note: Data for total nonfederal short-term general and other special hospitals.

Source: Data from American Hospital Association. 2007. *Hospital Statistics*, 2007 edition, Table 1. Chicago: Health Forum LLC, an affiliate of the AHA.

most prestigious hospital. Hospitals competed for physicians by offering them all of the services available at other hospitals so that the physician's productivity and convenience of caring for patients would be increased and physicians would not have to refer patients to another hospital. This wasteful form of nonprice competition was characterized as a "medical arms race" and resulted in rapidly rising hospital expenditures.

As the costs of nonprice competition increased, federal and state governments attempted to change hospitals' behavior. Regulations were enacted to control hospital capital expenditures; hospitals were required to have certificate-of-need (CON) approval from a state planning agency before they could undertake large investments. According to proponents of state planning, controlling hospital investment would eliminate unnecessary and duplicative investments. Unfortunately, no attempts were made to change hospital payment methods, which would have changed hospitals' incentives to undertake such investments.

Numerous studies concluded that CONs did not have any effect on limiting the growth in hospital investment. Instead, CONs were used in

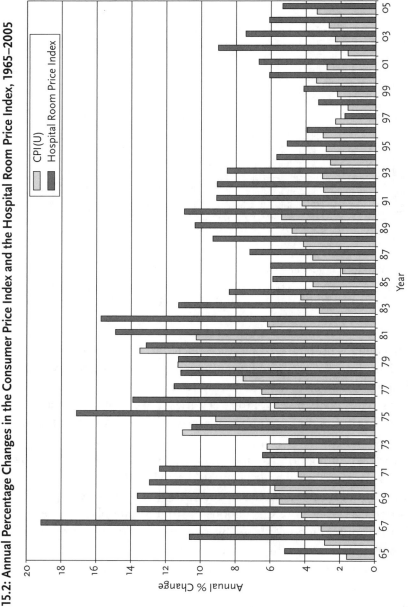

Figure 15.2: Annual Percentage Changes in the Consumer Price Index and the Hospital Room Price Index, 1965–2005

Note: Due to changes in BLS coding, data after 1996 are for hospital services.

Source: U.S. Department of Labor, Bureau of Labor Statistics. 2006. [Online information.] http://www.bls.gov.

an anticompetitive manner to benefit existing hospitals in the community, which ended up controlling the CON approval process. Ambulatory surgery centers (unaffiliated with hospitals) did not receive CON approval for construction because they would take away hospital patients; HMOs such as Kaiser found entering a new market difficult because they could not receive CON approval to build a new hospital; and the courts found that the CON process was used in an "arbitrary and capricious manner" against for-profit hospitals attempting to enter the market of an existing nonprofit hospital.

TRANSITION TO PRICE COMPETITION

Until the 1980s, hospital competition was synonymous with nonprice competition, and its effect was wasteful and rapidly rising expenditures.

During the 1980s, hospital and purchaser incentives changed. Medicare began to pay hospitals a fixed price per admission (which varied according to the type of admission). This new payment system, referred to as DRGs, was phased in over five years starting in 1983. Faced with a fixed price, hospitals now had an incentive to reduce their costs of caring for aged patients. In addition to becoming more efficient, hospitals reduced lengths of stay for aged patients, which caused declines in hospital occupancy rates. For the first time, hospitals became concerned with their physicians' practice behavior. If physicians ordered too many tests or kept patients in the hospital longer than necessary, the hospital lost money given the fixed DRG price.

As employers became concerned with their employees' rising medical expenses, they pressured their insurers to reduce the cost of the largest and fastest-growing component of medical expenditures, hospital services. As a result, insurers changed their insurance benefits to encourage patients to have diagnostic tests and minor surgical procedures performed in an outpatient setting. Insurers instituted utilization review to monitor the appropriateness of inpatient admissions, and this further reduced hospital admissions and lengths of stay. These changes in hospital and purchaser incentives further reduced hospital occupancy rates from 76 percent in 1980 to 67 percent by 1990; as of 2005, the rate was about 67 percent. The decline in occupancy rates was much more severe for small hospitals, falling to below 50 percent.

As hospital occupancy rates declined, hospitals were willing to negotiate price discounts with insurers and HMOs that were able to deliver a large number of patients to their hospitals. As a result, price competition started among hospitals by the late 1980s.

Price competition does not imply that hospitals compete only on the basis of which hospital has the lowest price. Purchasers are also interested in other characteristics of a hospital, such as its reputation, the hospital's location in relation to its patients, which facilities and services are available, patient satisfaction, and treatment outcomes.

PRICE COMPETITION IN THEORY

How did hospitals respond to this new competitive environment in which purchasers demand lower prices? Let us examine two hypothetical situations. In the first situation, only one hospital exists in an area; it has no competitors, and no substitutes for inpatient services are available. The hospital is a monopolist in providing hospital services and has no incentive to respond to purchaser demands for lower prices, quality information, and patient satisfaction. The purchaser has no choice but to use the only hospital available. If the hospital is not efficient, it can pass on the resulting higher costs to the purchaser. If the patients are dissatisfied with the hospital's services or the hospital refuses to provide outcomes information on its open-heart surgery facility, the purchaser and patients have no choice but to use the only hospital in town. (Obviously at some point it becomes worthwhile for patients to incur large travel costs to go to distant hospitals.)

When only one hospital serves a market, that hospital is unlikely to have good performance. The hospital has little incentive to be efficient or respond to purchaser and patient demands.

The second hypothetical scenario consists of many hospitals, perhaps ten, serving a particular geographic area. Now assume a large employer in the area is interested in lowering its employees' hospital costs and is also interested in the quality of and satisfaction with the care received. Furthermore, for simplicity, each of the ten hospitals is equally accessible to the firm's employees (with regard to distance and staff appointments for the employees' physicians). How are hospitals likely to respond to this employer's demands?

At least several of the hospitals would be willing, in return for receiving a greater number of patients from that employer, to negotiate lower prices and accede to the employer's demands for information on quality and patient satisfaction. As long as the price the hospital receives from that employer is greater than the direct costs of caring for its patients, the hospital will make more money than if it did not accept those patients. Furthermore, unless each hospital is as efficient as its competitors, it cannot hope to win such contracts. A more efficient hospital would always be able to charge less.

Similar to competing on price is the competition that would occur among hospitals regarding their willingness to provide information on treatment outcomes. As long as the hospitals have to rely on purchaser revenues to survive, they will be driven to respond to purchaser demands. If a given hospital is not responsive to purchaser demands, other hospitals would be, and the first hospital would soon find that it had too few patients to remain in business.

When hospitals compete on price, quality, and other purchaser requirements, their performance is opposite that of a monopoly provider of hospital services. Hospitals have an incentive to be efficient and respond to purchaser demands in price-competitive markets.

What if, instead of competing with one another, the ten hospitals decided to agree among themselves not to compete on price or provide purchasers with any additional information? The outcome would be similar to a monopoly situation. Prices would be higher, and hospitals would have less incentive to be efficient. Patients would be worse off because they would pay more, and patient quality and patient satisfaction would be lower because employers and other purchasers would be unable to select hospitals based on patient quality and satisfaction information.

The benefits to consumers are greater the more competitive the market. For this reason, society seeks to achieve competitive markets through its antitrust laws. Although competitive hospitals might be harmed and driven out of business, *the evaluation of competitive markets is based on their effect on consumers rather than on any competitors in that market.*

The antitrust laws are designed to prevent hospitals from acting anticompetitively. Price-fixing agreements, such as those described, are illegal because they lessen competition among hospitals. Barriers that prevent competitors from entering a market are also anticompetitive. If two hospitals in a market are able to restrict entry into that market (perhaps through the use of regulations such as CON approval), they will have greater monopoly power and be less price competitive and less responsive to purchaser demands. Mergers may be similarly anticompetitive. For example, if the ten hospitals merged so that only two hospital organizations remained, the degree of competition would be less than when there were ten competitors. For this reason, the FTC examines hospital mergers to determine whether they will lessen competition in the market.

PRICE COMPETITION IN PRACTICE

The above discussion provides a theoretic basis for price competition. To move from price competition's theoretic benefits to reality we must consider two questions. First, does any market have enough hospitals for price competition to occur? Second, is there any evidence on the actual effects of hospital price competition?

The number of competing hospitals in a market is determined by the cost–size relationship of hospitals (economies of scale) and the size of the market (the population served). A larger-sized hospital, for example, 200 beds, is likely to have lower average costs per patient than a hospital with the same set of services that has only 50 beds. In a larger hospital, some costs can be spread over a greater number of patients. For example, some costs will be the same whether there are 50 or 200 patients, such as those for an administrator, an x-ray technician, and x-ray equipment, which can be used more fully in a larger organization. These economies of scale (size), however, do not continue indefinitely; at some point the higher costs of coordination of services begin to exceed the gains accruing from a larger size. Studies have generally indicated that hospitals in the size range of 200 to 400 beds have the lowest average costs.

If the population in an area consists of only 100,000, only one hospital of 260 beds is likely to survive (assuming 800 patient days per 1,000 and 80 percent occupancy). If more than one hospital is in the area, each will have higher average costs than one larger hospital; one of the hospitals will expand, achieve lower average costs, and be able to set its prices lower than the other hospital. An area with a population of 1 million is large enough to support three to six hospitals.

Hospital services, however, are not all the same. The economies of scale associated with an obstetrics facility are quite different from those associated with organ transplant services. Patients are also less willing to travel great distances for a normal delivery than for a heart transplant. The travel costs of going to another state for a transplant represent a smaller portion of the total cost of the service (and the travel time is less crucial) than for giving birth. Thus, the number of competitors in a market depends on the particular service. For some services the relevant geographic market served may be relatively small, whereas for others the market may be the state or region.

As of 2005, approximately 82 percent of hospital beds were located in metropolitan statistical areas (MSAs). An MSA may not necessarily be indicative of the particular market in which a hospital competes. For some services the travel time within an MSA may be too great, whereas for other services (organ transplants) the market may encompass multiple MSAs. However, the number of hospitals within an MSA provides a general indication of the number of competitors within a hospital's market. As shown in Figure 15.3, 200 MSAs (47 percent) have fewer than four hospitals, and 75 MSAs (18 percent) have four or five hospitals. The remaining MSAs (35 percent) have more than six hospitals; however, that 35 percent of MSAs contain almost 75 percent of the hospitals located in metropolitan areas. Therefore, the large majority of hospitals in MSAs (75 percent) are located in MSAs with six or more hospitals. Even within an MSA with few hospitals, substitutes are often available to the hospitals' services, for example, outpatient surgery, which decreases those hospitals' monopoly power.

When few providers of specialized facilities exist in a market (because of economies of scale and the size of the market), the relevant geographic market is likely to be much larger because the demand for highly specialized services is generally not of an emergency nature and patients are more willing to travel. Insurers negotiate prices for transplants, for example, with several regional "centers of excellence," hospitals that perform a high number of transplants and have good outcomes.

Thus, price competition among hospitals appears to be feasible. As insurers and large employers have become concerned over the costs of hospital care and are better informed on hospital prices and patient outcomes, hospitals are being forced to be responsive to purchaser demands and compete according to price, outcomes, and patient satisfaction. Data shown in Figures 15.1 and 15.2 show how competition has lowered the rate of increase in hospital expenditures and prices. As hospitals had to compete to be included in provider panels of managed care plans, they had to become more efficient and discount their prices.

A number of studies on hospital price competition have been published in the past several years. This research provides further support for traditional economic expectations regarding competitive hospital markets. The change to hospital price competition was not uniform throughout the country. Price competition in California developed earlier and more rapidly than in other areas. Within California, hospitals were classified according to whether they were in high- or low-competition markets. Hospitals in more competitive markets (controlling for other factors) were found to have a much lower rate of increase in the costs per discharge and per capita than were hospitals in less-competitive markets.

Figure 15.3: Number of Hospitals in MSAs, 2005

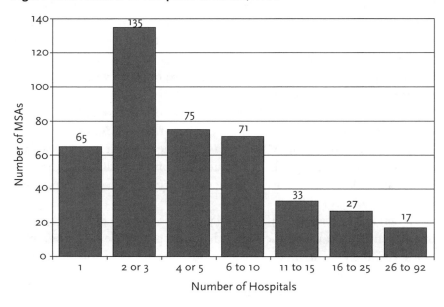

Source: Data from American Hospital Association. 2007. *Hospital Statistics*, 2007 edition, Table 8. Chicago: Health Forum LLC, an affiliate of the AHA.

Bamezai et al. (1999) classified hospitals according to whether they were in a high- or low-competition market and whether the managed care penetration was high or low. The authors found that an increase in managed care penetration reduced the rise in hospital costs (Table 15.1). The reduction in costs, however, was much greater for hospitals in more competitive markets. Also, regardless of the degree of managed care penetration, hospital competition was important in lowering hospital cost increases. These findings imply that hospital mergers that decrease competition are likely to result in higher hospital prices.

Other studies have found similar results using different methods and data on specific types of hospital treatment. For example, Kessler and McClellan (2000) analyzed Medicare claims data for Medicare patients admitted to the hospital with a primary diagnosis of a heart attack for the period 1985 to 1994. They found that before 1991, competition led to higher costs and, in some cases, lower rates of adverse health outcomes. After 1990, hospital price competition led to substantially lower costs

Table 15.1: Hospital Cost Growth in the United States, by Level of Managed Care Penetration and Hospital Market Competitiveness, 1986–1993

Level of Managed Care Penetration	Level of Hospital Competition		% Difference
	Low	High	
Low	65	56	16*
High	52	39	33*
% difference	25*	44*	67**

*% difference = [(high − low)/low].

**[low/low (65) − high/high (39)]/[high/high (39)].

Source: Calculations by Glenn Melnick, RAND.

and to significantly lower rates of adverse outcomes. Patients had lower mortality rates in the most competitive markets.

SUMMARY

The controversy over whether hospital competition results in higher or lower costs is based on studies from two different periods. When hospitals were paid according to their costs, nonprice competition occurred and resulted in rapidly rising hospital costs. Medicare's change to fixed-price hospital payment and managed care plans' change to negotiated prices also changed hospitals' incentives. Hospitals now have incentives to be efficient and compete on price to be included in managed care plans' provider panels. Consequently, hospital costs and prices have risen less rapidly in more competitive hospital markets. Public policy, such as the antitrust laws, that encourages competitive hospital markets will be of greater benefit to purchasers and patients than policies that enable hospitals to increase their monopoly power.

As enrollment in managed care plans increased, the demand for hospital care decreased. Hospital consolidation is occurring as fewer hospitals are needed and hospitals seek the cost savings that accrue in a larger hospital system. Although intense price competition still takes place among hospitals, mergers are reducing excess hospital capacity and creating fewer hospital competitors. These trends suggest that as fewer hospitals compete with one another, they are better able to increase their prices.

DISCUSSION QUESTIONS

1. Why did hospital expenditures rise so rapidly after Medicare and Medicaid were introduced in 1966?

2. What changes did Medicare DRGs cause in hospital behavior?

3. What is the likely response of hospitals when the hospital is the only one in the market compared with when ten hospitals are competing for a large employer's employees?

4. What determines the number of competitors in a market? Apply your answer to obstetrics and to transplant services.

5. What are some anticompetitive hospital actions that the antitrust laws seek to prevent?

REFERENCES

Bamezai, A., J. Zwanziger, G. Melnick, and J. Mann. 1999. "Price Competition and Hospital Cost Growth in the United States: 1989–1994." *Health Economics* 8 (3): 233–43.

Dranove, D., M. Shanley, and W. White. 1991. "How Fast Are Hospital Prices Really Rising?" *Medical Care* 29 (8): 690–96.

Kessler, D., and M. McClellan. 2000. "Is Hospital Competition Socially Wasteful?" *Quarterly Journal of Economics* 115 (2): 577–615.

Chapter 16

The Future Role of Hospitals

HOSPITALS HAVE TRADITIONALLY been the center of the health care system. Before Medicare and Medicaid were implemented in 1965, hospital expenditures represented 40 percent of total health expenditures. During the late 1960s and the 1970s, the growth of Medicare, Medicaid, and private insurance stimulated the demand for hospital services. By 1975, 46 percent of health expenditures were for hospital services. Although hospital expenditures have continued to increase, hospitals' share of total health expenditures has declined, falling to 30.8 percent in 2005. Will the role of the hospital continue to decline, or will the aging of the population and technologic developments reestablish the central role of hospitals in the delivery of medical services?

FROM MEDICARE TO THE PRESENT

During the post-Medicare period (from 1966 to the early 1980s), hospitals were reimbursed for their costs, hospitals engaged in nonprice competition to attract physicians, new technology was quickly adopted, hospital facilities and services grew rapidly, and hospitals were the largest and fastest-increasing component of health care expenditures.

Starting in the mid-1980s, the financial outlook for hospitals changed. Medicare introduced DRGs, which changed Medicare payment from a cost basis to a fixed price per admission (by type of admission). Hospital incentives changed as hospitals realized that by reducing their costs and patients' lengths of stay, they could keep the difference between the DRG price and their cost of caring for Medicare patients. Insurers, under pressure from employers, introduced managed care, with its cost-containment measures, such as utilization review, second surgical opinions, and lower-cost substitutes to inpatient care, including ambulatory surgery and outpatient diagnostic testing. To reduce treatment costs, managed care shifted services out of the hospital, the most expensive setting. Greater use occurred in outpatient facilities and step-down facilities, such as skilled nursing facilities, rehabilitation units, and home health care.

Hospitals developed excess capacity as they reduced Medicare patients' lengths of stay and private cost-containment measures reduced hospital use. With excess capacity, hospitals were willing to compete on price to be included in managed care PPOs.

Managed care competition, hospitals' excess capacity, and the resultant pressures for hospitals to compete on price led to hospital bankruptcies, mergers with failing hospitals, falling hospital profit margins, and, in general, a distressed hospital industry. The DRG Medicare payment system and managed care's utilization management methods left the industry with too much excess capacity. The financial survival of many hospitals was in doubt.

Table 16.1 describes the changes that occurred in the hospital industry. The number of hospitals, beds, admissions, average length of stay, and occupancy rates all declined. In the past several years, hospital admissions and occupancy rates started to rise. Throughout this entire period, outpatient visits sharply increased.

To increase physician referrals, hospitals bought physicians' practices. Hospitals eventually abandoned this strategy, however; employed physicians were less productive than previously, hospitals were not adept at managing physicians' practices, and physicians were suspicious of working too closely with hospitals. Hospital–physician relationships have been a continual concern to hospitals, especially as physicians have become competitors in physician-owned outpatient surgery centers.

Slowly, hospital profitability returned. To survive and even prosper, hospital strategies emphasized monopolization of the market. Mergers among competing hospitals increased. Large multihospital systems developed. The number of hospital competitors in a market decreased. The FTC, concerned that mergers were creating monopoly power enabling hospitals to raise their prices, brought several antitrust suits against mergers that resulted in increased hospital market power. The FTC, however, lost every hospital merger case. The judges believed nonprofit hospitals were different and would not exploit their market power and raise prices.

Table 16.1: U.S. Community Hospital Capacity and Utilization, 1975–2005

Year	Number of Hospitals	Number of Staffed Beds (Thousands)	Inpatient Admissions (Thousands)	Average Length of Inpatient Stay (Days)	Average Inpatient Occupancy Rate (%)	Outpatient Visits (Thousands)
1975	5,875	942	33,435	7.7	74.9	190,672
1980	5,830	988	36,143	7.6	75.6	202,310
1985	5,732	1,001	33,449	7.1	64.8	218,716
1990	5,384	927	31,181	7.2	66.8	301,329
1995	5,194	873	30,945	6.5	62.8	414,345
2000	4,915	824	33,089	5.8	63.8	521,404
2005	4,936	802	35,239	5.6	67.3	584,429

Source: Author's analysis based on data from American Hospital Association. 2006. *Hospital Statistics*, 2007 ed., Tables 2 and 3. Chicago: Health Forum LLC, an affiliate of the AHA.

The managed care backlash, which occurred in the late 1990s, resulted in MCOs having to expand their provider networks; this limited the insurers' ability to extract price discounts from hospitals by guaranteeing them increased patient volume. The weakening of managed care's cost-containment methods further increased hospitals' bargaining power over health insurers.

Hospital consolidation, the reduction in hospital bed capacity, and the demise of managed care's limited provider networks led to higher prices for hospital services and increased hospital profitability. As shown in Figure 16.1, hospital profit margins reached a high in 1996 and 1997. Profit margins then declined for several years as Medicare reduced hospital payments to postpone bankruptcy of the Medicare Trust Fund. In recent years, as inpatient admissions have begun increasing, with a consequent increase in hospital occupancy rates, hospital profit margins have started to rise again.

Currently, hospitals have gained greater market power as a result of mergers, decreased excess capacity, and the broad provider networks of insurers. These actions have enabled hospitals to increase their prices,

Figure 16.1: Aggregate Total Margins and Operating Margins for U.S. Hospitals, 1980–2004

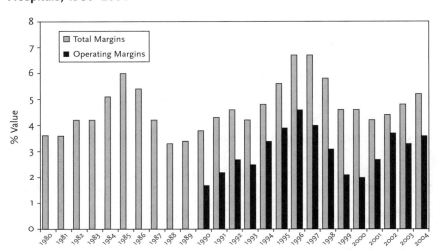

Note: Total hospital margin is calculated as the difference between total net revenue and total expenses divided by total net revenue. Operating margin is calculated as the difference between operating revenue and total expenses divided by operating revenue. Data on operating margin before 1990 are not available.

Sources: 1990–2004 data from Lewin Group analysis of the AHA Annual Survey data presented in Lewin Group. 2006. *Trends Affecting Hospitals and Health Systems.* April, Chart 4.2. [Online information.] http://www.ahapolicyforum.org/ahapolicyforum/trendwatch/chartbook2006.html; 1980–1989 data are author's calculations based on data presented in *Hospital Statistics,* various editions. Chicago: AHA.

and hospital profitability has increased. Will these higher profit margins continue, and will they provide sufficient funds to allow hospitals to access the capital markets to replace aging buildings, upgrade their facilities, and purchase the latest technology?

HOSPITAL REVENUES

How hospitals will fare in coming years depends on likely revenues and costs, the difference being profitability. With regard to the revenue side, hospital revenues are simply price multiplied by quantity, namely utilization. Several of the factors likely to affect trends in hospital utilization are considered, followed by a discussion of likely changes in hospital payments.

Hospital Utilization

Hospital utilization in coming years will be affected by several diverging trends. Before managed care began in 1980, hospital utilization rates in the United States were 1,312 patient days per 1,000 persons; in New York and California the rates were 1,500 and 967 patient days, respectively. Managed care and the change to a fixed price per admission in Medicare's hospital payment system reduced hospital use. By 2004, patient days per 1,000 declined to 666 (United States), 950 (New York), and 505 (California). Medical practice is likely to continue in the direction of shorter lengths of stay, thereby reducing hospital utilization.

Population growth and an aging population, however, are likely to increase hospital use. The population is increasing slowly, about 0.9 percent per year. As the population ages, the baby boomers become eligible for Medicare starting in 2011, and life expectancy increases, use of medical services should be greater than previously. The aged have the highest hospital use rates of any population group. Health expenditures for those aged 65 years and older are more than three times greater than for those aged 34 to 44 years; health expenditures for those aged 75 years and older are five times greater. Although there are large differences in use of services by age, the aging of the population is gradual and is estimated to increase medical expenditures by only 0.5 percent per year (Reinhardt 2005). Demographic change is likely to have a relatively small effect on the overall medical expenditure growth rate.

Two additional factors affecting the demand for medical services and hospitals are per capita income and health status. As incomes increase, expenditures on medical services increase by a slightly greater proportion; on average, a 1 percent increase in income leads to more than a 1 percent increase in medical spending. (Medical care is income "elastic.") Additional medical expenditures as a result of increased incomes, however, are unlikely to be for hospital services; spending is likely to be increased for procedures that are more elective and performed in an outpatient setting, such as joint replacements, cosmetic surgery, and diagnostic and imaging services.

Health status is an important determinant of medical care use. Over time, population health has improved and disability has decreased; however, in recent years there have been reports of an obesity epidemic, which results in more chronic illnesses and higher hospital use.

The above factors affecting medical services use, demographic change, increased incomes, and changes in health status are gradual and unlikely to affect hospital use in a notable way in the short term. Hospital use, however, is likely to be significantly affected by trends in physician competition and technologic advances.

Physician Competition

Physician behavior can significantly affect hospital utilization, prices, and revenues. Many hospital services, such as diagnostic imaging and surgical procedures, are routinely performed in an outpatient facility. These outpatient facilities are substitutes for the same services performed in a hospital and are all or in part owned by physicians who view such services as a means of increasing their incomes. (Physician convenience and patient satisfaction are additional reasons for the development of physician-owned outpatient facilities.) When price markups (over cost) are relatively high for certain hospital services, physician entrepreneurs enter the market by starting competing services, thereby lowering hospital use and prices.

A more recent form of physician competition with community hospitals is the development of specialty hospitals. These specialty hospitals primarily focus on profitable services, such as cardiology and orthopedic surgery.

Proponents of specialty hospitals claim that patients are offered greater choice and market competition for those services is increased, which forces hospitals to increase their efficiency, improve their quality, and be more responsive to patients. Competition also pressures hospitals to invest in new equipment and make operating schedules more flexible for their physicians. Critics claim that physicians on the hospital's staff refer less severely ill patients to the specialty hospital in which they have a financial interest and concentrate on providing only the most profitable procedures. Community hospitals are adversely affected when they lose high-margin services, which they say are used to underwrite charity care and money-losing services.

Self-referral laws are meant to limit physicians' incentives to increase the demand for services for which they receive a referral fee. Physician ownership of specialty hospitals, however, does not appear to violate these laws.

As part of the Medicare Modernization Act enacted in December 2003, hospital associations were successful in having a moratorium imposed on the development of new specialty hospitals. That moratorium has since expired, and new specialty hospitals are being planned to compete with community hospitals.

Evidence suggests that physicians with an ownership interest in specialty hospitals are more likely to refer to their own facilities, and that these facilities treat a smaller percentage of severely ill patients than general hospitals (Guterman 2006; U.S. GAO 2003). Community hospitals therefore were disadvantaged by receiving the same payment for treating more costly patients.

Part of the concern with specialty hospitals involves the price hospitals receive for treating a patient with a particular diagnosis. Currently, Medicare DRG payments are not adjusted for severity of illness or for changes in productivity (which reduces the cost of providing a treatment). Consequently, patients who are less severely ill and procedures that have become less costly to perform are more profitable (i.e., have a higher price markup) than others. These distortions in the regulated pricing system provide physicians with an incentive to shift these patients and procedures to their own facilities. The solution for these price distortions is to adjust the payment for severity of illness and to update the cost for performing particular surgical procedures more frequently. (The payment system should be further improved by also paying for higher quality, thereby incurring fewer readmissions.)

Adjusting prices for severity of illness and productivity changes will force specialty and community hospitals to compete on how efficiently they can provide patient care and on patient satisfaction. Once these price distortions are corrected, the marketplace will determine whether specialty hospitals are better able to innovate in the delivery of medical services by concentrating on specific surgical procedures or specializing in particular diseases using coordinated treatment, as proponents claim. (Prohibiting specialty hospitals so as to preserve a hospital's ability to cross-subsidize the uninsured is less efficient—that is, more costly—than allowing competition to occur and providing direct subsidies to the uninsured, who can choose the facility they prefer.)

Experience has shown that entrepreneurial physicians will shift hospital services to an outpatient facility to enhance their incomes and to improve physician convenience and patient satisfaction. Price distortions inherent in a regulated pricing system have served to accelerate the movement of care out of the traditional hospital setting. Advances in medical technology have enabled services previously provided in a general hospital to be provided in an outpatient facility and specialty hospitals (Shactman 2005). These technologic trends are likely to continue. A hospital's competitors are not just other hospitals. Competition from physician-owned facilities is likely to limit the growth in hospital utilization.

Technologic Developments

Over time, technologic change is considered to be the most important determinant of rising health expenditures. Early advances in medicine increased the role of the hospital; anesthesia and control of surgical infections changed the hospital from an institution where little could be done for patients to a curative institution. Hospitals became the physician's workshop, and central to the delivery of medical services. Additional advances in technology, such as cardiac surgery and organ transplants, further enhanced the role of the hospital.

Starting in the 1980s, the development of new technology enabled many services that previously had to be performed inpatient to be performed in an outpatient facility, such as diagnostic imaging services and less-invasive surgeries. In contrast with previous technologic advances, these developments, including new drugs and disease management techniques, decreased the demand for hospital inpatient care. Physicians shifted these diagnostic services and less-invasive surgeries to outpatient centers, which they controlled, and thereby increased their incomes. To avoid losing the revenue from these new outpatient services, hospitals also developed their own ambulatory care facilities. Hospitals' service mix changed as a greater share of hospital revenue came from the provision of outpatient services (Goldsmith 2004).

Hospitals do not appear to have a competitive advantage over physician-owned facilities in providing these outpatient services. Consequently, more of what was previously hospital inpatient revenue has become outpatient revenue and is being increasingly received by physicians.

Will emerging new technologies once again provide hospitals with the central role in the delivery of medical services, or will new technologies continue to shift inpatient services to an outpatient setting, to be provided in physician-controlled facilities?

Goldsmith lists three emerging technologies that are likely to affect the role of the hospital. The first is "personalized" medicine, that is, the use of genetic profiling to better target drug treatments. Genetic testing will improve the clinical effectiveness of drug therapies by enabling practitioners to identify, for example, which types of cancer cells will be resistant to or more affected by different chemotherapy choices. Genetic testing will also be able to identify those who will not benefit from some drugs and those who will suffer an adverse drug reaction (almost 2 million people each year).

The second emerging technology, "regenerative" medicine (i.e., culturing and grafting human cells to repair or replace damaged tissue), may someday allow practitioners to use stem cells to replace damaged tissue and repair spinal cord injuries. Patients with Alzheimer's disease and other irreversible conditions may become functional once again.

Monitoring systems, Goldsmith's third emerging technology, which includes voice, visual images, and telemetry data, enable specialists to monitor large numbers of patients in remote locations. Thus, patients who are not acutely ill but have some clinical risk can be discharged from the hospital and monitored in their homes or in other, less-costly settings. Sensor monitoring will track a patient's physiologic condition, such as blood pressure and heart rate, and global positioning systems will track their physical movements, such as lying down or walking. Intelligent clinical information systems that integrate all of these measures will enable a patient care team to monitor large numbers of patients and intervene when a patient's clinical measurement reaches a certain threshold.

These emerging technologies are likely to decrease hospital admissions, readmissions, lengths of stay, and emergency department visits, which are hospitals' traditional product lines. Along with improved patient outcomes, hospital use and costs, the most expensive components of medical expenditures, will be reduced. Hospital revenue from traditional hospital services will decline. Does this mean hospitals will have a reduced role in patient care? The potential demand for these emerging technologies will be huge. The elderly are just one market segment; an aging population that is living longer will result in a great many frail, chronically ill patients. The cost of caring for the elderly using current medical practice would be very large; with the new technologies, however, it will be possible to greatly reduce the use of labor and substitute remote monitoring technologies.

Developing and implementing these technologies will require large sums of money. Skilled clinical teams will be needed to use the technologies, respond to patient needs, and be able to serve a large population base over a wide geographic area. Will hospitals, multispecialty medical groups, or other providers be better able to capitalize on this evolving technology? As revenue from hospitals' traditional services declines and these, and other, new technologies generate huge new sources of revenue, those with entrepreneurial skills will be better able to anticipate and benefit from serving this potential market. It is too early to know whether there are any economies of scale or scope in restorative therapy that will provide hospitals with a competitive advantage over free-standing, specialized firms in providing such services.[1]

Hospitals, in conjunction with their medical staffs, may be well-suited to capitalize on these new technologies and increase their role in patient care. If, however, hospitals are too slow to move from their traditional service lines and are unable to develop the necessary physician relationships, large multispecialty medical groups and other entrepreneurial firms are likely to seize the opportunity presented by these new technologies. The managed care movement, HMOs, PPOs, and utilization management companies were not started by hospitals, practicing physicians, or traditional insurers but by entrepreneurs who were able to anticipate and capitalize on the employer demand for cost containment. A redistribution of revenues occurred, away from traditional providers and insurers to the new market entrants. Whether the same occurs with the new technologies will determine the future role of hospitals and their revenues.

Hospital Payment

How hospitals are paid, and how much, has a significant effect on hospital revenues. Hospitals are paid by the government for Medicare and Medicaid patients and by insurers for privately insured patients. Hospitals cannot negotiate with the government over the price Medicare pays for hospital services. Instead, hospital associations negotiate politically with legislators who determine Medicare's annual rate increases. Negotiation with private insurers over hospital prices depends upon their relative bargaining power. Thus, hospital prices are determined in both a competitive and a political marketplace.

Figure 16.2 describes how hospital payment sources have changed over time; government now accounts for about 56 percent of hospital revenue.

---

1. Economies of scale occur when a firm's output increases by a greater proportion than the increase in its input cost; average total cost per unit therefore decreases as output increases. Larger firms will have lower unit costs than smaller firms. Economies of scope occur when it is less costly for a firm to produce certain services (or products) jointly than if separate firms produced each of the same services independently. An example is when the physician who undertakes stem cell research also provides stem cell therapy. In this case, it is less costly when the research and therapy are provided together than when each is provided separately by different firms. When economies of scope exist, multiproduct (service) firms will be more efficient than single-product (service) firms. Economies of scale are unrelated to economies of scope.

Figure 16.2: Sources of Hospital Revenues, by Payer, Selected Years, 1965–2005

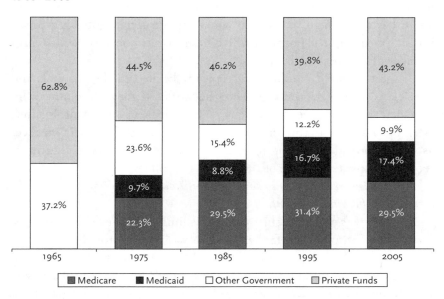

Note: Medicaid includes SCHIP and Medicaid SCHIP expansion. Other government includes worker's compensation, Department of Defense, maternal/child health, Veterans Administration, vocational rehabilitation, temporary disability, state/local hospitals, and school health.

Source: Author's calculations based on data from Centers for Medicare & Medicaid Services, Office of the Actuary, National Health Statistics Group. 2007. [Online information.] http://www.cms.hhs.gov/NationalHealthExpendData/.

Hospital Prices: Private Payers

Hospital prices are referred to as *charges*. However, few purchasers of hospital services pay full, or 100 percent of, charges.[2] Discounts from charges are given to almost all payers. Hospitals may discount their charges by up to 50 percent. Insured patients are insensitive to the prices

2. Although few payers pay full charges, hospitals will attempt to collect 100 percent of their charges from those who have not previously negotiated a discounted price. Those most likely to be billed full charges are those who are uninsured and those who are brought to the hospital by an ambulance as a result of an auto accident. At that point neither the accident victim nor his auto insurance company is in a position to negotiate a discounted rate from the hospital. Billing auto insurance companies full charges can be very profitable for hospitals.

charged by hospitals because they typically do not pay any out-of-pocket costs when they are admitted to the hospital.[3] (Only about 3 percent of hospital revenue is paid out of pocket by patients, which is lower than any other component of medical care.) The insurer negotiates a prearranged price with the hospital, which has separate contracts with a large number of different health plans.

Privately insured enrollees are typically limited to the hospitals and physicians in their insurers' provider networks. If they use nonnetwork providers, patients have to pay a large out-of-pocket copayment. Insurers attempt to include in their network providers preferred by their enrollees as well as providers willing to give larger price discounts in return for receiving a greater volume of the insurer's enrollees.

It is the insurer's ability to shift patients to competing hospitals that determines its hospital discount.

The insurer's ability to shift patients is limited in the following ways. First, when consumers prefer health plans with broad provider networks, the plan's bargaining power is weakened because hospitals that are unwilling to give a discount cannot be excluded. Second, enrollees who are willing to switch health plans to have access to certain hospitals, for reasons of location or reputation, or because it is where the patient's physician practices, provide those hospitals with greater bargaining power than hospitals less differentiated from others. To the extent that an insurer needs a particular hospital in its provider network for any of these

---

3. Instead of price sensitivity, economists use the term *price elasticity of demand*, which is the percentage change in quantity demanded with a 1 percent change in price. When the percentage change in quantity demanded exceeds the percentage change in price, the good or service is considered to be price "elastic." For example, if the price decreases by 5 percent and the quantity demanded increases by 10 percent, the price elasticity equals −2. If the percentage change in price is greater than the percentage change in quantity, the service is price "inelastic" (price increases by 5 percent and quantity demanded decreases by 2 percent). Price elasticity is important in determining the effect of a change in price on revenue. When a service is price inelastic, increasing price will increase total revenue; decreasing price will decrease total revenue. Conversely, when the demand for a service is price elastic, increasing price decreases total revenue. Price elasticity is mainly determined by the closeness of substitutes. A hospital with good substitutes (i.e., comparable hospitals) will have a price-elastic demand curve; if it raises price its, total revenue will decrease. By merging, hospitals decrease the number of substitutes the insurer can contract with, and their new demand curve will be less price elastic, enabling them to increase price and increase their total revenue.

reasons, the greater is that hospital's market power, and hence the higher its markup. Third, hospitals that are capacity constrained have more leverage over insurers than those that are not; they are less in need of the insurer's enrollees. Fourth, and most important, is the degree of hospital competition in a market ("hospital market structure"). Markets with only one hospital are monopolists and can charge more than hospitals in markets where there are five similar hospitals. In competitive hospital markets, insurers will be able to shift their enrollees to lower-cost (equal-quality) hospitals. The greater the number of hospitals competing on price, the lower will be the hospital's price markup and the greater the hospital discount. Hospital price markups depend on the relative bargaining power between hospitals and insurers (Ho 2005).

Hospital mergers in concentrated markets reduce the number of hospitals (substitutes) with which the insurer can contract; the insurer has a reduced ability to shift enrollees.

Recently, the FTC brought (and won) an antitrust suit against a hospital that had merged several years earlier. This lawsuit was the first time the FTC challenged a hospital merger based on how the hospitals behaved *after* they merged, rather than challenging a hospital merger based on what the hospitals might do *if* they merged. The FTC's retrospective analysis of the hospital merger convinced the judge that the merged hospitals used their market power to increase prices more than would have been possible without the merger. The judge ruled that the merger had to be dissolved.

Although this merger case is being appealed, it is likely that the FTC's success at reexamining hospital mergers that lessen price competition will be a constraint on hospitals' use of their market power to increase prices.

Hospital Prices: Public Payers

Medicare and Medicaid pay about 56 percent of total hospital expenditures; this percentage varies greatly among hospitals. Hospitals receive about 90 percent of their average costs for Medicaid patients and 92 percent for Medicare patients. These percentages have varied over time and have a major effect on hospital profitability.

Under the Medicare DRG system, Congress annually decides the percentage increase in the DRG price. Although this annual DRG update is supposed to be based on technical reasons, such as hospital input price increases and productivity changes, Congress is also influenced by politics (such as the number of senators representing rural states who are protective of rural hospitals' solvency) and concern with the projected bankruptcy of the Medicare Trust Fund, which pays for hospital services. The method Medicare uses to control hospital spending is to limit the rate of increase in the annual update of DRG prices (Scanlon 2006). The Medicare Trust Fund is financed by a payroll tax of 2.9 percent on all earned income (employers and employees each pay half the tax). The Medicare Trust Fund is projected to be bankrupt by 2020. The declining number of workers per Medicare beneficiary contributes to this financing problem.

Previously, when the Medicare Trust Fund was projected to be bankrupt, payroll taxes were increased and hospitals received lower payments. It has been estimated that a 10 percent decrease in Medicare's hospital payments will be needed to extend the solvency of the Medicare Trust Fund from 2020 to 2025 (Altman, Shactman, and Ellat 2006). At this point Medicare's DRG prices will fall much further below average costs and have a large adverse effect on hospitals.

Medicaid is also likely to be constrained in its payments to hospitals. States, which pay about half the costs of Medicaid, must balance their budgets each year. As medical costs increase and an increasingly large number of aged require long-term care, states will be pressured to limit Medicaid expenditures.

Thus, hospital revenue growth is likely to be reduced by the FTC's opposition to mergers that lessen price competition, by the growth of physician-owned outpatient and specialty facilities that reduce hospital use, and by lower hospital payments for Medicare and Medicaid patients.

COST OF PROVIDING HOSPITAL CARE

Rising demand for hospital services and greater revenue for such services do not necessarily mean hospitals will be profitable. Profit is the difference between total revenue and total costs. If hospitals are to have the capital to expand their facilities and invest in new equipment and additional services, hospitals must be able to earn a profit. Understanding trends in hospital costs therefore is important.

Salaries and benefits are the largest component of hospital costs, comprising 53 percent of hospitals' overall expenses. Registered nurses (RNs) represent 24 percent of hospital personnel, and RN wages are likely to rise more rapidly in coming years. As the baby boomers become eligible for Medicare and increase their demand for medical services and as the number of the old-old aged increases, the demand for RNs will increase. Although RNs are used predominantly in hospital settings, RNs are increasingly being used in lesser care settings, from outpatient facilities, to home health care, to hospices. The likely supply of RNs, in addition to increased RN demand, determines RN wages. The RN workforce is aging, and unless a greater number of RNs are recruited from overseas or a greater number of men enter nursing, RN wages, relative to other occupations, will likely increase more rapidly, increasing hospital costs.

Legislation enacted in several states, and being considered in many other states, would mandate minimum RN–patient ratios, which will further increase hospital labor costs.

The aging of the population also affects the supply of labor. The number of workers per retiree is declining. As this occurs, the relatively smaller workforce will result in higher wages, hence increased labor costs to hospitals.

As RN wages and labor costs increase, hospitals will attempt to substitute capital, such as monitoring equipment, for RNs, delegate more RN tasks to less-trained personnel, seek additional ways to increase labor productivity, and increase overseas recruiting. How successful hospitals are in reducing their labor costs, constrained by state laws that limit the tasks that health professionals are permitted to perform and regulations on RN ratios, will have an important effect on their profitability.

Productivity increases in a service industry such as health care have been more difficult to achieve than in manufacturing.

Hospitals will be making large investments in information technology, such as electronic medical records, which capture patient information as patients visit their physicians, see specialists, take laboratory tests, fill prescriptions at pharmacies, and use hospitals and outpatient facilities in their communities. Hospitals will also be making huge investments in clinical information technology to streamline clinical decision making, promote quality, and reduce medication errors. These investments, while likely to improve quality and reduce some costs, will require nonprofit hospitals to incur debt, which will add to their cost structure.

Whether hospitals will have the revenue to cover these costs, which will likely increase more rapidly than economy-wide inflation, depends on future utilization and their pricing ability.

HOSPITAL SPENDING

Figure 16.3 illustrates annual rates of growth in hospital spending (adjusted for inflation) since the 1960s. Medicare and Medicaid led to a large increase in spending growth rates in the late 1960s. Thereafter, annual growth rates have been in a generally downward trend. In the last several

Figure 16.3: Annual Rate of Increase in Hospital Expenditures, Actual and Trend, GDP Price Deflated, 1961–2005

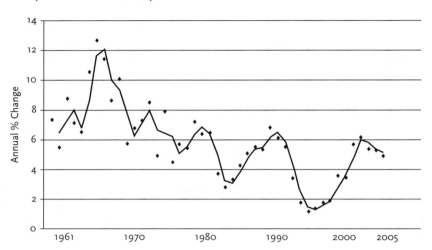

Note: Line represents two-year moving average.

Sources: Author's calculations based on data from Centers for Medicare & Medicaid Services, Office of the Actuary, National Health Statistics Group. 2007. [Online information.] http://www.cms.hhs.gov/NationalHealthExpendData/; GDP data from Executive Office of the President of the United States. 2007. *Budget of the United States Government: Historical Tables Fiscal Year 2007*, Table 10.1. [Online information.] http://origin.www.gpoaccess.gov/usbudget/fy07/pdf/hist.pdf.

years, spending growth rates have increased, as high as in the pre–managed care period. Will the upward trend in expenditure growth rates continue, or will they decline, together with a diminished role for hospitals?

The future offers both threats and opportunities for hospitals. In recent years, mergers, the weakening of managed care, and reduced capacity have enabled hospitals to increase their bargaining power over health plans, enabling them to increase their prices and profitability. The population is aging and the first of the baby boomers become eligible for Medicare in 2011; demographics should increase hospital use.

Offsetting these positive hospital developments is the movement by physicians of inpatient services to outpatient facilities and the development of physician-owned specialty hospitals. An important unknown is new technology: Will hospitals or physician entrepreneurs be better able to develop and offer new diagnostics and treatments? The growing reliance of hospitals on government payment, at a time when the Medicare Trust Fund is projected to be insolvent by 2020, is another uncertainty. Finally, the current emphasis on "consumerism" in health care, high-deductible health plans, greater patient price sensitivity, price "transparency" (i.e., making information on hospital prices, quality, and report cards available on the Internet), is likely to create price and value competition among hospitals and physician-owned facilities, limiting hospitals' ability to charge high price markups.

Given these uncertainties, it is doubtful that current annual spending rates of 7 percent are sustainable. Furthermore, not all hospitals are alike. Safety-net hospitals, which provide a significant amount of care to low-income and uninsured populations, and whose emergency departments attract patients who do not have a regular physician, are likely to experience greater financial pressures.

SUMMARY

Hospital fortunes have changed over time. Managed care and Medicare DRG payment greatly reduced hospital utilization, created excess capacity, and weakened hospitals' bargaining power with insurers. Over time, hospital capacity was reduced, mergers occurred, and managed care broadened its provider networks; hospitals used their increased bargaining power over insurers to increase their prices. Hospital spending in recent years has sharply increased.

Hospitals face several threats to their revenues in coming years. Technology has enabled a greater number of complex procedures to be performed in an outpatient setting. Physician entrepreneurs have been able to use these medical advances to establish physician-owned outpatient services and specialty hospitals, both to enhance their incomes and gain greater control over their medical practices. Competition between physician-owned facilities and hospitals has increased. Furthermore, to forestall bankruptcy of the Medicare Trust Fund, greater emphasis will be placed on caring for the aged in less-costly facilities, such as the patient's home, and reducing the annual percentage increase in Medicare DRG prices. These Medicare strategies will reduce the rate of increase in hospital revenues.

DISCUSSION QUESTIONS

1. What are several trends that are likely to increase hospital use?

2. What is the likely effect of physician-owned outpatient facilities and specialty hospitals on hospital expenditures?

3. How will emerging technologies likely affect hospital use?

4. Why do hospital mergers increase hospitals' bargaining power over insurers?

5. How will the projected insolvency of the Medicare Trust Fund affect DRG prices?

REFERENCES

Altman, S., D. Shactman, and E. Ellat. 2006. "Could U.S. Hospitals Go the Way of U.S. Airlines." *Health Affairs* 25 (1): 11–21.

Goldsmith, J. 2004. "Technology and the Boundaries of the Hospital: Three Emerging Technologies." *Health Affairs* 23 (6): 149–56.

Guterman, S. 2006. "Specialty Hospitals: A Problem or a Symptom?" *Health Affairs* 25 (1): 95–105.

Ho, K. 2005. *Insurer-Provider Networks in the Medical Care Market.* Working Paper No. 11822, p. 54. Cambridge, MA: National Bureau of Economic Research.

Reinhardt, U. 2005. "Does the Aging of the Population Really Drive the Demand for Health Care?" *Health Affairs* 24 (3): 27–39.

Scanlon, W. 2006. "The Future of Medicare Hospital Payment." *Health Affairs* 25 (1): 70–80.

Shactman, D. 2005. "Specialty Hospitals, Ambulatory Surgery Centers, and General Hospitals: Charting a Wise Public Policy Course." *Health Affairs* 24 (3): 868–73.

U.S. General Accounting Office. 2003. *Specialty Hospitals.* Publication No. GAO-04-167. Washington, DC: U.S. GAO.

Chapter 17

Cost Shifting

EMPLOYERS AND INSURERS believe one reason for the rise in employees' health insurance premiums is *cost shifting*. When one purchaser, whether it is Medicare, Medicaid, or the uninsured, does not pay its full charges, many believe hospitals and physicians raise their prices to those who can afford to pay, namely those with private insurance. Cost shifting is believed to be unfair, and its elimination is an important reason why large employers, whose employees have health insurance, favor mandating that all employers provide their employees with health insurance. "All-payer" systems, whereby each payer pays the same charges for hospital and medical services, are also favored by those who believe cost shifting increases their medical prices.

Evidence of cost shifting is based on the observation that different payers pay different prices for similar services (Figure 17.1). Private payers have always had higher payment–cost ratios than Medicare and Medicaid, and Medicare has generally paid more than Medicaid. The payment–cost ratios for all three payers have changed over time.

Although the logic of cost shifting may seem straightforward, it raises a number of troubling questions. For example, can a hospital or physician merely increase prices to those who can pay to recover losses from those who do not pay? If the provider is able to shift costs, why do hospitals complain about the uncompensated care they are forced to provide? Furthermore, if providers are able to offset their losses by increasing prices to those with insurance, why have they not done so previously and thereby earned greater profits?

Figure 17.1: Aggregate Hospital Payment–Cost Ratios for Private Payers, Medicare, and Medicaid, 1980–2004

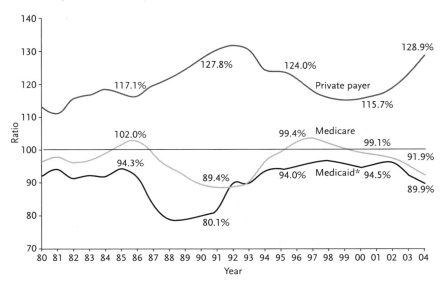

*Includes Medicaid disproportionate-share payments.

Source: American Hospital Association/The Lewin Group. 2006. *Trends Affecting Hospitals and Health Systems,* April, Chart 4.6. [Online information.] http://www.ahapolicyforum.org/ahapolicyforum/trendwatch/chartbook2006.html.

To better understand cost shifting, we must discuss (1) the provider's objective when it prices its services and (2) how different objectives result in different pricing strategies.

SETTING PRICES TO MAXIMIZE PROFITS

Firms typically price their services to maximize profits, that is, to make as much money as possible. This objective is the simplest one to start with for analyzing hospital and physician price setting. Assume that the hospital has two sets of patients, those who can pay and those who cannot pay for their services. Table 17.1 illustrates how a profit-maximizing price is set for the insured group of patients. The relationship between price (P) and quantity (Q) is inverse, meaning the lower the price the more units are likely to be purchased. Total revenue (TR) is price multiplied by quantity. As the price is reduced, more units will be sold and TR will increase; after some point, however, the increased number of

Table 17.1: Determining the Profit-Maximizing Price

Price (P)	Total Quantity (Q)	Total Revenue (TR)	Total Cost (TC)	Profit	TC₂	Profit₂
11	1	11	9	2	11	0
10	2	20	13	7	17	3
9	3	27	17	10	23	4
8	4	32	21	11	29	3
7	5	35	25	10	35	0
6	6	36	29	7	41	−5
5	7	35	33	2	47	−12
4	8	32	37	−5	53	−21
3	9	27	41	−14	59	−32

units sold will not offset the lower price per unit and TR will actually decline. The effect on TR when price is decreased and more units are sold is shown by the TR curve in Figure 17.2.

To determine the price and output that results in the largest profit we must also know the costs for producing that output. Total cost (TC) consists of two parts: fixed costs, which do not vary as output changes (e.g., rent for an office or depreciation on a building), and variable costs, which do vary. For this example fixed costs are assumed to be $5, and variable costs are constant at $4 per unit. The difference between TR and TC is profit. According to Table 17.1, the largest amount of profit occurs when the price is $8 and output equals four units. At that price TR is $32, TC is $21 ($5 fixed cost plus $16 variable costs), and profit is $11. According to Figure 17.2, the greatest difference between the total cost line (TC) and TR (profit) occurs at four units of output.

Raising or lowering the price will only reduce profits. If the hospital lowers its price from $8 to $7, it will have to lower the price on all units sold. The hospital's volume will increase; TR will rise from $32 to $35, or by only $3. Because the variable cost of the extra unit sold is $4, the hospital will lose money on that last unit. The profit at a price of $7 will be $10. Similarly, if the hospital raises its price from $8 to $9, it will sell one less unit, reducing its variable cost by $4 but forgoing $5 worth of revenue

Figure 17.2: Profit-Maximizing Price With and Without a Change in Variable Cost

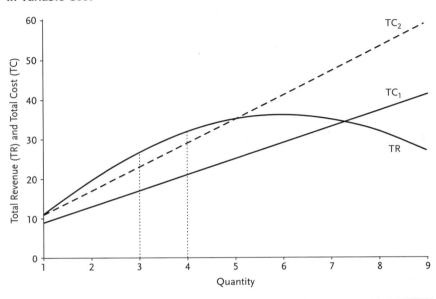

(Figure 17.3).[1] Raising the price once it is at the profit-maximizing price lowers the hospital's profit.

Table 17.1 illustrates several important points. First, *establishing a profit-maximizing price means the price is set so that the additional revenue received is equal to the additional cost of serving an additional patient.* When the change in TR is equal to the change in TC, choosing any other price will result in less profit.

Second, if the hospital's fixed costs increase from $5 to $11, the hospital should not change its price; if it did, it would make even less profit. With an increase in fixed costs, profit would decline by $6 at every quantity

---

1. Figure 17.3 is another way to illustrate how a change in price affects TR. Price is shown along the vertical axis, and quantity, or number of units sold each month or year, is shown along the horizontal axis. When the price is $9 per unit, three units are sold. When price is reduced to $8, four units will be sold. Reducing the price from $9 to $8 results in a decrease in TR of $1 for each of the three units that would have been sold at $9. This loss of $3 is shown by area A. However, lowering the price to $8 gains $8 for that additional unit sold, shown as area B. The difference between area A (loss of $3) and area B (gain of $8) is $5, which is the increase in TR from selling one additional unit. Increasing the price from $8 to $9 has the opposite effect, a loss of $5 in TR.

Figure 17.3: Effect on Total Revenue of a Change in Price

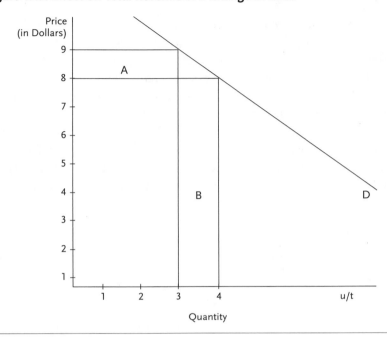

sold. At a price of $8 the hospital would make a total profit of $5; TR is $32, while TC is now $27 ($11 plus $16). If the hospital raised its price to $9 to compensate for the rise in its fixed costs, TR would be $27, TC would be $23 ($11 plus $12), and total profit would fall to $4. Thus, *changes in fixed costs should not affect the hospital's profit-maximizing price.*

Third, *if the hospital's variable costs changed, perhaps because nurses' wages or the cost of supplies increased, the hospital would find it profitable to change its price.* For example, if variable costs increase by $2 and the price–quantity relationship is unchanged, the largest profit will occur at a price of $9 (TR − TC_2 = $profit_2$ in Table 17.1). The higher variable cost is shown in Figure 17.2 as TC_2. The distance between TR and TC_2, which is profit, is greatest at three units of output. If the price per unit remains at $8 when variable costs increase to $6 per unit, the addition to TR from producing four rather than three units is only $5. The hospital will lose money on that last unit, the cost of which is $6. Thus, by raising price and producing fewer units, the increase in TR slightly exceeds the additional cost of producing that last unit. Hospitals therefore would be expected to raise their prices as their variable costs increased. Similarly, if variable costs decline, the hospital will realize more profit by lowering its price.

Fourth, *hospitals would also be expected to change their prices if the relationship between price and quantity were to change.* The price–quantity relationship is a measure of how price sensitive purchasers are to changes in the hospital's price. When the price is changed and quantity changes by a smaller percentage, purchasers are not very price sensitive; the demand for the hospital's service is *price inelastic.* Conversely, when quantity changes by a greater percentage than the change in price, purchasers are said to be more price sensitive; the demand is *price elastic.* As the demand for the hospital's services becomes more price sensitive (price elastic), a hospital would be expected to lower its price, even if there is no change in its costs.[2]

---

2. The effect of price sensitivity (economists use the term *price elasticity*) on hospital prices and markups is based on the following formula:

$$\text{markup} = \frac{MC}{\left[1 - \dfrac{1}{\text{price elasticity}}\right]}$$

MC is marginal cost of producing an additional unit and is assumed to be equal to average variable cost. For simplicity, assume MC = \$1,000.

Thus, if a hospital believes the price sensitivity of a particular employee group is such that a 1 percent increase (decrease) in the hospital's price leads to a 2 percent decrease (increase) in admissions, the hospital's markup, applied to its average variable costs, would be 100 percent:

$$\frac{\$1,000}{\left[1 - \dfrac{1}{2}\right]} = \frac{\$1,000}{\dfrac{1}{2}} = \$1,000 \times \frac{2}{1} = \$2,000$$

If use of services were more price sensitive, such that a 1 percent price increase (decrease) leads to a 3 percent decrease (increase) in admissions, the markup would be 50 percent:

$$\frac{\$1,000}{\left[1 - \dfrac{1}{3}\right]} = \frac{\$1,000}{\dfrac{2}{3}} = \$1,000 \times \frac{3}{2} = \$1,000 \times 1.5 = \$1,500$$

If the hospital's variable costs of serving the patients were the same in both examples, the prices charged to each employee group could vary greatly depending on their price sensitivity. Even those hospitals that have few good substitutes and a less price-elastic demand for their services will always price in the elastic portion of their demand curve. For an explanation see Browning and Zupan (2006).

For example, if five hospitals exist in a market and each hospital is considered to be a relatively good substitute for the others in terms of location, services, reputation, medical staff, and so on, each hospital's demand is considered to be very price sensitive. In competing to be included in different HMO and insurer provider networks, each of the hospitals will compete on price. If just one hospital lowers price, it will cause large increases in that hospital's patient volume. Similarly, raising its price when the other hospitals do not will cause that hospital to lose a large portion of its market share. Conversely, a hospital that is a sole community provider or that has the only trauma unit, for example, faces a less price-sensitive demand for its services or its trauma unit. That hospital's prices will be higher than if good substitutes were available for its services.

If the hospital is already charging a profit-maximizing price to its paying patients and the variable costs of serving paying patients have not changed, the hospital will make even less profit by further increasing prices to paying patients. Referring to Table 17.1, if the hospital raises its price from $8 to $9 simply because other patients did not pay, the hospital will forgo profit. Assuming the hospital wants to make as much money as possible from those who can afford to pay, the hospital will not raise its price to those patients unless there is a change in variable costs or in their price–quantity relationship. Because neither factor changes when another group of patients pays less, it will not make sense for the hospital to charge its paying patients more.

Based on the above explanation of how a profit-maximizing price is set, *changes in prices can be explained by changes in the variable costs of caring for patients or by a change in the price-sensitivity relationship facing a hospital (or a physician).*

Contrary to what many people believe, when the government lowers the price it pays for Medicare or Medicaid patients, physicians will likely *lower* the prices they charge to higher-paying patients. For example, assume that a physician serves two types of patients, private patients and Medicaid patients. The government determines the price charged to Medicaid patients, whereas the physician sets the price for private patients. Traditionally, the price received by the physician for treating private patients is higher than that received for Medicaid patients. The physician presumably allocates his time so that revenues per unit of time are the same regardless of the types of patients served. To produce equal returns when the prices for Medicaid and private patients are different, the physician may spend less time on the Medicaid patient.

If the government further reduces the price it pays for Medicaid patients, the physician is likely to decide that she can earn more by shifting some time away from Medicaid patients and toward caring for more private patients. As more physicians reduce the time they spend with Medicaid patients and reallocate their time toward the private market, the supply of physician time in this market increases. With an increase in supply, physicians would be willing to reduce their prices to receive an increased number of private patients. Assuming limited demand creation by physicians, a lower price for Medicaid patients is likely to result in lower physician fees for private patients.

Assuming that the objective of both hospitals and physicians is to make as much money as possible, these two examples suggest that prices for private patients will either be unchanged or reduced when another payer pays the provider less.

ORIGINS OF CLAIMS OF COST SHIFTING

Based on the previous discussion, why do private purchasers claim that they are being charged more to make up for the lower prices paid by government? The belief that cost shifting is occurring may simply be an artifact of rising trends over time in both hospital prices and uncompensated care. Hospitals may appear to be raising prices to compensate for lower prices charged to other patients, but in actuality hospital prices to private payers have increased for two reasons: (1) variable costs have been increasing as expenses for wages and supplies have risen, and (2) changes in the hospitals' payer mixes (an increase in the proportion of patients who are less price sensitive) may have enabled them to increase their markups on certain types of private patients. This association of rising prices and uncompensated care does not necessarily indicate a causal relationship.

There does exist, however, a logical explanation, unrelated to cost shifting, why some purchasers pay more for the same service than other purchasers: Some purchasers might be more price sensitive than others. Previously, private patients had either indemnity insurance or BlueCross hospital coverage; because hospitals had a close relationship with BlueCross (hospitals started and controlled BlueCross), BlueCross was charged a lower price than indemnity insurers. The price–quantity relationship for those with indemnity insurance represented the average relationship for everyone in the indemnity plan. However, as employers began offering different types of health plans, such as HMOs, PPOs, and managed care, in addition to the traditional indemnity plan, and as employees had to pay different premiums and copayments under these different plans, the price–quantity relationships of these plans differed. Those with indemnity insurance could choose whatever hospital and physician they desired. Other plans, however, were more restrictive in deciding which providers their subscribers could use. HMOs and PPOs were likely to bargain with providers for lower prices in return for directing their subscribers to these approved providers.

Faced with different price–quantity relationships with different purchasers, hospitals began charging different prices to each type of payer. These prices take into consideration the price sensitivity of each of these different insurance plans. Patients remaining in the traditional indemnity plan are charged the highest prices because they are not restricted in their use of providers. Their insurers cannot promise to direct their subscribers to particular hospitals and are least able to negotiate lower hospital prices.

PRICE DISCRIMINATION

Charging according to what the market will bear is not really cost shifting but rather simply charging a profit-maximizing price to each group; this is *price discrimination*. Services for which purchasers are willing to pay more have higher markups. Airlines charge higher prices for first-class seating and lower prices for 21-day advance purchases, for example. Movie theaters charge lower prices for matinees and to senior citizens. Each of these industries is pricing according to different groups' willingness to pay; each group has a different price–quantity relationship. Hospital pricing is no different. Hospitals placing a proportionately higher markup over costs on laboratory tests or drugs used by inpatients than on the room-and-board fee are engaging in price discrimination. Patients who have to pay part of the bill themselves can more easily compare hospital room-and-board rates before they enter the hospital; hospitals therefore have to be price competitive on their room rates. Once a patient is hospitalized, however, patients have little choice in what they pay for services rendered in the hospital. The price–quantity relationships for inpatient services are quite insensitive to prices charged. Hospitals do not face any competition for laboratory tests or other services provided to their inpatients. Thus, their markup for these services is much higher.

Price discrimination is an important reason why some purchasers are able to pay lower hospital prices than others. A large employer or an

HMO that is willing to direct its employees or enrollees to a particular hospital will receive a lower price for the same service than a single patient negotiating with the same hospital. The hospital's price–quantity relationship will be more price sensitive when the hospital negotiates with a large purchaser than when the hospital deals with a single insured patient. The single insured patient does not pay higher prices because the large purchaser pays a lower price. The hospital is less concerned with losing one patient's business than with losing 1,000 patients from a large purchaser.

Even if the government increased its payments to hospitals for treating Medicare patients, the price to the single insured patient would not be reduced because the price–quantity relationship for these patients, which is less price sensitive, would be unchanged. Only if the patient with indemnity insurance becomes part of a larger purchasing group, which is willing to offer a hospital a greater volume of patients in return for lower prices, can the indemnity patient receive a lower hospital price. Different prices to different purchasers are related to how price sensitive they are rather than to what other purchasers are paying. As the insurance market has become more segmented with HMOs, PPOs, self-insured employer groups, traditional indemnity-type insurance plans, and so on, hospitals have developed different pricing strategies for each group.

Empirical evidence supports the view that hospital prices are not raised to other purchasers when prices are reduced to large purchasers. Dranove and White (1998) found that hospitals that had a higher proportion of Medicaid patients (20 percent or more of their budgets) did not raise prices to other paying patients when Medicaid reduced its reimbursement; if anything, hospitals lowered their prices to private payers. Instead, the hospital reduced the service levels for Medicaid patients relative to those for privately insured patients. The amount of free or uncompensated care provided has also been found to be reduced, such as by reducing access to the emergency department, which serves a high proportion of uninsured patients.

CONDITIONS UNDER WHICH COST SHIFTING CAN OCCUR

Under certain circumstances, however, cost shifting may occur. Some hospitals may have a different pricing objective—they do not price to maximize their profits. These hospitals may voluntarily forgo some profits to maintain good community relationships. When hospitals do not set profit-maximizing prices, increases in uncompensated care or fixed costs may cause the hospital to raise its prices to those groups who have a greater ability to pay. For example, "average cost" pricing occurs when a hospital sets its price by relating it to the average cost of caring for all of its patients. If one payer (e.g., the government) decides to pay the hospital less, the average price becomes higher for all other payers. For cost shifting to occur, the purchasers of hospital (or physician) services would also have to be relatively insensitive to the higher prices. If the purchasers switch to other providers or use fewer services as a result of the provider's cost shifting, the provider's revenues and profits will decline.

How likely is it that cost shifting is an important reason why private patients are paying higher medical prices today? Purchasers have become more price sensitive since the mid-1980s. Given the increased competitive market in which providers find themselves, it is unlikely that providers are willing to forgo profits by not setting profit-maximizing prices. Forgoing profits means the hospital has no better use for those funds. Several ways in which the hospital could use those higher profits are to purchase new equipment or start new services to increase its revenues. The medical staff, an important constituency within the hospital, also desires new equipment and facilities. Paying higher wages also makes it easier to attract needed nursing and technical personnel. Hospitals could enhance their community image and market themselves by providing screening and health awareness programs to their communities. Furthermore, additional funds could always be used to provide care to those in the community who are unable to afford it and who are not covered by public programs.

The benefits to the hospital of forgoing profit on some payer group are unlikely to exceed the benefits to the hospital of using that forgone profit in other ways. By not setting profit-maximizing prices, the hospital's decision makers are placing a greater weight on benefiting some purchaser group than on using those funds for other constituencies.

One type of cost shifting occurs when the government pays hospitals a fixed price for Medicare patients' use of the hospital but reimburses outpatient services on a cost basis. If the hospital has $100 in indirect administrative costs to allocate between inpatient units (paid according to a fixed-price DRG) and outpatient units (paid on a cost basis), the hospital will select a cost-allocation method that optimizes its payment from the government, namely the method that allocates a greater portion of the $100 to outpatient units.

Another type of cost shifting occurs when the government shifts its costs to employers, as when requirements that would otherwise cost the government money are imposed on employers. For example, if the government required all employers to buy health insurance for their employees, the government's Medicaid expenditures for low-income employees and their dependents would be reduced.

Payment–cost ratios for all three payers—private, Medicare, and Medicaid—have fluctuated over time (see Figure 17.1). During the early 1980s, the payment–cost ratios for private payers, Medicare, and Medicaid were relatively close. Private payer payment–cost ratios have been affected by the rise and decline of managed care. Managed care had its greatest effect in the latter part of the 1990s, reducing premiums and negotiating large price discounts from hospitals. In recent years, the effect of hospital mergers, decreased hospital capacity, and broadened managed care provider networks resulted in hospitals having greater market power; their price markups increased rapidly, returning to what existed before the managed care period.

Medicare and Medicaid hospital payments are related to federal and state budget deficits and surpluses. In the mid-1980s, the new Medicare DRG system led to higher hospital markups on Medicare patients. As hospital Medicare profit margins increased, Congress reduced annual percentage increases in DRG prices. As the solvency of the Medicare Hospital Trust Fund became a concern in the late 1990s, Congress reduced annual DRG price increases, and hospital Medicare markups declined.

The economic expansion that occurred during the 1990s led to state budget surpluses, enabling Medicaid to pay hospitals a greater percentage of their costs. In recent years, Medicaid payment ratios declined as the size of the Medicaid population and Medicaid expenditures have increased rapidly.

Although payment–cost ratios by payer type have changed over time, the ratios for Medicare and Medicaid have been similar in the past several years to the ratios that existed in the early 1980s; however, private-payer ratios are much greater currently than in the earlier period. Changes in ratios for each payer should be examined with regard to trends in hospital market power, solvency of the Medicare Trust Fund, and the burden of Medicaid expenditures on state budgets.

SUMMARY

Previously, when insurance premiums were paid almost entirely by the employer and managed care was not yet popular, hospitals were probably less interested in making as much money as possible. Many hospitals were reimbursed according to their costs, and they could achieve many of their goals without having to set profit-maximizing prices. However, as occupancy rates declined and left hospitals with excess capacity, price competition increased, HMOs and PPOs entered the market, and hospitals could no longer count on having their costs reimbursed regardless of what those costs were. Hospital profitability declined. Those hospitals that did not price to make as much money as possible began to do so. Some cost shifting occurred during this transition period.

Differences in hospital prices for different payer groups today are more likely the result of price discrimination than cost shifting. The difference between these two explanations is significant. Cost-shifting proponents believe that unless government payments to hospitals and physicians are increased, private payers, such as insurers and employers, will have to pay higher prices for health care. Economists, however, predict that with lower government provider payments, medical prices to private payers will instead decrease, not increase. As the payment for one type of patient decreases and becomes less profitable, physicians can earn more money by shifting some time away from less-profitable patients. The supply of physician time in the private market will increase, resulting in lower prices to private payers.

DISCUSSION QUESTIONS

1. Explain why an increase in a hospital's fixed costs or an increase in the number of uninsured cared for by the hospital will not change the hospital's profit-maximizing price.

2. Why would a change in a hospital's variable costs change the hospital's profit-maximizing price?

3. Why are hospitals able to charge different purchasers different prices for the same medical services?

4. Under what circumstances can cost shifting occur?

5. How does cost shifting differ from price discrimination?

REFERENCES

Browning, E., and M. Zupan. 2006. *Microeconomics: Theory and Applications*, 9th ed., 318. New York: John Wiley & Sons.

Dranove, D., and W. White. 1998. "Medicaid-Dependent Hospitals and Their Patients: How Have They Fared?" *Health Services Research* 33 (2, Part I): 163–85.

ADDITIONAL READINGS

Morrisey, M. 1994. *Cost Shifting in Health Care: Separating Evidence from Rhetoric.* Washington, DC: American Enterprise Institute Press.

————. 2003. "Cost Shifting: New Myths, Old Confusions, and Enduring Reality." *Health Affairs* Web exclusive, October 8, W3-489–W3-491. [Online publication; retrieved 11/15/06.] http://content.healthaffairs.org/cgi/reprint/hlthaff.w3.489v1.

Robert Wood John Conference. 2002. "When Public Payment Declines Does Cost-Shifting Occur? Hospital and Physician Responses." Washington, DC, November 13. [Online information; retrieved 11/15/06.] http://www.hcfo.net/costshiftingslides.htm.

Chapter 18

Can Price Controls Limit Medical Expenditure Increases?

IN THE DEBATE over health care reform, proponents of regulation, such as those who favor a single-payer system, have proposed placing controls on the prices physicians and hospitals charge to limit the rise in medical expenditures. To prevent hospitals and physicians from circumventing such controls by simply performing more services, they would also impose an overall limit (a *global budget*) on total medical expenditures.

Price controls and global budgets may seem to be obvious approaches for limiting rising medical expenditures, but the potential consequences should be examined before placing one-sixth (16 percent) of the U.S. economy (more than $1.9 trillion a year) under government control. The health care industry in the United States is larger than the economies of most countries. An announcement in any country that price controls would be imposed on the entire economy would seem incredible to all who have observed the previous communist economies of Eastern Europe and Russia. Widespread shortages occurred, many of the goods produced were of shoddy quality, and black markets developed. In these countries the inherent failures of a controlled economy have been recognized, and now their task is to try to develop free markets.

Why should we think health care is so different that access to care, high quality, and innovation can be achieved better by price controls and regulation than by reliance on competitive markets? What consequences are likely if price controls are imposed on medical services?[1]

---

1. For a more complete discussion of this subject see Haislmaier (1993).

EFFECT OF PRICE CONTROLS IN THEORY
Imbalances Between Supply and Demand

Imbalances between demands for care and supply of services will occur. The demand for medical services and the cost of providing those services are constantly changing. Prices bring about an equilibrium between the demanders and suppliers in a market. Prices reflect changes in demands or in the costs of producing a service. When demands increase (perhaps because of an aging population or rising incomes), prices increase. Higher prices will cause some of the demand to decrease, but suppliers will respond to the higher prices by increasing the quantity of their services. Higher prices provide a signal (and an incentive) to suppliers that greater investment in personnel and equipment will be needed to meet the increased demand (Baumol 1988).

When regulators initially place controls on prices, they are assuming that the conditions that brought about the initial price, namely the demands for service and the costs of producing that service, will not change. However, these conditions do change for many reasons. Thus, the controlled price will no longer be an equilibrium price. The problem with price controls is that demand is constantly changing, as is the cost of providing services. Although regulators often allow some increases in prices each year to adjust for inflation, seldom if ever are these price increases sufficient to reflect the changes in demand or costs that are occurring. When prices are not flexible, an imbalance between demand and supply will occur.

Not only do the demands and costs of producing services change, but the "product" itself, that is, medical care, is also continually changing, which complicates the picture for regulators. For example, the population is aging. Thus, if the hospital treats more seriously ill patients, the hospital is forced to spend more resources on those patients, such as providing more nursing time and more tests. Relatively new diseases, such as AIDS, require extensive testing, treatment, and prolonged care. Technology is continuing to improve. Since the mid-1990s, transplants have become commonplace, and they are occurring more frequently. Diagnostic equipment has reduced the need for many exploratory surgeries. Low-birth-weight infants can now survive. Such continuing advances increase the demands for medical services and require a greater use of skilled labor, expensive monitoring equipment, and new imaging machines. Unless regulators are aware of these changes in the medical product and technology, their controlled prices will be below the costs of providing these services. How will these demands be met? Imbalances will undoubtedly occur because regulators cannot anticipate all of the changes in demands, costs, and technology.

Shortages

Shortages are the inevitable consequence of price controls. Demands for medical services are continually increasing, yet price controls limit increases in supply. To expand its services a hospital or a medical group must be able to attract additional employees by increasing wages to lure skilled and trained employees away from their current employers. Similarly, as wages increase, trained nurses who are not currently employed as nurses will find returning to nursing financially attractive, and more people will choose nursing careers as wages become comparable to those in other professions. However, if hospitals cannot raise wages because they cannot raise their prices, they will not be able to hire the nurses needed to expand their services.

Price controls not only limit increases in medical services but actually cause a reduction in such services, which exacerbates the shortage over time. As prices and wages continue to increase throughout the economy, price controls on the health sector make it difficult for hospitals and medical groups to pay competitive wages and rising supply costs. Hospitals must hire nurses and technicians, buy supplies, pay heating and electric bills, and replace or repair equipment. A hospital that cannot pay competitive wages will be unable to retain its employees. If the wages of hospital accountants are not similar to those of accountants working in nonhospital settings, fewer accountants will choose to work in hospitals (or those who do accept lower wages may not be as qualified). As medical costs increase faster than the permitted increases in prices, hospitals and medical groups will be unable to retain their existing labor forces and provide their current services.

As costs per patient rise faster than government-controlled prices, hospitals, outpatient facilities, and physician practices are faced with two choices: They can either care for fewer, more costly patients, or they can care for the same number of patients but devote fewer resources to each patient.

Eliminating all of the waste in the current system would merely result in a one-time savings. If rising expenditures were caused by new technologies, aging of the population, and new diseases, and not by waste, medical costs would still rise faster than the rate at which hospitals and other providers were being reimbursed under price controls. Providers would then be faced with the same two choices, that is, either caring for fewer patients or devoting fewer resources to each patient and thus providing lower-quality service.

Price controls on medical services cause the demand for medical services to exceed the supply. The out-of-pocket price the patient pays for a physician visit, an MRI, an ultrasound, or laboratory tests will increase more slowly than it would if the price were not controlled. (The "real," or inflation-adjusted, price to the patient is likely to fall.) Consequently, although patient demand for such services increases, suppliers cannot increase their services if the cost of doing so exceeds the fixed price. In fact, over time the shortage will become even larger because the fixed price will cover the cost of fewer such services. We have seen this occur when rent controls are imposed on housing, such as in New York. The demand for rent-controlled housing continually exceeds its supply, and the supply of existing housing decreases as the costs of upkeep exceed the allowable increases in rent and cause landlords to abandon entire city areas.

Shift of Capital Away from Price-Controlled Services

Furthermore, as profitability is reduced on services subject to price control, capital investment will eventually be shifted to areas that are not subject to control and in which investors can earn higher returns. Less private capital will be available to develop new delivery systems, invest in computer technology for patient care management, and conduct research and development toward breakthrough drugs. Price controls on hospitals cause hospital investment to decline and capital to move into unregulated outpatient services and home health care services. Should all health services become subject to controls, capital would move to nonhealth industries and to geographic regions without controls.

EFFECT OF PRICE CONTROLS IN PRACTICE
Medicaid

Price controls have been tried extensively in the United States and other countries. Shortages and decreased access to care, which typify the Medicaid program, are caused by price controls. Once a patient is eligible for Medicaid, the price he has to pay for medical services is greatly reduced, thus increasing his demand for such services. Government Medicaid payments to physicians are fixed, however, and below what physicians could earn by serving non-Medicaid patients. Low provider payments have decreased the profitability of serving Medicaid patients and resulted in a shortage of Medicaid services. As the difference in prices for Medicaid and private patients increases, more of the physician's time is shifted toward serving private patients, thereby increasing the shortage of medical services faced by Medicaid patients.

Medicare

Hospitals are also subject to price controls on the payments they receive from Medicare. When fixed prices per diagnostic admission were introduced in 1984, hospitals began to "up-code" their Medicare patients' diagnoses to maximize their reimbursements. Medicare hospital payments increased sharply, and 75 percent of the increase was attributed to "code creep." Eventually, the government reduced Medicare payments so much that more than two-thirds of all hospitals lost money on their Medicare patients. After a few years of losses, payments were increased. Indications are that Medicare reform will again reduce hospital payments to save money.

The failure of Medicare DRG payments to accurately measure patient severity of illness has led some hospitals to "dump" on other hospitals those Medicare patients whose costs exceed their payments. Congress has enacted legislation to penalize hospitals that engage in dumping.

In the early 1970s, Medicare limited how rapidly physician fees could increase under Medicare. As the difference between Medicare and private fees became greater, physicians stopped participating in Medicare and billed their patients directly. To prevent this, Congress changed the rules in the 1990s. Physicians are no longer able to participate for some of their patients and not others; instead physicians must participate for all (or none) of their Medicare patients.

When price controls and actual fee reductions were imposed on Medicare physician fees in 1992, physicians whose fees were reduced the most showed the largest increases in volume of services. For example, radiologists' fees declined by 12 percent, while their volume increased by 13 percent. Similarly, urologists' fees declined by 5 percent, while their volume increased by 12 percent. These specialists were apparently able to "create demand" among their Medicare fee-for-service patients.

Several years ago, Medicare limited the rise in premiums for Medicare HMOs. Consequently, a number of HMOs dropped out of the Medicare HMO market.

Rationing

Under price controls, as demands for medical services exceed supplies, what criteria will be used to ration the supplies that are available? Undoubtedly emergency cases would take precedence over elective services, but how would elective services be rationed? In some countries where age is a criterion, those above a certain age do not have access to hip replacements, kidney dialysis, heart surgery, and other services. Both quality of life and life expectancy are reduced.

Waiting Lists

Typically, waiting lists are used for rationing elective procedures. In countries that rely on this approach, waiting times for surgical procedures, whether for cataracts or open-heart surgery, may vary from six months to two years.[2] Delays are costly in terms of reduced quality of life and life expectancy. When resources are limited, acute care has a higher priority than preventive services. Women over the age of 50 years have a lower use rate of mammograms in Canada, where price controls and global budgets are used, than in the United States. (More than 60 percent of women aged 50 to 69 in the United States had a mammogram in the previous 12 months, compared with 48 percent in Canada [Sanmartin et al. 2004].)

Those who can afford to wait, that is, those with lower time costs, such as the retired, will be more likely to receive physician services than those with higher time costs. Access to nonemergency physician services will be determined by the value patients place on their time. Waiting is costly in that it uses productive resources (or enjoyable time). A large, but less visible, cost is associated with waiting. Suppose the out-of-pocket price of a physician's office visit is limited to $10, but the patient must take three hours off work to wait and see the physician. If the patient earns $20 an hour, the effective cost of that visit is $70. The "lower" costs of a price-controlled system never explicitly recognize the lost productivity to society or the value of that time to the patient. Patients with high time costs would be willing to pay not to wait, but they do not have that option. They cannot buy medical services the value of which exceeds what they would be willing to pay.

---

2. The Fraser Institute (http://www.fraserinstitute.ca) collects data annually on waiting times in each of the Canadian provinces by procedure and on waiting time for a referral from a general practitioner to a specialist.

The effects of price controls are often a greater burden on those with low incomes and those who do not know how to "work the system." Specialists frequently see those with connections more quickly, and those with higher incomes can travel elsewhere to receive care. For example, in 1990, the premier of Quebec received cancer treatment in the United States at his own expense (Wood 1990).

Deterioration of Quality

As the costs of providing medical services increase faster than the controlled price, providers may reduce the resources used in treatment, resulting in a deterioration of quality. A physician may prefer a highly sophisticated diagnostic test such as an MRI, but to conserve resources she may order an x-ray instead. The value to the patient of a diagnostic test may exceed its cost, but an overall limit on costs will preclude performing many cost-beneficial tests or procedures. Experience with Medicaid confirms these concerns with quality of care. Large numbers of patients are seen for very short visits in Medicaid "mills." Such short visits are more likely to lead to incorrect diagnosis and treatment. Similarly, in Japan, where physicians' fees are controlled, physicians see many more patients per day than U.S. physicians and spend 30 percent less time with each patient.[3]

When controlled prices do not reflect quality differences among hospitals or physicians, suppliers have less incentive to provide higher-quality services. If all physicians are paid the same fee, the incentive to invest the time to become board certified is reduced. In a price-controlled environment with excess demand, even low-quality providers can survive and prosper. Similarly, drug and equipment manufacturers have no incentive to invest in higher-quality products if such products could not be priced to reflect their higher value.

"Gaming" the System

Price controls provide incentives for providers to try to "game" the system to increase their revenues. For example, physicians paid on a fee-for-service basis are likely to decrease the time they devote to each visit,

---

3. In 1991, Japanese physicians saw an average of 49 patients a day, and 13 percent saw 100 patients a day (Ikegami 1991). The U.S. average was 22 patients per day in 1996. A more recent study (Othaki, Othaki, and Fetters 2003) analyzed the amount of time spent by Japanese and U.S. physicians and found that Japanese physicians spent 30 percent less time with each patient.

which enables them to see more patients and thus bill for more visits. Less physician time per patient represents a more hurried visit and presumably lower-quality care. Physicians are also likely to "unbundle" their services; by dividing a treatment or visit into its separate parts they can charge for each part separately. For example, separate visits may be scheduled for diagnostic tests, to receive the results of those tests, and to receive medications. Price controls also provide physicians and hospitals with an incentive to "up-code" the type of services they provide, that is, to bill a brief office visit as a comprehensive exam.

Gaming the system results in increased regulatory costs because a larger bureaucracy is needed to administer and monitor compliance with price controls. C. Jackson Grayson (1993), who was in charge of price controls imposed in the United States in 1971, stated, "We started Phase II [from 1971 to 1973] with 3½ pages of regulations and ended with 1,534."

Gaming is also costly to patients. Multiple visits to the physician, which enable the physician to bill for each visit separately, increase patient travel and waiting times, an inefficient use of the patient's time that may discourage patients from using needed services.

GLOBAL BUDGETS
To ensure that gaming does not increase total expenditures, an expenditure limit (global budget) is often superimposed on price controls. Included in a global budget are all medical expenditures for hospital and physician services, outpatient and inpatient care, health insurance and HMO premiums, and consumer out-of-pocket payments. Unless the global budget is comprehensive, expenditures and investments will shift to unregulated sectors. Additional controls will then be imposed to prevent expenditure growth in these areas, and monitoring compliance with the controls becomes even more costly.

What happens under global budgets when demand for certain providers or MCOs increases? The more efficient health plans cannot increase their number of physicians and facilities to meet increased enrollment demands. Thus, the public is precluded from choosing the more efficient, more responsive health plans that are subject to overall budget limits. Limiting a physician's total revenue discourages the use of physician assistants and nurse practitioners who could increase the physician's productivity, because the physician would prefer to receive the limited revenue rather than share it. Once a physician has reached the overall revenue limit, what incentive does she have to continue serving patients? Why not work fewer hours and take longer vacations? What incentives do hospitals or physicians have to develop innovative, less-costly delivery systems, such as managed care, outpatient diagnostics and surgery, or home infusion programs, if the funds must be taken from existing programs and providers? Efficient providers are penalized if they cannot increase expenditures to expand, and patients lose the opportunity to be served by more efficient providers.

To remain within their overall budgets, hospitals will undertake actions that decrease efficiency and access to care. Hospitals adjust to stringent budget limits by keeping patients longer, as long-stay patients require fewer resources than does performing procedures on more patients. Strict budget limits will result in greater delays in admitting patients, and patients will have less access to beneficial but costly technology.

Global budgets are based on the assumption that the government knows exactly the "right" amount of medical expenditures for the nation. However, a correct percentage of GDP that should be spent on medical care has never been determined, and the fact that other countries spend less than the United States does not tell us which country we should emulate or what we should forgo. Medical expenditures increase for many reasons. No accurate information exists as to how much of the rise in expenditures is attributable to waste, new diseases (such as AIDS), an aging population, and new technology. The quality of health care will deteriorate, and long waiting times for treatment will result if price controls and global budgets are set too low.

Whether politicians would permit a strict global budget to continue in the face of shortages and complaints about access to medical services is questionable. More likely, politicians would respond to their constituents' complaints and relax the budget limit. This has in fact occurred in other countries when access to medical services became too limited because of price controls and global budgets. Great Britain, for example, permits "buyouts." A private medical market is allowed to develop, and those with higher incomes who can afford to buy private medical insurance jump the queue to receive medical services from private providers. To the extent that buyouts are permitted, medical expenditures will increase more rapidly, and a two-tier system will evolve. If a buyout is envisaged, the rationale for price controls and global budgets is questionable.

SUMMARY

Price controls and global budgets provide the appearance of controlling rising prices and expenditures, but in reality, they lead to cheating and a reduction in quality, impose large costs on patients and providers, and do little to improve efficiency.

If the purpose of regulation is to improve efficiency, eliminate inappropriate services, and decrease the costly duplication of medical technology, government policies should provide incentives to achieve these goals. Such incentives are more likely to occur in a system in which purchasers make cost-conscious choices and providers must compete for those purchasers. Competitive systems provide both purchasers and providers with incentives to weigh the benefits and costs of new medical technology. When patients are willing to pay not to wait and to have access to new technology, medical expenditures will increase faster, but the rate of increase will be more appropriate.

DISCUSSION QUESTIONS

1. Why do price controls cause shortages, and why do these shortages increase over time?

2. Why do price controls require hospitals to make a trade-off between quality of medical services and number of patients served?

3. What are the various ways in which a provider can "game" the system under price controls?

4. What "costs" do price controls impose on patients?

5. What are the advantages and disadvantages of permitting patients to "buy out" of the price-controlled medical system?

REFERENCES

Baumol, W. 1988. "Containing Medical Costs: Why Price Controls Won't Work." *Public Interest* 93 (Fall): 37–53.

Grayson, C. J. 1993. "Experience Talks: Shun Price Controls." *The Wall Street Journal* March 29, A14.

Haislmaier, E. F. 1993. *Why Global Budgets and Price Controls Will Not Curb Health Costs*. Washington, DC: The Heritage Foundation.

Ikegami, N. 1991. "Japanese Health Care—Low Cost Through Regulated Fees." *Health Affairs* 10 (3): 87–109.

Ohtaki, S., T. Ohtaki, and M. Fetters. 2003. "Doctor-Patient Communication: A Comparison of USA and Japan." *Family Practice* 20 (3): 276–82.

Sanmartin, C., E. Ng, D. Blackwell, J. Gentleman, M. Martinez, and C. Simile. 2004. *Joint Canada/United States Survey of Health, 2002–03.* [Online publication; retrieved 11/15/06.] http://www.cdc.gov/nchs/data/nhis/jcush_analyticalreport.pdf.

Wood, N. 1990. "Missing, but Not Forgotten." *McLean's* 103 (10): 14.

Chapter 19

The Evolution of Managed Care

AN IMPORTANT POLICY debate concerns the organization and delivery of medical services—namely, should this country rely on regulation or on market competition to achieve efficiency in the provision of medical services? Market competition can take different forms; one such form was the emergence and rapid growth of MCOs during the 1980s and 1990s. What effect has managed care competition had? Has managed care improved efficiency and reduced the rate of increase in medical expenditures? What happened to patient satisfaction and quality of care? To discuss these issues we must discuss what is meant by "managed care," why it came about, the evidence on how well it has performed, how it is evolving, and the recent development of CDHC.

WHY MANAGED CARE CAME ABOUT

Managed care was a market response to the wasteful excesses of the past, resulting in rapidly rising medical costs in a system widely believed to be inefficient. Traditional indemnity health insurance, with its comprehensive coverage of hospitals and small patient copayments for medical services, lessened patient concerns with hospital and medical expenses. Physicians were paid on a fee-for-service basis and were not fiscally responsible for hospital use, which they prescribed. New medical technology was introduced rapidly because the insurer paid for its use and cost; insurers merely passed the higher cost onto employers.

The lack of insurer, patient, physician, and hospital incentives to be concerned with cost led to rapidly rising costs. Insured patients demanded "too many" services (moral hazard), physicians paid on a fee-for-service basis had an incentive to supply more services (supplier-induced demand), and hospitals competed for physicians by making available to them the latest technology so their patients would not have to be referred to other hospitals and physicians. Advances in medical technology and the lack of cost incentives led to nonprice competition among hospitals; technology was adopted no matter how small its medical benefits. This not only led to higher costs but also lowered quality, as studies demonstrated that hospitals that performed fewer complex procedures had worse outcomes than hospitals that performed more such procedures (Hughes, Hunt, and Luft 1987).

As large employers sought to reduce the rapid increases in health insurance premiums, physicians, hospitals, and traditional health insurers were not responsive to their cost concerns. Instead, entrepreneurs recognized the potential for reducing medical system inefficiencies and started HMOs, utilization review firms, and PPOs. These innovators, who aggressively marketed their approaches to large employers, were richly rewarded for their efforts.

WHAT IS MANAGED CARE?

Managed care embodies a variety of techniques and types of organizations. Financial incentives, negotiation of large provider discounts, limited provider networks, physician gatekeepers, utilization management, and drug formularies are some of these techniques.

Managed care health plans were successful in interfering with the traditional physician–patient relationship because employees were willing to switch from traditional insurers in return for lower premiums. Managed care plans contracted with those physicians and hospitals willing to discount their prices, which was a precondition for joining the plan's limited provider network. Given the excess capacity that existed among physicians and hospitals, they were willing to discount their prices in return for increased patient volume. The patient's choice of physician was restricted to only those in the plan's provider panel, as were the specialists to whom the patient could be referred and the hospitals in which the patient could stay. Decisions about whether to hospitalize a patient, length of stay, specialist referrals, and types of drugs prescribed—which were formerly made by the physician—were now influenced by the managed care plan.

Managed care techniques have changed over time. First-generation approaches were quite restrictive. Managed care plans relied on "selective contracting," which limits the provider panel to those who are willing to discount their prices and are appropriate users of medical services, a gate-keeper model, and stringent utilization review. An enrollee in a managed care plan chose a primary care physician from among a panel of physicians who would manage that patient's care and control diagnostic and specialist referrals. The primary care physician would often do some tasks previously performed by specialists. Utilization review includes prior authorization for hospital admission, concurrent review (i.e., the patient's length of stay is reviewed to make sure the stay does not exceed what is medically necessary), and retrospective review (to ensure that appropriate care was provided).

The initial sources of managed care savings were lower hospital use (the most expensive component of care) and deep provider price discounts. The HMOs were able to shift large numbers of their enrollees to those providers who competed to be included in the HMO's provider panel and were able to achieve cost savings relatively easily and without changing the practice of medicine.

To achieve further reductions in medical costs, managed care had to become more innovative and effective in managing patient care. So-called second-generation managed care approaches relied more on changing physicians' practice patterns, such as identifying high-risk enrollees early, decreasing the variation in physicians' utilization patterns, reducing inappropriate use of services, and substituting less-costly in-home services for continued care in the hospital. Managed care plans are relying more on "evidence-based medicine" to achieve their savings. By having access to large data sets on physicians' treatment patterns from around the country and information technology to analyze those data, health plans can determine which treatment decisions have better outcomes. Integrated and coordinated care and disease management can decrease medical costs as well as improve patient outcomes.

Some managed care plans (particularly in California) shifted more of the capitation payment, hence risk, to physicians and hospitals; providers were thereby given an incentive to innovate in the delivery of medical services. Furthermore, with the shifting of risk from employers to HMOs, large employers placed greater emphasis on report cards. Because managed care plans and their providers have a financial incentive to provide fewer services under capitation, both the plans and their providers have to be continuously monitored for patient satisfaction and medical outcomes. Health plans and their providers are being held accountable for the health status of their enrolled populations.

TYPES OF MANAGED CARE PLANS

Managed care health plans vary in the degree to which they use a select network of providers and limit access to specialists. Typically, the more restrictive the managed care plan, the lower its premium. The most restrictive type of managed care plan is an HMO, which offers the most comprehensive health benefits. An HMO relies on a restricted provider network, and the patient is responsible for the full costs of going to nonnetwork providers. Cost control by an HMO is achieved through stringent utilization management, financial incentives to physicians, and limited access to providers.

Managed fee-for-service indemnity insurance plans include a PPO, which is a closed provider panel. Providers are paid on a fee-for-service basis, and enrollees have a financial incentive (lower copayment) to use the PPO providers versus "going out of network." Specialist referrals also vary. In an HMO, the primary care physician must recommend specialist referrals. In a PPO setting the patient may self-refer to a specialist, but the copayment is lower if the specialist is in the PPO. Costs are controlled through utilization management, patient copayments, and discounted fees from PPO providers.

Traditional HMOs began to offer a point-of-service option to counter the growing popularity of PPOs. A point-of-service plan is an HMO that permits its enrollees to use nonparticipating providers if the enrollees are willing to pay a high copayment (e.g., 40 percent) each time they use such providers.

Figure 19.1 shows the market share of each type of managed care plan and how that share has changed over time. In the early 1980s, managed care was just beginning to grow. Traditional indemnity insurance, with free access to all providers ("unmanaged care"), was the dominant form (95 percent) of health insurance. Since that time, the distribution of different types of health plans has changed rapidly. By 2005, traditional insurance had virtually disappeared, and various types of managed care had become the predominant form of insurance.

The premium in a typical managed care plan is allocated as shown in Figure 19.2. In this example, the ABC Managed Care Health Plan retains 15 percent of the premium to cover expenses associated with marketing, administration, and profit. About 35 percent of the premium is allocated for hospital and other medical facility expenses, 40 percent is set aside for physician services, and 10 percent is allocated for pharmacy and ancillary services. Use of services by enrollees outside the plan's area

Figure 19.1: The Trend Toward Managed Care

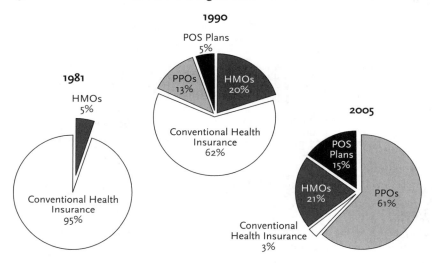

Health maintenance organization (HMO): An organization that provides comprehensive health care services to a voluntarily enrolled membership for a prepaid fee. HMOs control costs through stringent utilization management, payment incentives to physicians, and restricted access to providers.

Preferred provider organization (PPO): A third-party payer contracts with a group of medical providers who agree to furnish services at negotiated fees in return for prompt payment and increased patient volume. PPOs control costs by keeping fees down and curbing excessive service through utilization management.

Point-of-service (POS): An HMO that permits its enrollees access to nonparticipating providers if the enrollees are willing to pay a high copayment each time they use such providers.

Conventional health insurance: Patients are permitted to go to any provider, and the provider is paid on a fee-for-service basis. The patient normally pays a small annual deductible plus 20 percent of the provider's charge, up to an annual out-of-pocket limit of $3,000.

Sources: Kaiser Family Foundation and Health Research and Educational Trust. *Employer Health Benefits: 2005 Annual Survey.* [Online information.] http://www.kff. org/insurancce/7315/upload/7315.pdf; *KPMG Survey of Employer-Sponsored Health Benefits: 1981, 1990.*

and certain catastrophic expenses may also be included in the health plan's percentage.

Providers within each of these budgetary allocations may be paid in several ways. Some managed care plans place their physicians on a salary (e.g., Kaiser Health Plan), others pay discounted fee for service, and still

Figure 19.2: How an HMO Allocates the Premium Dollar

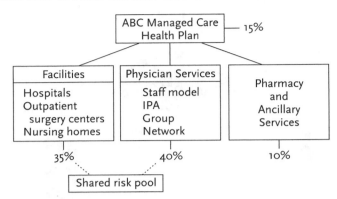

Types of HMOs:

Staff model: An HMO that delivers health services through a physician group that is controlled by the HMO unit.

IPA: An HMO that contracts directly with physicians in independent practices.

Group: An HMO that contracts with one independent group practice to provide health services.

Network: An HMO that contracts with two or more independent group practices.

others may capitate their physicians (pay an annual amount to the physician group for each enrollee for whom they are responsible). (Capitated medical groups are primarily in California.) Within each of these payment arrangements, the organization that is at financial risk withholds a certain percentage of the budget allocation to ensure that sufficient funds are available to provide all of the necessary services. Funds remaining at the end of the year are divided among the members of that provider group.

When medical groups and hospitals were capitated, a "shared risk pool" existed between them. Part of the hospital's capitated payment was set aside to be shared among the hospital and medical group to provide the medical group with an incentive to reduce use of the hospital.

HOW HAS MANAGED CARE PERFORMED?

Managed care did not spread equally to all parts of the country or to all population groups. It moved more rapidly into those areas that had high health care costs, where the potential for cost reductions were greatest. Managed care plans were more likely to enter urban than rural areas.

The West, particularly California, introduced managed care earlier and had a greater percentage of its population enrolled in managed care than did the East or Southeast. Those employed in large firms moved more rapidly into managed care than did those on Medicare and Medicaid, who had limited price incentives to enroll in managed care plans.

A significant portion of the population is still not subject to managed care. As of 2005, only 14.2 percent of the 43 million aged were in managed care plans (referred to as Medicare Advantage plans). In 2005, 46.6 million people were uninsured. Only since the early 2000s has Medicaid managed care increased. By 2005, 63 percent of the 45.4 million on Medicaid were in managed care. Managed care systems, therefore, have not competed for the approximately 100 million people, or 33 percent of the U.S. population, who rely on the unmanaged fee-for-service system.

To determine the performance of managed care competition we must examine the population groups subject to managed care, namely the remaining 67 percent of the population. (For example, using total health care expenditures, which include Medicare and Medicaid, rather than employer-paid health insurance premiums, will not provide as accurate a description of the effect of managed care.)

The Issue of Biased Selection

Managed care plans initially attracted younger enrollees, persons new to an area, and fewer persons who were chronically ill—people who did not have long-standing physician relationships. If HMOs and managed care plans enrolled a healthier population group, a comparison of their performance relative to traditional health insurers would be biased. Better health outcomes and lower health care costs in an HMO would be more related to the population enrolled than to its performance. Thus, crucial to any study determining whether managed care plans are better at controlling growth in costs and improving treatment outcomes is the ability to control for lower-risk groups enrolled in managed care.

A large number and variety of studies have been conducted on the performance of HMOs, managed care plans, and traditional insurers (Glied 2000). Following is a brief summary of the results of these studies (which have controlled for biased selection).

Rise in Health Insurance Premiums

Managed care competition works in the following manner. As managed care plans entered a market and enrolled a significant number of members, hospitals and physicians competed on price to be included in the managed care plan's provider network. Given their excess capacity and need for more patients, providers were also willing to accept utilization review, which decreases hospital use. These cost savings (discounted prices and lower hospital use rates) enabled the managed care plan to lower its premium relative to those of non–managed-care health plans. When employees are required to pay the additional cost of more expensive health plans, studies show that premium differences as small as $5 to $10 a month will cause 25 percent of a health plan's employees to switch. Employees are very price sensitive. Health plans therefore have to be very price competitive.

To prevent further losses in their market share, indemnity, non–managed-care insurers adopted managed care techniques like utilization review and PPOs to limit the rise in their premiums. Managed care plans not only reduced their own medical costs but, by their competitive effect, forced other insurers to adopt managed care techniques to reduce their costs to remain price competitive.

Managed care competition dramatically slowed the rise in health insurance premiums. Figure 19.3 shows the national trend in employer-paid health insurance premiums and the annual percentage change in the CPI. Also included are premium data from California, where managed care competition started earlier and was more extensive than in the rest of the country. Clearly, as managed care market share increased (see Figure 19.1), insurance premiums rose more slowly. (In California, the managed care effect was even more pronounced; it occurred earlier and included a greater percentage of the population. For several years, health insurance premiums in California actually declined.)

A major source of the early savings from managed care was reduced hospital use, which is shown in Figure 19.4. Hospital patient days per 1,000 population declined from 1,302 in 1977 to 666 by 2005. Also shown is the earlier and larger decline in hospital use rates in California; rates there declined from 996 to 505 per 1,000 population over that same period. New York, which had a hospital use rate higher than the national average, also saw a decline, although at 950 in 2005 it was still much higher than the national average and almost twice as high as in California.

Hospital admissions per 1,000 population have also fallen, although not as dramatically as patient days. Admission rates in 1978 were 162 nationally, 147 in New York, and 141 in California. By 2005, these rates had declined to 119, 132, and 95, respectively.

Figure 19.3: Annual Percentage Increase in Health Insurance Premiums for the United States and California, and the CPI, 1988–2005

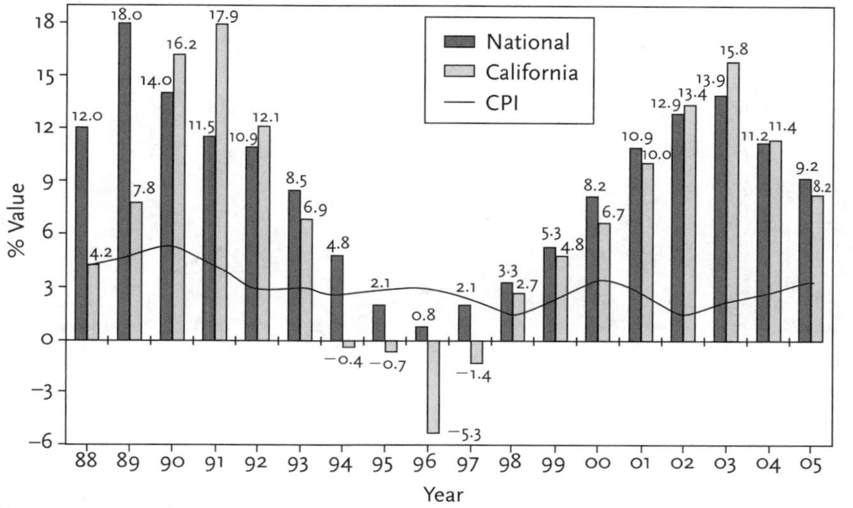

Sources: National data: 1988–1998, Gabel, J. *KPMG Surveys of Employer-Sponsored Health Benefits, HIAA Survey of Employer-Sponsored Health Benefits*; 1999–2005, *Kaiser/HRET Survey of Employer-Sponsored Health Benefits*. 2005. [Online information.] http://www.kff.org/insurance/7148/upload/Employer-Health-Benefit-Survey-2004-Chartpack.pdf. California data: California Public Employees Retirement System (CALPERS) and California Health Care Foundation/HRET. 2005. *California Employer Health Benefit Survey*. [Online information.] http://www.chcf.org/documents/insurance/EmployerBenefitSurvey05.pdf. CPI data: Bureau of Labor Statistics. 2006. [Online information.] http://data.bls.gov.

As a consequence of managed care, hospitals' share of total medical expenditures declined. The decline in hospital use rates that occurred in California indicates the reductions in hospital use that are still possible in other parts of the country.

ONE-TIME VERSUS CONTINUAL COST SAVINGS

Managed care achieved the easiest cost reductions, such as decreased hospital days, substitution of less-costly settings for costly inpatient stays, and lower provider prices. These reductions, however, are one-time cost savings, although they occur over a period of years and are instituted at different times in different parts of the country. An important policy question is whether managed care competition is only

Figure 19.4: Trends in Hospital Utilization per 1,000 Population: United States, California, and New York, 1977–2005

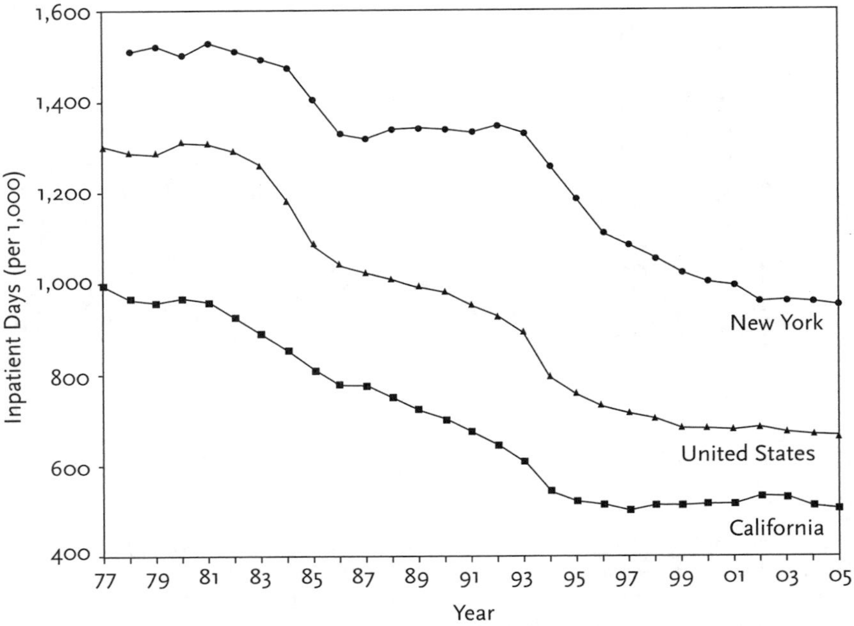

Sources: Population data from U.S. Census Bureau. [Online information.] http://www.census.gov. Data as of July 1, except 1980, 1990, and 2000, as of April 1. Utilization figures from American Hospital Association. 2007. *Hospital Statistics,* various years. Chicago: Health Forum LLC, an affiliate of the AHA.

able to produce these one-time savings or whether it can achieve continual cost reductions.

The two most important factors that determine the rate at which medical expenditures will increase are demographics—the aging of the population with more costly care needs—and the development and adoption of new medical technology. Whether managed care is able to achieve continual cost reductions will depend on whether it is able to innovate in the management of care of the aged and the chronically ill and whether it can reduce the rate of new technology diffusion while encouraging the development of cost-reducing technology.

Under unmanaged fee-for-service indemnity insurance new technology was adopted as long as it provided some additional benefit, no matter how small, regardless of its cost. There was little financial incentive to develop cost-reducing technology. For managed care to produce continual savings new technology must be justified on its costs as well as its benefits. To the extent that investment in technology can be directed to reducing the use of more-costly procedures, using less-invasive procedures, enabling care to be provided in the home or an outpatient setting, and preventing costly acute care from occurring, continual reductions in medical costs are possible.[1]

Based on a limited number of studies, managed care slowed the rate at which new technology is adopted. Furthermore, as managed care penetration increased in an area, capacity use of the equipment increased; consequently, fewer facilities were needed than under the unmanaged fee-for-service system. Managed care appears to have been able to achieve continual reductions in the cost of medical care.

Managed care achieved one of the main goals it was meant to accomplish: It reduced the rise in health care expenditures. Without managed care, insurance premiums would have increased more rapidly. Higher insurance premiums make health insurance less affordable; consequently, the number of uninsured would have been greater because the demand for insurance is inversely related to its price. Furthermore, the lower rate of increase in insurance premiums resulted in a *redistribution of income* from hospitals and physicians (an important reason for their opposition to managed care) to employees. Lower health insurance premiums meant that employees had greater take-home pay. Lower premiums also meant, however, that less revenue was available for physicians, hospitals employed fewer people, and their wages increased more slowly.

Patient Satisfaction and Quality of Care

An evaluation of managed care performance should be broader than just examining whether it results in lower insurance premiums. Managed care competition (as well as any system for organizing the delivery of medical services) should also be evaluated on whether it promotes efficiency (the rate at which premiums increase), desired treatment outcomes, and patient satisfaction.

---

1. On balance, new technology has led to increased, not decreased, medical expenditures. However, increased medical expenditures resulting from new technology are not the same as inflation in medical costs. The medical treatment the patient receives is different and improved. Furthermore, as long as the public is willing to pay for those increased benefits, it is appropriate for medical costs to increase.

Many studies have examined member satisfaction in managed care plans, such as HMOs and non-HMOs. (These studies typically compare the most restrictive form of managed care, an HMO, to less-restrictive forms or to non–managed-care insurance plans.) Member satisfaction typically includes waiting times for an appointment, referrals to a specialist, and travel times to a panel provider. These results typically show a very high degree of member satisfaction in HMOs. Such studies, however, have limited usefulness because most people do not have health problems and therefore do not make costly demands on the HMO.

More recent surveys attempt to measure patient satisfaction by those who are chronically ill and have serious health problems. Such studies have examined access to care by those with low incomes, those who are HIV positive, and those who are chronically ill. The results of these studies are mixed. Either there are no significant differences between the health plans, or in some HMOs patient satisfaction is better, whereas in others it is not. On one hand, in traditional unmanaged health plans, the patient has easier access to specialists and fewer restrictions on hospital use. In managed care plans, however, coordination of care becomes important in caring for those with chronic illness; otherwise a chronically ill patient can be hospitalized multiple times, increasing the managed care plan's costs. Early managed care plans were not experienced in caring for those with chronic illness and as a result of anecdotal stories of access problems, regulatory restrictions were placed on managed care plans; this has since changed in most managed care plans.

With regard to quality of care in managed care versus traditional insurance, the empirical literature suggests little difference between the two. Some studies indicate that traditional insurance may perform better for those who have serious health conditions, particularly those with low incomes. Given the large number of managed care plans and the different types of such plans, generalizations as to whether one type of health plan results in greater or worse patient satisfaction and treatment outcomes are difficult to make. How the providers are paid (fee for service, salary, or capitation), who is at financial risk, the type of decision-making structure, and the managed care culture of the medical group are likely to be more important determinants of patient satisfaction and outcomes than the type of health plan.

To the extent that risk-adjusted premiums are used to pay for high-risk patients and those who have serious illnesses, a higher capitation rate paid by the employer to the health plan for such groups provides managed care plans with an incentive to compete for such patients, improve their access to care, and innovate in devising new treatment methods.

THE CHANGE IN MANAGED CARE

Managed care underwent a change starting in the late 1990s. Several events occurred that resulted in a loosening of managed care's more restrictive cost-containment measures.

Economic Prosperity of the 1990s

In the late 1990s, the U.S. economy was expanding, the stock market was reaching new highs, "dot-com" companies were the craze, and firms had difficulty attracting and retaining skilled employees. In that prosperous period, employees wanted health plans that were less restrictive on specialist referrals and that offered broader provider networks to enable greater choice of provider. Given the tight labor market, employers were more concerned with keeping their employees than with the costs of health care; employers were willing to pay higher insurance premiums for more generous health plans. Enrollment growth in HMOs, the most restrictive type of plan, began to decline, and PPO plans became more popular.

As health plans restructured themselves to accommodate employees' demands, the health plans had more difficulty controlling medical costs. Changing from limited to broad provider networks meant that health plans had less leverage over the provider to negotiate large price discounts. The removal of physician gatekeepers meant an increase in self-referrals to specialists and more procedures. Less utilization review by health plans also led to greater use of medical services. Greater use of specialists, more procedures, and reliance on fee-for-service payment over a broad provider network not only made coordinating and monitoring patient care more difficult but also increased the cost of care and, consequently, premiums.

Furthermore, to the extent that managed care plans have broader provider networks and providers participate in multiple health plans, holding the health plan accountable for the performance of its providers is difficult. Similarly, a single health plan has difficulty collecting data from providers, monitoring their performance, and changing their practice patterns. The broader the provider network and the fewer the restrictions on specialist referrals, the less control health plans have over providers.

Higher Prices for Hospitals, Physicians, and Prescription Drugs

The industry structure was also changing during the late 1990s. To improve their bargaining power with fewer but larger health plans, hospitals and physicians began merging and consolidating into fewer, larger organizations. Hospital mergers within a market meant fewer competitors among which the health plan could negotiate discounts; hospitals were therefore able to charge the health plans higher prices. Drug costs also began increasing sharply as new, more effective drugs became available and pharmaceutical companies were successful in stimulating demand with direct-to-consumer advertising. Health plans had to increase their premiums to pay for these higher costs.

Regulation of Managed Care

By the end of the 1990s, a backlash by providers and patients forced many managed care plans to abandon the strict cost-containment methods such as gatekeepers and specialist referral requirements, and adopt less-restrictive options. Increased government regulation of managed care occurred for several reasons:

- Widespread media attention was given to certain cases of denial of care by HMOs.
- The public wanted increased access to specialists (without paying more).
- The American Medical Association wanted to redress the balance of power between managed care plans and physicians; physicians' bargaining power would be increased if limited provider networks could be opened to all physicians, thereby allowing patients greater choice of physician ("any willing provider" laws).
- Some were opposed to managed care because they wanted a single-payer system and regulation would eliminate managed care's success in reducing medical costs.

Legislators saw an opportunity to gain visibility by holding hearings on HMO practices and receive the public's support by enacting legislation making certain managed care practices (e.g., outpatient mastectomies and "drive-through deliveries") illegal.

Legislators did not discuss the trade-offs between legislating freer access to care and the increased premiums that would result. The public was led to believe increased access would come at no additional cost.

Congress and the states increased regulation of managed care plans. To the extent that government intervenes in the practice of medicine (establishing minimum lengths of stay and determining which procedures can be performed in an outpatient setting) and regulates how managed care plans structure their delivery systems, treatment innovation is inhibited and health insurance premiums will increase by more than they would otherwise.

Also, in October 1999, a class-action lawsuit requesting billions of dollars in damages was filed against a managed care firm (Humana), alleging that by using cost-containment methods the firm reneged on its promise to pay for all medically necessary care. Although the lawsuit was dismissed three years later, along with similar ones against other managed care plans, managed care plans relaxed their cost-containment methods.

RECENT DEVELOPMENTS IN MANAGED CARE

As managed care's stringent cost-containment methods and limited provider networks were loosened, premiums began increasing rapidly in the late 1990s. Employers and their employees once again became concerned with rising premiums. Employers started shifting a greater portion of the insurance premium to their employees and pressured managed care firms to better control rising health care costs.

New Cost-Containment Approaches

Managed care's cost-control approaches have evolved from restricting access to developing innovative approaches for managing care and reducing medical costs. Approaches being used today include the early management of diseases such as diabetes, hypertension, and congestive heart failure, as these diseases can lead to catastrophic medical expenses. Managing chronic illness includes developing clinical guidelines or protocols, clinical integration and coordination of care, and early identification and treatment of high-risk patients. With the aging of the population, managed care firms are learning how to manage chronic care needs for which they are at financial risk.

Assisting in the development of innovative approaches will be computer information systems and large databases, which can revolutionize treatment patterns (known as "evidence-based medicine"). Large data sets that track specific diseases over long periods will enable providers to determine which variations in treatment methods have the most desired patient outcomes; this information could be used for promoting changes in physicians' practice patterns. Information technology and large amounts of data will also enable managers to increase efficiency by better understanding their enrollees' medical costs as well as improve clinical outcomes and quality of care. Provider performance will be evaluated in terms of patient outcomes, satisfaction, and cost of care.

In addition to these approaches, some managed care plans are re-instituting some previously used methods, such as preapproval for certain surgical procedures and specialist referrals (Mays, Claxton, and White 2004).

Report Cards

Previously, consumers had little or no information by which to judge the quality of different providers or the quality of care they received. The development of managed care made it possible to evaluate patient satisfaction and treatment outcomes of enrolled population groups. By having limited provider panels of physicians and hospitals, together with a defined group of enrollees, a managed care plan is able to develop information on the practice patterns of and patient satisfaction with its providers and the care received by its enrollees.

Under pressure from employer coalitions for more information by which their employees can judge different managed care plans and their participating providers, managed care plans have provided data to independent organizations for developing "report cards." These report cards include information on patient satisfaction, quality process measures, and outcomes data on health plans and their participating providers. When these report cards are made available to employees during open enrollment periods, the additional information influences their choice of health plan (Wedig and Tai-Seale 2002). Public information increases the pressure on health plans and their providers to compete on satisfaction and outcome measures as well as on premiums. Employees can then make a more informed trade-off between lower premiums and easier access for referrals.

Pay for Performance

A recent development is incentive-based provider payments, referred to as *pay for performance*. Insurers typically pay physicians and hospitals for providing services, and little if any attempt has been made to reward providers who provide higher-quality services or who reduce treatment costs. This is beginning to change. Although quality of medical care is difficult to measure, medical experts agree that certain standards should be met for preventive care and for specified diagnoses (Rosenthal et al. 2005). Although the measures used for incentive payments are not standardized across different health plans, three types of measures are being used: (1) clinical quality, including childhood immunizations, breast cancer and cervical cancer screening, and measures related to the management of chronic diseases, such as diabetes and asthma; (2) patient satisfaction measures; and (3) measures related to investment in information technology that enables clinical data integration.

The pay-for-performance experiments have been started by those managed care plans having a large market share (therefore greater bargaining power over their providers). Currently, incentive payments paid to providers represent a small percentage of a provider's total revenue, 1 percent to 5 percent. Pay for performance is in its early stages. Medical societies have generally been opposed on grounds that the quality measures are not fully developed and there is an implication that providers are not providing high-quality care. Health plans using pay for performance claim there has been an improvement in the quality measures for which providers are being rewarded. Pay-for-performance programs will continue to evolve; the size of the incentive payment will likely increase, standards for judging providers will become uniform across health plans, and medical groups will have to invest more in information technology to be able to provide the data by which they will be measured.

CONSUMER-DRIVEN HEALTH CARE

An approach gaining in popularity for lowering rising insurance premiums is CDHC. More of the financial risk and responsibility for controlling cost, such as seeking lower provider prices and using fewer services, is placed on the consumer. A CDHC plan relies on a large-deductible insurance policy, making the enrollee responsible for large out-of-pocket payments. The Medicare Modernization Act of 2003 provided tax advantages to employees who establish a health savings account (HSA). An HSA has two parts: the first is a high-deductible health insurance policy; the second is a tax-free savings account for the employee, to which her contribution can be as large as the size of her deductible. Each year, funds in the savings account that are not spent on medical services can be accumulated. When the employee retires, the accumulated funds and the earnings on those funds belong to the employee.

A number of Internet web sites provide information on hospital and physician quality rankings and prices for different treatments to help employees with high-deductible plans choose their providers.

Although only about 3 million people have CDHC plans, they are achieving greater acceptance among employees and are likely to continue increasing (Claxton et al. 2005). Enrollment in managed care plans appears to have stabilized, and more managed care plans have begun marketing CDHC plans; managed care plans are also partnering with financial institutions to manage the tax-free savings accounts. It is too early to judge how CDHC plans will affect enrollment in more traditional managed care plans.

SUMMARY

As a consequence of the economic prosperity that led to employee demands for less-restrictive health plans in the 1990s, hospital mergers and physician consolidations that led to higher provider prices, increased drug prices, regulations imposed on managed care plans, and advances in medical technology, health insurance premiums once again began to increase sharply. Managed care plans have demonstrated less ability to control costs today than they had previously.

Employers and employees are searching for new approaches to limit their premium increases. Employers are shifting more of the insurance premium to their employees, and health plans are developing new cost-containment strategies, such as disease management and evidence-based medicine. Under pressure from employers, health plans are using report cards to enable employees to make more informed choices of health plans and participating providers. Health plans are also beginning to use incentive-based payment to encourage their participating providers to improve quality of care, patient satisfaction, and the use of information technology to integrate clinical data.

A recent trend affecting the growth of managed care plans is CDHC. These high-deductible plans, sold at lower premiums, shift more of the financial risk to consumers and require them to become more informed about their purchases of health care services and their choice of providers.

The market is responding to rising premiums by offering a variety of health plans, as consumers have different preferences and abilities to pay. Increased emphasis is being placed on consumer cost sharing to hold down costs and use of services.

DISCUSSION QUESTIONS

1. What is managed care, and what are managed care techniques?

2. When managed care enrollment increases in a market, how does it affect other insurers and providers?

3. Why did managed care occur?

4. What are the different types of managed care plans?

5. What are report cards, and what effects are they expected to have on managed care competition?

6. How has the growth of managed care affected the performance of the medical sector?

REFERENCES

Claxton, G., J. Gabel, I. Gil, J. Pickreign, H. Whitmore, B. Finder, S. Rouhani, S. Hawkins, and D. Rowland. 2005. "What High-Deductible Plans Look Like: Findings from a National Survey of Employers, 2005." *Health Affairs* Web exclusive, September 14, W5-434–W5-441. [Online publication; retrieved 11/15/06.] http://content.healthaffairs.org/cgi/content/abstract/hlthaff.w5.434v1.

Glied, S. 2000. "Managed Care." In *The Handbook of Health Economics*, edited by J. P. Newhouse and A. J. Culyer, 707–53. New York: North-Holland Press.

Hughes, R., S. Hunt, and H. Luft. 1987. "Effects of Surgeon Volume and Hospital Volume on Quality of Care in Hospitals." *Medical Care* 25 (6): 489–503.

Mays, G., G. Claxton, and J. White. 2004. "Managed Care Rebound? Recent Changes in Health Plans' Cost Containment Strategies." *Health Affairs* Web exclusive, August 11, W4-427–W4-436. [Online publication; retrieved 11/15/06.] http://content.healthaffairs.org/cgi/reprint/hlthaff.w4.427v1.

Rosenthal, M., R. Frank, Z. Li, and A. Epstein. 2005. "Early Experience with Pay-for-Performance." *Journal of the American Medical Association* 294 (14): 1788–93.

Wedig, G., and M. Tai-Seale. 2002. "The Effect of Report Cards on Consumer Choice in the Health Insurance Market." *Journal of Health Economics* 21 (6): 1031–48.

ADDITIONAL READINGS

Dranove, D. 2000. *The Economic Evolution of American Health Care: From Marcus Welby to Managed Care*. Princeton, NJ: Princeton University Press.

Draper, D., R. Hurley, C. Lesser, and B. Strunk. 2002. "The Changing Face of Managed Care." *Health Affairs* 21 (1): 11–23.

Robinson, J. 2004. "Reinvention of Health Insurance in the Consumer Era." *Journal of the American Medical Association* 291 (15): 1880–86.

Chapter 20

Has Competition Been Tried— And Has it Failed—to Improve the U.S. Health Care System?

CRITICS CLAIM THAT market competition has been tried but it has failed to improve the U.S. health care system. Once again, health care costs are rising rapidly, per capita health care spending is the highest in the world, and yet more than 15 percent of Americans—about 47 million people—are without health insurance. More of the middle class are finding that health insurance has become too expensive, life expectancy is lower than in other countries, and the U.S. infant mortality rate is higher than in some countries with lower per capita health care expenditures. In other words, is it time to try something different? Namely, is it time for more government regulation and control of the health care system?

"Some say that competition has failed, I say that competition has not yet been tried." Alain Enthoven wrote that statement in 1993, and it continues to be correct today (Enthoven 1993, 28).

This chapter discusses how medical markets differ from competitive markets, why making medical markets more competitive is desirable, the changes needed to bring about greater competition, whether competitive markets are responsible for the growing numbers of uninsured, and the role of government in a competitive medical care environment.

CRITERIA FOR JUDGING PERFORMANCE OF A COUNTRY'S MEDICAL SECTOR

The health of a population, as measured by life expectancy or infant mortality rates, is not solely the consequence of the country's medical system. How people live and eat are more important determinants of life expectancy than whether they have good access to medical services once they become ill. Life expectancy is related to a number of factors, such as smoking, diet, marital status, exercise, drug use, and cultural values. Although universal access to health insurance is desirable, studies have shown that medical care has a smaller effect on health levels than personal health habits and lifestyle (see Chapter 3).

Therefore, it is inappropriate to compare the medical care system on measures that are more affected by lifestyle factors. Instead, the financing and delivery of medical services has been based on treating people once they are ill. Several health care organizations in the United States have gone beyond treating people when they become ill and have tried to lower costs by preventing costly illnesses. Reducing hip fractures among the elderly and instituting monitoring mechanisms for diabetes patients, for example, have been shown to prevent more costly expenditures later. The financial incentives of these organizations differ from the typical fee-for-service payment methods predominantly used in the United States and other countries.

Assuming the purpose of a medical care system is more narrowly defined, that is, treating those who become ill, what criteria should be used to evaluate how well that system performs? The criteria should be the same as those used to evaluate the performance of other markets, such as housing, food, automobiles, electronics, markets that produce necessities, and luxuries. The following are performance criteria of a medical care system.

1. *Information:* Do consumers have sufficient information to choose the quantity and type of services based on price, quality, and other characteristics of the services being supplied?
2. *Consumer incentives:* Do consumers have incentives so that the value of the services used is not less than the cost of producing those services?
3. *Consumer choices:* Does the market respond to what consumers are willing to pay? If consumers demand more of some services, will the market provide more of those services? If consumers differ in how much they are willing to spend or want different types of services, will the market respond to those varied consumer demands?
4. *Supplier incentives:* Do the suppliers of the goods and services have an incentive to produce those services (for a given level of quality) at the lowest cost?

5. *Price markups:* Do the prices suppliers charge for their services reflect their costs of production? (This occurs when suppliers compete on price to supply their services.)
6. *Redistribution:* Do those who cannot afford to pay for their medical services receive medically necessary services?

To the extent that the medical sector approximates the first five criteria, the system will produce its output efficiently, and medical costs will rise at a rate that reflects the cost of producing those services.[1] The type of services available, as well as the new medical technology adopted, will be based on what consumers are willing to pay.

Competitive markets, compared with monopoly or government controls on prices and investment, come closest to achieving the first five criteria. Competitive markets are the yardstick by which all markets are evaluated and underlie the antitrust laws. Proponents of competition believe the same benefits can be achieved by applying competitive principles to medical care.

Competitive markets, however, do not help those unable to afford the goods and services produced. It is government's role, not the market's, to subsidize those with low incomes so they can receive the necessary amounts of food, housing, and medical services. When provided through a competitive market, however, the value of the subsidies will be greater; providers have incentives to produce them efficiently, and patients have greater choice when exercising them.

Market forces are very powerful in motivating purchasers and suppliers. The search for profits provides an incentive to suppliers to invest a great deal of money to satisfy purchaser demands. Suppliers innovate to become more efficient, develop new services, and differentiate themselves from their competitors, thereby increasing their market share and becoming more profitable.

Incentives exist in both competitive and regulated markets. The incentives appropriate to a competitive market are those where both the purchaser and the supplier bear the cost and receive the benefits of their

---

1. Increases in demand may result in temporary increases in prices (high price markups over cost), which serve both to equilibrate demand and supply so shortages do not occur and signal suppliers to increase their production to meet the increased demand. Over time, as supply is increased, prices will again reflect the cost of providing those services.

actions. When a purchaser's (or supplier's) costs and benefits are not equal, the market diverges from that of a competitive market and its performance is lessened.

HOW MEDICAL MARKETS DIFFER
FROM COMPETITIVE MARKETS
The Period Before Managed Care

Prior to the start of managed care in the 1980s and into the 1990s, health insurance coverage was predominantly traditional indemnity insurance; patients had little or no out-of-pocket cost when they used medical services, and hospitals and physicians were paid on a fee-for-service basis. Information on providers was nonexistent, as it was prohibited by medical and hospital associations, and accrediting agencies such as the Joint Commission on Accreditation of Healthcare Organizations did not make their findings public. Insurance companies merely passed higher provider costs on to employers, who paid their employees' insurance premiums. Medicare and Medicaid greatly reduced their beneficiaries' concern with medical prices. Medicare paid hospitals according to their costs, and physicians were paid on a fee-for-service basis. Medicaid paid hospitals and physicians fee for service.

Regulatory policies at both the state and federal levels, enacted at the behest of provider groups, led to greater market inefficiency. Restrictions were imposed on any form of advertising, on the tasks different health professionals were permitted to perform, on entry by new hospitals and free-standing outpatient surgery centers into hospital markets, on requiring HMOs to be not-for-profit, and on which health care providers would be eligible for payment under Medicare, Medicaid, and even BlueCross and BlueShield.

Neither patients nor physicians had any incentive to be concerned with the use or cost of services. Comprehensive health insurance results in a "moral hazard" problem; patients use more services because their insurance has greatly reduced the price they have to pay. The additional benefit of using more services is much lower than if the patient had to pay more of the cost. Figure 20.1 illustrates how payment for medical services has changed since 1960. Private insurance and government currently pay for most medical services; out-of-pocket payments by patients have declined from almost 50 percent of total medical expenditures to just over 10 percent. Furthermore, physicians, because they are paid on a fee-for-service basis, have a financial incentive to provide more services

Figure 20.1: Trends in Payment for Medical Services, 1960–2005

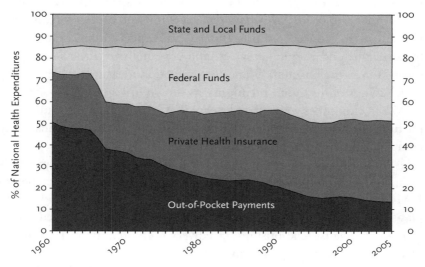

Note: The private health insurance category includes other private funds.

Source: Centers for Medicare & Medicaid Services, Office of the Actuary, National Health Statistics Group. 2007. [Online information.] http://www.cms.hhs.gov/NationalHealthExpendData/.

("supplier-induced demand"). Given the lack of patient and provider incentives to be concerned with the cost and use of services, "too many" services were provided; wide variations in care occurred because reasons other than clinical value were used in deciding on the services provided; and rapid increases occurred in the growth of medical spending.

To control rapidly rising medical costs during the late 1960s to the early 1980s, federal and state governments used regulatory approaches. The medical sector was placed under wage and price controls from 1971 to 1974, health-planning legislation placed controls on hospital investment, many states used hospital rate regulation, and Medicare instituted hospital utilization review and limited physicians' fee increases. Medicaid simply reduced payments to hospitals and physicians. These regulatory approaches failed to limit rising medical costs.

Managed Care

Managed care was the reaction of large employers against a medical care system that was out of control and had resulted in rapidly rising health insurance premiums. Under pressure from large employers and unions, health insurers and providers became adversaries. Health plans negotiated price discounts with providers and instituted cost-containment measures that reduced use of services (gatekeepers, prior authorization for specialist and hospital services, and covering care in less-expensive settings than the hospital). These cost-reduction measures achieved very large savings in insurance premiums, as shown in Figure 19.3.

When employees were offered a choice of health plans and had an opportunity to save on their monthly premiums, they switched plans. Price competition penalized higher-cost plans.

A backlash against managed care and its cost-containment methods occurred by the end of the 1990s. As more low-risk low users switched to HMOs for lower premiums, those remaining in traditional indemnity plans, patients with chronic illnesses and those with established physician and specialist relationships, faced very high premiums. They joined HMOs to reduce their premiums and were very dissatisfied with restrictions on access to their providers. The backlash against managed care was likely driven by those forced to join HMOs.

Managed care was, at most, a partial example of market competition. Although managed care competition achieved large private-sector cost savings for a limited time, much of the previous regulatory and economic framework under which competition occurred was unchanged. Any framework includes a set of consumer and supplier incentives. Market performance responds to these incentives. When, as a result of these incentives, consumers and suppliers consider the full costs and benefits of their decisions, market outcomes will be efficient. At times, however, the legal and economic framework within which consumers and producers make their choices distorts their costs and benefits, in which case markets perform inefficiently.

Following are examples of how the medical care market's legal and economic framework has distorted consumer and producer incentives, hence their choices, leading to inefficient market outcomes.

DEMAND-SIDE MARKET FAILURES
Tax-Exempt Employer-Paid Health Insurance
When an employer purchases health insurance on behalf of employees, these contributions are not considered taxable income to the employee. Compared with other employee purchases paid for with after-tax income, the purchase of insurance is subsidized; employees do not pay the

full price of their insurance as they would if they had to buy the same amount with after-tax income. When the price of a good or service is reduced, consumers will purchase an increased quantity of that service (known as the *law of demand*).[2] The price of insurance, when purchased by the employer, is not the same for all employees. Those in the highest income tax brackets receive the largest tax subsidies. On average, changes in the out-of-pocket price of health insurance result in an approximate proportional change in the quantity demanded of insurance. (A 5 percent decrease in price leads to about a 5 percent increase in the quantity demanded of health insurance.[3])

The tax subsidy for health insurance results in employees purchasing more comprehensive health insurance coverage with fewer deductibles and cost sharing (and additional benefits such as vision and dental care) than they would if they had to pay the entire premium themselves.

Consumer incentives have been distorted because they do not pay the full cost of health insurance or of their use of medical services. When consumers pay only a small fraction of the provider's price out of pocket, they are less aware of and concerned with the prices charged by medical providers.

Health Plan Choices

Health plan competition could have been stronger for several reasons. First, many employers limited their employees' choice to only one health plan.[4] For competition to occur among plans, employees must be offered a choice. Yet almost 80 percent of insured employees were offered only one health plan (Marquis and Long 1999). When employees are unable to choose among substitutes, the single plan being offered has less incentive to respond to employees' preferences or to lower prices.

---

2. Not every consumer necessarily purchases more when the price is reduced but, on average, there will be an increase in the quantity demanded of that product.

3. The tax exclusion for employer-purchased health insurance is unfair because employees in a higher tax bracket receive a greater subsidy (Figure 6.2). It is also unfair to individuals who are not part of an employer group; they do not qualify for the tax exclusion. Individual coverage is more expensive, not only because of higher marketing costs and insurer concern with adverse selection, but also because it is paid for with after-tax dollars.

4. Many small and medium-sized businesses were unable to offer their employees a choice of health plans; the indemnity plan was concerned that it would receive a higher-risk group. Thus, small businesses were typically offered only one plan for all of their employees.

Second, many employers offering their employees a choice of health plans either contribute more to the more expensive health plan or contribute a fixed *percentage* of the premium to the plan chosen by the employee. A fixed-percentage contribution provides a greater dollar subsidy to the more expensive plan, thereby decreasing the employee's incentive to choose the less-costly health plan. (If the employer pays 80 percent, the employee choosing the more expensive plan pays only 20 percent of the price difference, not 100 percent.) The more efficient health plan is at a competitive disadvantage because the more expensive competitor is more heavily subsidized.

When employees are offered a choice of plans, and the employer pays a fixed-dollar contribution to the chosen plan, most employees will select a more restrictive plan such as an HMO. "For example, 70–80 percent of active employees and dependents covered by the University of California, CalPERS, and Wells Fargo in California choose HMOs" (Enthoven and Tollen 2005, W5-429). (Each organization makes a fixed-dollar contribution.)

Third, when competing managed care plans offer broad networks with overlapping providers, the plans are not sufficiently differentiated and do not offer employees real choices. Overlapping provider networks make it difficult for the plan to control costs (because it cannot exclude providers) and for employees to observe quality differences. The plans are not competing on their ability to manage care, on the quality of their providers, or on patient satisfaction and have little incentive to invest resources to do so, as all plans with the same providers will benefit. Consumers should be able to choose among health plans that vary in their premiums, quality of care, access to providers, provider network, and so on.

Fourth, few employers pay insurers "risk-adjusted" premiums for their employees. Paying the same premium for an employee who is older and has more risk factors than a younger employee with less likelihood of incurring a large medical expense provides the insurer with an incentive to engage in risk selection by seeking out younger employees. Paying risk-adjusted premiums provides an insurer with an incentive to compete on price for higher-risk employees. Insurers would then also have to compete on how well they can manage the care of high-risk enrollees, rather than on which insurer can entice lower-risk employees to join their plans.

Lack of Information

Historically, health care providers have been opposed to being compared with one another. The FTC's antitrust suit against the American Medical

Association, affirmed by the U.S. Supreme Court in 1982, concerned the association's prohibitions on advertising. A consumer seeking information on a provider's prices and quality was unable to find it. Lack of information on how good a substitute one competitor is for another enables each competitor to charge higher prices or produce lower quality of care than if consumers were informed on the prices and quality of both.

One of the tenets of a competitive market is not only that consumers bear the cost of their choices, but also that they are informed purchasers. If consumers do not have access to information on provider quality, providers have little incentive to invest in higher-quality care, as they receive the same fee as those who do not.

In more recent years, quality and patient satisfaction measures on providers have been collected and disseminated in report cards to employees when they choose their health plans. One recent study found that after the publication of a report card, surgeons with the highest mortality rates were much more likely than other surgeons to retire or relocate (Jha and Epstein 2006).

Tax subsidies for purchasing health insurance have led to a demand for more comprehensive insurance—with lower out-of-pocket payments, limited choice of health plans, and larger employer subsidies for more expensive health plans—and have lessened consumer incentives to choose more efficient health plans. Subsidies and a lack of choice, combined with a lack of information on health plans and providers, have resulted in a medical care market where purchasers have insufficient incentives and limited opportunity to make informed choices.

Medicare and Medicaid

Almost half of all medical expenditures are made by federal and state governments. Incentives for those beneficiaries and Medicare and Medicaid's provider payment policies have a similarly important effect on the market's performance. Most Medicare beneficiaries have supplementary health insurance to cover their Medicare cost-sharing requirements. Because low-income persons are covered by Medicaid, there is no cost sharing. Thus, neither Medicare nor Medicaid beneficiaries have any incentive to be concerned with provider prices or their use of medical services.

Although Medicare allows beneficiaries a choice of health plans, the aged have little financial incentive to choose lower-cost, restrictive plans. Only if Medicare were to provide a fixed-dollar contribution, with the aged paying the additional cost of a more expensive health plan, would beneficiaries have an incentive to switch from the more costly, traditional fee-for-service Medicare plan. Medicaid enrollees are not provided with a choice of health plans. Instead, Medicaid may enroll some of its (young, low-cost) enrollees in a health plan, but most Medicaid expenditures on behalf of the aged and disabled are paid on a fee-for-service basis to hospitals, physicians, and nursing homes.

These market failures on the demand side have limited the expansion of more competitive managed care firms.

SUPPLY-SIDE MARKET FAILURES
Provider Consolidation
The greater the number of health care providers in a market, the greater the competition among them to respond to purchaser demands. Conversely, when only one provider is available in a market, the patient has no choice but to go to that provider. Providers respond when the purchaser has a substitute provider to choose from. A monopolist provider has no incentive to innovate, improve quality, respond to patients' needs, or offer lower prices.

A great deal of provider consolidation has been occurring. Insurers have fewer hospitals to negotiate with when hospitals merge in a market. The antitrust laws are meant to prevent suppliers, such as hospitals and physicians, from gaining market power. Unfortunately, the FTC has been unsuccessful in preventing hospital mergers that decrease competition. Federal judges, ruling in the merged hospitals' favor, believed merged not-for-profit hospitals would not exercise their market power as for-profit hospitals would. Consolidation of hospitals and single-specialty groups currently dominate certain markets (Nichols et al. 2004). Only recently has the FTC been successful in winning an antitrust suit against a nonprofit hospital merger that occurred years earlier.

As the number of competitors has declined, health plans have been forced to pay higher prices, which are passed on to consumers in the form of higher insurance premiums.

State Regulations
The states have enacted a number of anticompetitive regulations that limit price competition and result in higher health insurance premiums. These regulations address such areas as the training of health professionals and the tasks they are permitted to perform, entry into medical

markets, pricing of health insurance policies, health insurance benefit coverage, and rules covering provider networks.

More than 1,800 state mandates have been enacted that specify the benefits, population groups, and health care providers that must be included in health insurance policies. Large business firms are legally exempt from these state mandates when they self-insure their employees, which most large firms do. The higher cost burden of these state mandates falls predominantly on smaller businesses and individuals, raising the cost of insurance and thereby making health insurance unaffordable to those who prefer less-expensive health plans. Although some of these state mandates may be beneficial, many small businesses and individuals would prefer to have insurance they can afford rather than no insurance at all.

Many states regulate health insurance premiums charged to small businesses and individuals. *Community rating* includes all types of small businesses or individuals in a common risk pool, and all are charged the same premium. Firms whose employees are engaged in high-risk jobs are charged the same as those with employees who have low-risk jobs. Firms who provide incentives to employees to engage in healthy lifestyles are charged the same premium as others. Community rating eliminates price competition among insurers. Instead, insurers have an incentive to engage in favorable risk selection. Community rating increases the price of insurance to low-risk individuals, thereby leading many to drop their insurance.

CON laws prohibit competitors from entering a market. A CON protects existing providers from competition, thereby providing the existing hospital, home health agency, hospice, and nursing home with monopoly power.

Training of health professionals emphasizes process measures of quality as a prerequisite for licensure. Reexamination for relicensure is not used, and physicians are rarely evaluated on outcomes-based measures of quality. Innovative methods of training health professionals are inhibited when rigid professional rules specify training requirements. The *tasks health professionals are permitted to perform* are specified in state practice acts, based on political competition by different health associations over which profession is permitted to perform certain tasks. A greater supply of health manpower can be achieved and care can be produced in a less-costly manner when performance is monitored and flexibility is permitted in the tasks health professionals are qualified to perform.

Any-willing-provider (AWP) laws limit price competition among physicians (and dentists). Health plans were able to negotiate large price discounts from physicians by offering them exclusivity over their enrollees. The AWP laws enable any physician to have access to a health plan's enrollees at the negotiated price. As a result of AWP laws, physicians have no incentive to compete on price for a health plan's enrollees because they cannot be assured of a greater volume of patients in return for a lower price.

Lack of Physician Information

Competitive markets assume that both demand-side and supply-side participants are well-informed. Physicians, who act as the patient's agent and as a supplier of a service, are considered to be knowledgeable regarding their patient's diagnosis and treatment. Furthermore, the physician is assumed to act in the patient's best interest. If these assumptions are incorrect, medical services are not being provided efficiently, quality of care may be inappropriate, and the cost of medical services is higher than it would otherwise be.

Wide variations exist in the medical services provided by physicians in the same specialty, to patients with the same diagnosis, and across different geographic regions (Wennberg, Fisher, and Skinner 2002). These variations in medical services are likely attributable to two reasons. First, physicians are not equally proficient in their diagnostic ability and in their knowledge of the latest treatment methods. These wide variations have given rise to evidence-based medicine, whereby large insurers analyze large data sets to determine best practices and disseminate clinical guidelines to their network physicians.

Second, physicians have a financial interest in the quantity and type of care they provide. Most physicians are paid fee for service; thus, the more they do, the more they earn. Supplier-induced demand is the term economists use to explain physicians' financial incentive to increase their services. When combined with the lack of consumer incentives regarding prices and use of medical services and their lack of knowledge regarding physicians' practice methods, both the use and cost of medical services are greatly increased.

Medicare, where most aged have supplementary insurance to cover their cost sharing, is a prime example of how lack of patient price sensitivity and medical information, together with some physicians' own lack of knowledge and the incentives inherent in fee for service, have resulted in very large variations in both the cost and number of services provided to the aged.

Based on the preceding discussion, it is clear that market forces have been greatly weakened. Given the lack of effective market competition in medical markets, one cannot claim that competition has been tried and has failed.

HOW CAN MEDICAL MARKETS BE MORE COMPETITIVE?

Markets always exist but, depending on government rules, they can be efficient or inefficient. To improve market efficiency in medical care, several changes are needed in government regulations and in the private sector.

Government tax policy that excludes employer-paid health insurance from an employee's taxable income should be changed. Employer contributions should be treated as regular income; however, it would be more politically feasible to limit the amount that is tax free. This change will affect how much insurance consumers buy, their choice of health plans, and how much medical care they use. Additional needed government reforms include removing restrictions on market entry and on laws promoting anticompetitive behavior, such as CON and AWP laws; overriding state mandates that increase health insurance costs; eliminating state insurance regulations requiring community rating; enforcing antitrust laws; and reforming Medicare and Medicaid so that beneficiaries pay the additional cost of more expensive health plans, thereby giving these beneficiaries incentives to choose health plans based on their costs and benefits.[5] These policies should stimulate greater competition in both the private and public medical sectors.

With regard to the private sector, employers who subsidize their employees' health insurance should be encouraged to offer a choice of health plans, to give fixed-dollar contributions, and to use risk-adjusted premiums in making such payments. With more plan choices and employee

---

5. Recent unsuccessful legislative proposals seeking to lower insurance premiums in the individual and small-group markets included permitting "association health plans," which allow organizations, such as nonemployer groups, ethnic organizations, and small business associations, to form and negotiate with insurers on behalf of their members; these associations would have a more stable insurance pool as well as greater bargaining power with insurers. Furthermore, legislation permitting insurers to sell their products across state lines would enable them to bypass costly state mandates in those states requiring them.

incentives to be concerned with the cost as well as benefits of a health plan, information will become more available to help employees make choices. When consumers can choose, information has a value, and private sources will develop to provide it, as occurs in other markets.

In competitive markets, not all purchasers have to be informed or switch in response to changes in prices and quality for suppliers to respond and for markets to perform efficiently.[6] In competitive medical markets, as in other markets, the more responsive purchasers and suppliers drive the market toward greater efficiency.

WHAT MIGHT COMPETITIVE MEDICAL MARKETS LOOK LIKE?

If medical care markets were to become more like a competitive market, what might one observe? As consumers (and Medicare and Medicaid enrollees) have to pay the additional cost of more expensive health plans and become more cost conscious, the variety and number of plan choices will increase; plans will attempt to match purchasers' preferences and willingness to pay. Some people would prefer choosing among health plans, which is less "costly" than choosing and evaluating different providers.

Competitive markets might evolve in several ways. Integrated delivery systems, as articulated by Enthoven (2004), are organizations with their own provider networks that offer enrollees coordinated care. These integrated delivery systems might be built around large multispecialty medical groups with relationships to hospitals, as well as other care settings, and be paid a risk-adjusted annual capitation amount per enrollee. Health plans would compete for consumers on the basis of risk-adjusted premiums. These systems would select health care providers, be responsible for monitoring quality, examine large data sets to develop evidence-based medicine guidelines, reduce widespread variations in physicians' practice patterns, provide coordinated care for patients across different care settings (the physician's office, hospital, ambulatory care facilities, and the patient's home), have incentives to innovate in caring for patients with chronic conditions, and minimize total treatment costs, not just the costs of providing care in one setting while shifting costs to other settings. In addition, health plans would be responsible for evaluating new

---

6. In some markets, such as rural areas, competition among health plans is unlikely to be strong enough to achieve the same efficiency as in large urban areas. Rural populations do not have the same choices with regard to other services either.

technologies and would in turn be evaluated by how well they perform in improving the health of their enrolled populations, their premiums, and patient satisfaction.

At the other end of the spectrum of financing and delivering medical services is CDHC. Under this model, consumers purchase a high-deductible (catastrophic) plan, which provides them with the incentive to be concerned with both their use of medical services and the prices of different health care providers. The HSA approach combines a high-deductible plan with a savings account; money saved in the HSA belongs to the individual and can be accumulated year after year. Relying on information (such as risk-adjusted outcomes studies on coronary artery bypass graft surgery) provided on the Internet and from other sources, consumers are responsible for their care and in turn are not restricted in their choice of providers, who are paid fee for service.

Health plans preferred by consumers will expand their market share while others will decline. Health plans and large multispecialty medical groups will have an incentive to innovate in ways that reduce costs, improve quality and treatment outcomes, and achieve greater patient satisfaction, as by doing so they will differentiate themselves from their competitors and achieve a competitive advantage. Other health plans will copy methods used by more successful competitors; the process of innovation and differentiation will then start over again. (Economist Joseph Schumpeter referred to this as the process of "creative destruction.")

ARE THE POOR DISADVANTAGED IN A COMPETITIVE MARKET?

Opponents of competitive medical care markets claim that the poor will be unable to afford medical services. Competitive markets are meant to produce the most goods and services, for a given amount of resources, that consumers are willing to buy and to sell them at the lowest possible price. By doing so, goods and services will be more affordable to those with low incomes. However, competitive markets should not be evaluated on whether the poor receive all the medical services needed.

Achieving market efficiency has little to do with ensuring that everyone's needs are met or that everyone receives the same quantity of services. It is the role of government, based on voters' preferences, to subsidize the care of the poor, just as is done with regard to food and housing programs. Providing the poor with subsidies (e.g., vouchers for a health plan) to be exercised in a competitive market is more likely than any other approach to ensure that they receive the greatest value for those subsidies.

Competitive medical markets may be considered "unfair" because those with higher incomes are able to buy more than those with lower incomes. Those who are wealthy always have, and always will, be able to buy more than the poor. Even in the Canadian single-payer health system, those with more money are able to skip the waiting lines and travel to the United States for their diagnostics and surgery.

SUMMARY

Markets are evaluated by how closely they approximate a competitive market. The closer the approximation, the more likely the market will produce products efficiently and be responsive to consumer demands. Medical markets are not inherently different from other markets in their ability to efficiently allocate resources. It is the regulatory framework of medical markets that leads to inefficient outcomes.

Medical markets differ in significant ways from competitive markets. The tax treatment of health insurance lessens consumer incentives to be concerned with the price and use of medical services. Consumers lack the necessary information to make economic and medical choices; often they are not offered choices. Competition among suppliers is limited by laws barring market entry, restricting tasks health professionals are permitted to perform, preventing price competition, and regulating market prices.

These market failures have resulted in inefficiency, inappropriate care, less-than-optimal medical outcomes, and rapidly rising medical costs. Increasing government regulation is more likely to worsen than improve market performance. Several of the major inefficiencies in medical care markets are the result of government intervention. Government regulation to limit rising medical prices was tried in the 1970s and failed. Medicare, which controls hospital and physician fees, fails to limit overuse of services and gaming of the system; "up-coding" and "unbundling" of services are common.[7] Under a system of government regulation of prices, budgets, and entry restrictions, interest groups, such as hospitals, physicians, unions, and large employers, are more effective in representing their economic interests than, and at the expense of,

---

7. Unbundling occurs when a provider charges separately for each of the services previously provided together as part of a treatment. Up-coding occurs when the provider bills for a higher-priced diagnosis or service rather than the lower-cost service actually provided.

consumers. Organized interest groups are more effective than consumers in the political marketplace. Consumer interests are best served in competitive economic markets.

Government has an important role to play. Government sets the rules for competitive markets, such as eliminating practices that result in anti-competitive behavior, monitoring inaccurate information, and enforcing antitrust laws. It is also government's responsibility to raise the funds to subsidize those unable to afford medical care; those subsidies can be provided at lower cost and higher quality in a competitive market.

Market competition has not failed in medical care; it has not had a full opportunity to work. Consumer incentives must be changed so that consumers consider the costs as well as the benefits of their choices. Medicare enrollees should be offered a choice of health plans where they pay the additional cost of a more expensive plan. And restrictions on providers' ability to compete on price should be removed. Without competition, providers have no incentive to be efficient, innovate, invest in new facilities and services, improve quality, develop best practices and clinical guidelines, or lower prices.

DISCUSSION QUESTIONS

1. Why is it said that competition in medical care has failed?

2. What are the criteria for a competitive market?

3. How well does medical care meet the criteria of a competitive market?

4. Is it the responsibility of a competitive market to subsidize care for those with low incomes?

5. What changes are required for medical care to more closely approximate a competitive market?

REFERENCES

Enthoven, A. 1993. "Why Managed Care Has Failed to Contain Health Costs." *Health Affairs* 12 (3): 27–43.

———. 2004. "Market Forces and Efficient Health Care Systems." *Health Affairs* 23 (2): 25–27.

Enthoven, A., and L. Tollen. 2005. "Competition in Health Care: It Takes Systems to Pursue Quality and Efficiency." *Health Affairs* Web exclusive, September 7, W5-420–W5-433. [Online publication; retrieved 11/15/06.] http://content.healthaffairs.org/cgi/reprint/hlthaff.w5.420v1.

Jha, A., and A. Epstein. 2006. "The Predictive Accuracy of the New York State Coronary Artery Bypass Surgery Report-Card System." *Health Affairs* 25 (3): 844–855.

Marquis, S., and S. Long. 1999. Trends in Managed Care and Managed Competition, 1993-1997." *Health Affairs* 18 (6): 75–88.

Nichols, L., P. B. Ginsburg, R. A. Berenson, J. Christianson, and R. E. Hurley. 2004. "Are Market Forces Strong Enough to Deliver Efficient Health Care Systems? Confidence Is Waning." *Health Affairs* 23 (2): 8–21.

Wennberg, J., E. Fisher, and J. Skinner. 2002. "Geography and the Debate over Medicare Reform." *Health Affairs* Web exclusive, February 13, W96–W114. [Online publication; retrieved 11/15/06.] http://content.healthaffairs.org/cgi/reprint/hlthaff. w2.96v1.

ADDITIONAL READING

Butler, S. 2004. "A New Policy Framework for Health Care Markets." *Health Affairs* 23 (2): 22–24.

Chapter 21

How Will the Internet
Change Health Care?

THE INTERNET IS still relatively new, and its applications to health care are evolving. This technology is expected to have wide-ranging effects on all sectors of the economy. However, the Internet's full potential for health care, as well as for other industry sectors, is not yet completely understood. This chapter examines four issues related to the use of the Internet in health care. First is a discussion of how an innovation such as the Internet can create economic value. Second is an analysis of the types of e-commerce health care applications that are likely to offer gains in economic efficiency. Third is a discussion of why firms that have innovated in the use of the Internet will not necessarily profit from that innovation. Fourth is a discussion of how health care providers or health plans can use the Internet to increase their market power, hence profitability.

HOW THE INTERNET CREATES ECONOMIC VALUE

An innovation creates economic value or benefits when either consumers or producers are willing to pay to have access to or use that innovation. The total amount consumers or producers are willing to spend on that innovation (less its costs) is a measure of the value of the innovation.[1]

---

1. The total value of an innovation to a purchaser is defined by the total amount the purchaser is willing to pay; the value to consumers of the last unit purchased is reflected in the price they pay for that last unit. However, the value of an innovation to purchasers may not be reflected in the total amount they actually pay for its use, as the price they pay for each unit is determined by competition to supply that innovation and by willingness to pay, which determines price. When many firms compete to provide an innovation, the price is reduced and consumers will pay less than the maximum amount they were willing to pay.

The framework of a competitive market can be used to determine how the growth of the Internet creates value. Competitive markets, in contrast to monopoly markets, are considered to be the most economically efficient markets, that is, *competitive firms produce the maximum amount of goods and services for a given amount of resources (have the lowest production costs), and the output is sold at the lowest possible price to consumers.* An important outcome of a competitive market is that prices equal costs (which include a normal profit). The extent to which prices exceed costs is an indication of a firm's market power. The higher the price–cost ratio, the greater the firm's market (monopoly) power is.

The assumptions of a competitive health care market are that consumers have perfect information regarding their diagnoses, treatment needs, prices charged, and the quality/outcomes of different providers. To the extent that the patient relies on his physician, the physician is assumed to have this information and act in the patient's best interest. Another assumption is that the service the patient purchases is homogeneous, making the information assumption even more important, as medical services are not similar across all providers. Further assumptions are that many firms are competing and no entry barriers exist, allowing new firms to enter, compete with existing firms, and offer patients greater choice. Providers are also assumed to be knowledgeable regarding how best to produce medical services, such as the appropriate technology and the productivity and wages of various personnel used in the production process.

Obviously, many of these assumptions are not met in medical markets. Wide variations exist in prices charged for the same service, in treatment methods, and in production methods, and barriers to entry exist in the various professions (Table 21.1).

When the characteristics of an actual market differ from those of a (theoretic) purely competitive market, economic efficiency can be increased if the actual market is able to more closely resemble the competitive model. Deviations from economic efficiency that lead to higher price–cost ratios can occur because of inefficiencies (deviations from the

---

In fact, some firms might for strategic reasons provide free access to the innovation, such as publishing an article on a new surgical technique or providing free access to the Internet. In these cases, the users of that innovation benefit without having to pay (and determining how much people would have been willing to pay for the innovation becomes difficult).

Table 21.1: Comparison of Competitive Markets and Medical Care Markets

	Perfectly Competitive Markets	Medical Care Markets
Homogeneous or standardized service	Yes	No
Perfect information by consumers regarding their diagnoses, treatment needs, prices charged, and quality/ outcomes of different providers	Yes	No
Ease of entry into the industry by other firms	Yes	No
Large number of competitors	Yes	Yes
Perfect information by providers on how best to produce medical services; on appropriateness of care; and on technology, wages, and productivity of different professionals	Yes	No

competitive model) on either the demand side (buyers) or the supply side of a market.[2]

An important assumption with respect to medical markets is that patients and providers have full information. The lack of information on the part of patients (and the lack of a financial incentive on the part of physicians to act in consumers' best medical and financial interests) results in higher prices, a greater variation in prices paid (by patients and providers for the supplies they purchase), and lower quality of care than

---

2. It may not be possible to bring about all the conditions that exist in a textbook example of a competitive market, such as having a large number of competitive firms, as the least-cost size of firm in relation to the size of the market may be such that only several competitors can exist. The auto industry is one such example. However, even with few competitors, intense price and quality competition can occur among firms. Typically, the largest deviations from a competitive market are caused by regulatory barriers to entry and a lack of consumer information regarding prices charged and differences in quality of competing firms. To the extent that an existing market can more closely approximate a competitive market, economic efficiency is increased.

if patients had more complete information on the prices being charged by every physician and their medical and surgical outcomes. Because that information is not readily available and the time costs spent searching for lower-priced, higher-quality providers are high, consumers may visit more costly, lower-quality providers.

To the extent that all market participants have better information, economic efficiency is improved and prices for the products and services bought by consumers and the supplies and equipment bought by firms are closer to costs. Thus, innovations that improve information to patients or providers, such as making price and quality information easily available, have an economic value to consumers. Just as a consumer looking for a new automobile is willing to pay for information that reduces her "search costs" for finding the lowest price for a particular model of car, consumers would be willing to pay for information that improves their medical knowledge, on the prices charged by medical providers, and on the quality/outcome rankings of different providers. Information produces an economic benefit for which people are willing to pay.

INTERNET HEALTH CARE APPLICATIONS THAT INCREASE BENEFITS TO CONSUMERS

Two types of improvements in economic efficiency result from the Internet. First are "business-to-consumer" Internet applications, those that improve consumer efficiency, that is, affect the demand side of the market. Second are those directed to the supply side of the market, referred to as "business-to-business" applications.

Business-to-Consumer Internet Applications

Among the earliest and most popular web sites are those providing medical information on medical symptoms, descriptions of different diseases, treatment regimens, and general health information and suggestions for prevention. This type of information is eagerly sought by those who are newly diagnosed or who have chronic illnesses, as they can find out about the latest treatments for their diseases (Wagner et al. 2005). These health-related web sites also include chat rooms to provide community support for those with a specific illness. In addition, the worried well can keep up to date with the latest health news.

Some web sites also provide evaluations of hospitals, physicians, and health plans. Performance measures provided on these web sites include, for example, rankings of hospitals within a particular city according to medical outcomes for specific types of surgery, such as the volume of heart bypass surgeries performed in a year or the hospital's mortality rate by type of surgery. Each hospital receives a number of stars based on various quality measures. Some web sites contain similar information on surgeons.

Recently, major health insurers have created web-based pricing tools to enable consumers to comparison shop among providers. Aetna, for example, listed on its web site the prices it negotiated with physicians in certain geographic areas. Consumer health care web sites are used in a number of ways:

- gaining health information, including wellness, diagnosis, and chronic care;
- evaluating physicians, hospitals, and health plans;
- finding consumer medical supplies, such as durable medical equipment;
- purchasing drugs by consumers at prescription drug sites;
- shopping for health insurance;
- shopping for medical services;
- recruiting patients for clinical trials;
- reviewing defined-contribution plans for medical services, including PPOs;
- maintaining patient medical records;
- seeking second opinions;
- communicating with patients' physicians; and
- monitoring patient medical conditions.

A consumer can find the lowest price for medical supplies, such as durable medical equipment, prescription drugs, health insurance, and even medical services, from physician visits and cosmetic surgery to in-hospital surgical procedures. These web sites enable a consumer to compare different prices and contract for services using the Internet.

Patients with particular illnesses can use the Internet to find out whether they can enroll in clinical trials evaluating experimental drugs. Some web sites offer employers and their employees an HSA, in lieu of a traditional health plan, together with a list of providers from which employees can create their own PPOs. New Internet health applications for consumers continue to be developed and include seeking medical second opinions by electronically sending medical records and x-rays to specialists, communicating with providers (making appointments and receiving test results), and having medical conditions monitored by the physician's office. Furthermore, some web sites maintain patients' medical records online; ready access to these records by a physician could instantly supply a person's blood type, allergies, prescribed drugs, and past treatments, which could save the patient's life in a medical emergency.

These Internet applications have developed because they provide value to consumers. Many of these web sites have an important feature in common: They lower the consumer's/patient's search costs by providing information.

In purchasing services buyers incur certain search costs, which, in addition to the price paid, increase their cost of the transaction. Search costs typically incurred by purchasers include gathering information about the prices, service characteristics, and reputations of different providers/sellers, as well as out-of-pocket expenses such as transportation costs, telephone calls, and newspaper and magazine subscriptions. An important component of these search costs is the opportunity cost of the buyer's time spent searching, time that could have been spent working or being with family. It is rational from a cost-benefit perspective to continue searching for lower prices/higher quality as long as the savings/benefits, in terms of lower prices/increased quality, resulting from the search are greater than the additional costs of searching. Compared with visiting libraries or specialists, patients can save time by using the Internet to learn about alternative treatment methods for a particular diagnosis.

Lower search costs lead to lower prices; buyers can more easily comparison shop and find lower-cost sellers of given quality that more closely match their needs, resulting in an increase in economic efficiency, particularly when services are standardized or more homogeneous. Even in markets in which products and services are not standardized, such as open-heart surgeries or physician services, easier access to information on provider characteristics, quality rankings, and prices will result in a smaller variation in prices and quality rankings. It becomes more difficult for lower-quality, higher-priced providers to survive when purchasers have good information on competitive providers.

Not all purchasers need be well-informed for providers to compete on price and quality. In most markets, such as electronics, many consumers are not familiar with prices charged by different sellers or the quality of their products and services. A sufficient number of informed purchasers, however, will cause sellers to compete for their business, benefiting the remainder of the purchasers who are not as well-informed. Business will be shifted to higher-quality providers, increasing the average level of quality. As long as the seller must provide the same product and service to both informed and uninformed purchasers, those who are less informed also benefit. By increasing information, the Internet increases the number of informed purchasers. Online comparison shopping reduces supplier market power. Intense price competition among suppliers reduces their profits, as the lower prices are passed on to consumers.

Price dispersion results from imperfect information. Even when products are homogeneous, when consumers must incur search costs, prices will vary. The more frequent the purchase, the greater are the savings. Therefore, it pays for consumers to search more for repeated purchases. For example, prices for repeatedly purchased prescriptions (for which the expected benefits of search are highest) exhibit significant reductions in both price dispersions and supplier price–cost margins.

Quality competition would also be expected to increase as information regarding surgical outcomes of different hospitals becomes readily available on the Internet. Purchasers have greater choice when the Internet provides information on prices, quality, outcomes, accessibility, and so on for providers and health plans over a wider geographic area.

Lower search costs also enable new markets to develop. For example, lower search costs can enable patients in overseas markets to find specialists in the United States for particular medical and surgical treatments. U.S. specialists can also provide second opinions for overseas patients as transmitting data via the Internet becomes feasible and less costly. Similarly, U.S. patients can search the Internet for medical services in other areas, such as India or Europe.

The use of the Internet in medical care benefits consumers in a variety of ways. Some consumers may receive lower prices, some will have more choices, and many will benefit from easier access to health information.

Business-to-Business Internet Applications

The Internet and e-commerce can increase efficiency for both providers and health plans, while also improving patient care, in several ways.

The development of online markets, or exchanges, can reduce the search costs associated with finding suppliers of medical supplies, equipment, and so on. The search costs for hospital purchasing agents, for example, are greatly reduced by using online medical supply exchanges. These purchasing agents can quickly find suppliers and in general reduce their time costs by decreasing negotiations, particularly when the medical supplies and equipment can be easily standardized.

Negotiation occurs over product specifications and prices. The transaction costs of ordering, billing, making arrangements for transportation, and other factors must also be considered. E-commerce reduces the cost of procurement before, during, and after the transaction. Before the transaction, e-commerce lowers the costs of searching for suppliers or buyers and making price and product comparisons. These search costs can be particularly high for small purchases or sales. During the transaction, e-commerce reduces the costs of communicating, such as the need for travel, meetings, and paperwork. After the transaction, e-commerce reduces the costs of monitoring performance, confirming delivery, updating inventory, maintaining accounting records, and so on. The potential savings are very large. In short, online markets can reduce operating costs.

The availability of Internet supply exchanges for such items as medical supplies, drugs, and equipment enables providers to easily shop for the best price. These exchanges also enable providers with a small volume of patients to receive savings comparable to those of larger purchasers, reducing the scale advantages of providers with larger volumes.

Increased Internet connectivity among different providers and health plans, as well as with government agencies, should reduce provider and health plan transaction costs.[3] For example, any treatment prescriptions can be entered on the patient's electronic medical record, and this entry would generate requests for referrals, if necessary, as well as generate a claim for payment. Furthermore, increased government regulations related to patient care and government payment have required increases in staffing and paperwork to ensure compliance. These regulations can also be programmed on the patient's electronic medical record and claims payment to ensure that treatment patterns, referrals, payment, and so on are in compliance with the regulations. Providers would be immediately notified if certain actions did not conform with regulations. This interconnectivity will reduce costs by reducing staffing as well as fraud and abuse that may result from inadequate compliance with numerous regulations.

---

3. Walker and colleagues (2005) estimate that yearly savings of $77 billion are possible once a health care information exchange has been established and there is interoperability among providers (hospitals and medical groups), laboratories, pharmacies, and payers.

The Internet also offers promise for improving patient care by enabling physicians to better manage their patients' care. Large amounts of individual patient data can be stored online. When prescribing a drug, for example, and entering the prescription into a patient's medical record, the new prescription can be checked automatically against a large database of patients with similar medical conditions and combinations of drugs. As a result of software programs searching through large numbers of medical records and prescriptions, a physician can be immediately informed that a new drug he is prescribing may be in conflict with another drug that a patient is taking for a different chronic illness.

Inappropriate prescribing can cause patient deaths. For several reasons, many prescriptions currently require a call from the pharmacist to the physician. Both quality and cost control will be increased through Internet drug databases.

Similarly, with large data sets available online a physician can immediately receive likely results of prescribed treatments for patients with similar characteristics. The probable effects of a prescribed treatment would be presented so the physician could compare those likely outcomes to other prescribed treatments.

By having access to a patient's medical record online, different physicians will be able to determine which tests the patient has received. Previously, different specialists seen by the patient repeated tests because they did not have ready access to such information. Unnecessary duplication of tests will be eliminated.

Coordination of care will also be improved. Scheduling of tests, referrals, prescribed treatment, and follow-up services can all be accomplished automatically as the Internet connects all providers and is able to access their schedules. Patient reminder notices can also be prearranged. The primary care physician would receive results from all of a patient's providers, and follow-up appointments would be scheduled.

Patients with chronic illnesses can be better monitored through use of a combination of instruments such as monitoring devices that are connected to phone lines. This would enable continuous or frequent monitoring without the necessity of a physician visit. Data could be compared electronically to determine whether a nurse should contact the patient (possibly via the patient's interactive television) if certain monitoring signs deviate from a particular pattern.

PROFIT POTENTIAL OF HEALTH CARE INTERNET FIRMS

Although an innovation may create value to both consumers and suppliers within a market, innovative firms may not be able to capture that value in the form of increased profits. The effects of innovation in a market may be different from the effects on an innovative firm. Firms that introduce innovation and increase the efficiency of an industry do not necessarily become very profitable. If other firms can easily enter and provide a similar service, and the initial firm cannot differentiate itself from its competitors, intense price competition will occur and none of the firms will be able to sustain high profits.

Two types of Internet firms have arisen: those that establish an online market or exchange and those that offer a particular service such as information.

Internet Markets or Exchanges

Although online markets have few barriers to entry, eventually only one or two firms are likely to control online markets in each product or service category. Online markets are subject to economies of scale, which result from the fact that creating an Internet market involves primarily fixed costs, while the costs of adding market participants are close to zero. More important, online markets have "network" effects, that is, online markets with a large number of users will attract even more users. Having large numbers of users within an online market facilitates sharing of information with other users and allows for a greater variety of interests to be accommodated. Furthermore, as the number of users/buyers in a market increases, a larger number of sellers will also be attracted to those markets. Thus, both buyers and sellers have an incentive to trade on the highest-volume online markets or exchanges. Fewer online markets, hence greater concentration of such exchanges, are therefore likely to exist in each product/service market.

Innovative firms that have started an online market have found that survival is difficult if they cannot attract the major buyers and sellers to their marketplaces. To create a successful exchange, such as for hospital equipment, the Internet firm organizing that market must sign up both a large number of buyers (hospitals) and a majority of the suppliers. Unless the exchange can deliver both the purchasing power and the suppliers, neither group will be willing to rely on the exchange for its business. If an exchange does not have the participation of all or most of the suppliers of the service, transaction cost savings are limited, as the purchasers must seek other, nonparticipating suppliers.[4]

The ownership of online exchanges, particularly supply-type exchanges such as medical supplies and equipment, has evolved so that the major suppliers have started their own exchanges. These large suppliers have allied to establish their own supply exchanges (business to business) rather than merely participating with a new Internet company that would perform the function. Such exchanges have occurred in the automobile, airline, hospital supply, and health insurance industries.

An independent exchange is viable when no large buyers or sellers have significant market power. When several buyers or sellers do have a large market share, they can harm an independent exchange by refusing to participate. Because buyers/sellers want to participate in those exchanges that have the largest number of sellers/buyers, firms with large market shares are likely to join together to start their own exchange. Thus, the market structure of an industry will determine whether an independently established exchange is likely to survive.

Only when many small buyers and sellers exist can an independent firm maintain an online exchange. In these cases, the participation of any single buyer or seller is not important to the success of the exchange.

Internet Services

Internet firms that provide a particular service, such as medical information, have found earning a profit difficult because other organizations are willing to provide the same service for free. For example, health information web sites are among the most popular sites visited by consumers. Consumers would be willing to pay for access to health information, but well-known medical institutions, such as the Mayo Clinic and The Johns Hopkins medical school, have initiated their own health information web sites and offer them free of charge. These organizations use their Internet web sites as complements to the medical services for which they charge; their Internet sites are a form of advertising to attract patients to their medical institutions. Stand-alone Internet information sites have difficulty generating revenues other than advertising dollars.

---

4. Many suppliers/buyers are reluctant to join an exchange because they believe they have established relationships with purchasers/suppliers. These suppliers/buyers believe they could receive more favorable terms as a result of these relationships.

An additional problem for Internet firms is that the timing of new e-commerce products/processes is very important to their success. Most agree that physicians, hospitals, health plans, and pharmacies should be electronically connected. Medical care can be coordinated, costs reduced, and quality increased. However, if physicians are reluctant to use such electronic processes, firms providing such connectivity links are unlikely to become profitable for some time.

THE INTERNET AND HEALTH CARE FIRMS' STRATEGIC RESPONSE

Providing price information to purchasers has forced suppliers to reduce their prices; their markups have declined. The Internet has increased price competition among firms. When firms offer undifferentiated products and services, purchasers choose products or services based solely on price. When firms compete solely on price, they must become as efficient as possible; otherwise, more efficient firms can undercut their prices. Firms that compete solely on price are typically less profitable than firms that are able to differentiate themselves from their competitors. The strategic issue facing health care providers and health plans is how they can escape from what would otherwise become a very price-competitive environment.

Competitive advantage for a firm comes from (1) increasing operational efficiency, or having lower costs relative to competitors, and (2) differentiating products or services so consumers are willing to pay more for what they perceive as a higher-valued product.

The Internet can increase a firm's operational efficiency through on-line exchanges that enable it to purchase supplies and other products at lower prices, through electronic processing of claims, through better patient care management, and through greater coordination of patient care. Competitive pressures will force health care firms to use the Internet and e-commerce to increase operational efficiency.

If a firm is to become profitable, however, it must be able to differentiate itself from its competitors. Every firm strives to be able to have a high markup over its costs. The extent to which price exceeds cost is an indication of a firm's market (monopoly) power. The higher the price–cost ratio, the greater is the firm's market power. Some firms are able to have a high markup because few good substitutes (real or imagined) are available to the consumer. For example, a firm may be the only producer of a product because barriers prevent other firms from entering that industry, as occurs with a new, patented prescription drug.

Internet technology offers health care firms a way of differentiating themselves. When it becomes "costly" for patients to switch health care providers, perhaps because they already have a relationship with a particular provider, these "switching costs" differentiate their providers from competing providers. The patient does not view these competing providers as being a good substitute for her own provider. If a provider or health plan can create switching costs, it has market power and can charge more than its competitors.

Internet technology can create switching costs by providing customized information and services to patients, and it allows individual consumers to be identified and tracked both within an online web site and across web sites. Similar to programs that create customer loyalty (hence switching costs), such as frequent-flyer programs, Internet technology can provide consumers with customized information and services based on their individual preferences.

Using profiles of consumers and patients with similar likes and dislikes, consumers can be provided with health information on topics in which they are interested as well as appointment scheduling, reminders about annual tests, updates on drug interactions for their medicines, diet programs and recipes, the latest information on advances in treatment for their conditions, chat rooms for their illnesses, prescription renewals, "ask-the-physician" features by specialty, health risk appraisals, advice on how to reduce various risk factors, and information regarding preferred health plans or provider groups at open enrollment time. The patient can be provided with his medical records online, and records can be automatically updated with the latest information. The Internet enables a provider or health plan to personalize information and services to patients and enrollees.

The physician's manner of communicating with the patient, quality of care, and reputation are important in health care. The Internet enables a provider or health plan to personalize its relationships with patients/enrollees. The firm (health plan, hospital, or physician group) is able to respond quickly, through the Internet, to patient concerns.

By customizing services to the patient, the provider or health plan is able to provide the patient or enrollee with additional value. These services tie the patient or enrollee to the organization providing them. If the patient or enrollee leaves the provider/health plan, she will lose these services. Although other organizations may provide similar services, the patient/enrollee would have to take the time to provide the new organization with all of her information and learn to navigate a new system.

The organization providing its patients/enrollees with such customized services has increased patients' switching costs. The higher the switching costs, the lower is the patient's/enrollee's price sensitivity. Brand loyalty is created, providing the organization with market power that enables it to increase its prices.

The aged, who are heavy users of medical services, are also heavy users of the Internet. The Internet can be used to reach this growing population group and, by providing them with customized Internet services, tie them to the organization.

The Internet should be an integral part of a health care firm's strategy. Rather than forcing organizations to engage in intense price competition with other health plans, hospitals, or physician groups, the Internet can instead be used by the health care firm to differentiate itself from its competitors by providing its enrollees or patients with additional value.

SUMMARY

The Internet reduces search costs by providing the buyer with a wide range of choices over a wide geographic region. Reducing search costs lowers prices and decreases their variation. Lower search costs increase the competitiveness of an industry.

When economic efficiency in a market is increased, value is increased to either consumers or firms. Consequently, those who benefit from increased efficiency should be willing to pay for this increased value. The innovating firm, however, may not be able to profit from creating this value. Capturing the profit from innovation depends on (1) how easily other firms can replicate the organization's innovation and (2) whether the organization can charge for the service. For example, web sites offering health information cannot charge a price as long as other organizations are willing to provide the same service for free.

Traditional companies were slow to use the Internet as part of their company strategies. As traditional companies are able to incorporate Internet technology, however, stand-alone Internet companies will lose any competitive advantage they once had over traditional companies. Competition between firms is based on more than price, which is what the Internet has emphasized. Firms also compete on service, reputation, product choices, and other characteristics to differentiate themselves from their competitors. "Most buyers will value a combination of online services, personal services, and physical locations over stand-alone Web distribution. They will want a choice of channels, delivery options, and ways of dealing with companies" (Porter 2001, 78).

In the Internet marketplace, where search costs have been greatly reduced, greater price and quality competition are likely among health care providers and health plans. The challenge for firms in a very competitive industry is to learn how to decrease their customers' reliance on price when choosing providers (or health plans). If price competition can be reduced, the firm has greater flexibility in setting its prices, thereby increasing its profits.

Rather than view the Internet as a means of stimulating price competition, providers and health plans should recognize an opportunity to increase their patients'/enrollees' switching costs. The ability to individualize and customize information and services for patients/enrollees will make them more reluctant to switch firms, as they would be uncertain that a similar service would be available to them within a short period once they switched providers/health plans.

DISCUSSION QUESTIONS

1. What are the different ways the Internet can increase value to consumers and to health care providers and health plans?

2. What are the likely effects of the Internet on health care competition?

3. Why may innovative Internet firms be unable to make a profit?

4. What are network effects, and why do they occur?

5. How can health care firms (providers and health plans) use the Internet to gain a competitive advantage?

REFERENCES

Porter, M. 2001. "Strategy and the Internet." *Harvard Business Review* 79 (3): 63–78.

Wagner, T., M. Bundorf, S. Singer, and L. Baker. 2005. "Free Internet Access, the Digital Divide, and Health Information." *Medical Care* 43 (4): 415–20.

Walker, J., E. Pan, D. Johnston, J. Adler-Milstein, D. W. Bates, and B. Middleton. 2005. "The Value of Health Care Information Exchange and Interoperability." *Health Affairs* Web exclusive, January 19, W5-10–W5-18. [Online publication; retrieved 11/15/06.] http://content.healthaffairs.org/cgi/reprint/hlthaff.w5.10v1.

ADDITIONAL READINGS

Bakos, Y. 2001. "The Emerging Landscape for Retail E-Commerce." *Journal of Economic Perspectives* 15 (1): 69–80.

Lucking-Reiley, D., and D. Spulber. 2001. "Business-to-Business Electronic Commerce." *Journal of Economic Perspectives* 15 (1): 55–68.

Stigler, G. 1961. "The Economics of Information." *Journal of Political Economy* 69 (3): 213–25.

Chapter 22

U.S. Competitiveness and Rising Health Costs

ONE OF THE oft-cited reasons for controlling the rise in health care costs has been that it makes American business less competitive internationally. Automobile executives, for example, have complained that their competitors in other countries have lower health care costs per employee, enabling them to sell their products at a lower price than U.S. manufacturers.[1] After labor costs, health care is often the largest supplier to many firms. GM estimated that its employees' health care expenses were increasing faster than any other single cost incurred in producing a vehicle. Unless health care costs can be controlled, the executives claim, U.S. business will be priced out of international markets and foreign producers will increase their market share in the United States.

Do rising health costs really make U.S. industries less competitive than their foreign counterparts? To understand this controversy we must understand who actually bears the burden of higher employee medical costs—the employee, the firm, or the consumer?

---

[1]. At a meeting of the National Governors Association, former Ford Motor Company vice chairman Allan Gilmour stated that high health care costs could force Detroit automakers to invest overseas rather than in the United States to remain profitable. Ford spent $3.2 billion on health care in 2003 for 560,000 employees, retirees, and dependents. These costs added $1,000 to the price of every Ford vehicle built in the United States, up from $700 three years previously. Gilmour stated that their foreign competitors do not share these problems, and if health care costs are not controlled, investment will be driven overseas. He called on the states' governors to pass legislation to control health care costs (Mayne 2004).

WHO PAYS FOR HIGHER EMPLOYEE MEDICAL COSTS?

The market for labor is competitive. Large numbers of firms compete for different types of labor, and large numbers of employees compete for jobs. This competition among firms and employees results in a price for labor that is similar for specific types of labor. For example, if a hospital pays its nurses less than other hospitals in the area, the nurses will move to the hospital that pays the highest wages. Not all nurses have to change jobs to bring about similar pay among hospitals. Some nurses will move, and the hospital will find it difficult to replace them. The hospital will soon realize that its pay levels are below what nurses are receiving elsewhere. In reality, not all firms have the same working conditions, nor are they located next to one another. Employees are willing to accept lower pay for more pleasant conditions and require higher pay for traveling longer distances. The greater the similarity in how firms treat their employees, and the more closely they are located, the more quickly wage differences disappear.

When an employer hires an additional employee, the cost of that employee cannot exceed the value of that employee to the firm; otherwise, the firm will not profit from hiring the employee. The total cost to the firm of an employee consists of two parts: cash wages and noncash fringe benefits. The cost of hiring an additional worker is the total compensation—cash and noncash benefits—that the firm would have to pay to that employee. The employer does not care whether the employees want 90 percent of their total compensation in cash and 10 percent in noncash fringe benefits or a cash–noncash ratio of 60 to 40. The employer is only interested in an employee's total cost.

Employees working in high-wage industries typically prefer a higher ratio of fringe benefits to cash wages because of the tax advantages of having benefits purchased with pretax income. Low-wage industries typically provide their employees with few benefits; most of their compensation is in cash income. The combination of cash and noncash income reflects the preferences of employees, not employers. If an employer compensates its low-wage employees with a high proportion of fringe benefits, the employees will seek the same total compensation at another firm that pays them a higher ratio of cash wages.

What happens when the fringe benefits portion of total compensation rises sharply, as occurs when health insurance premiums increase? For example, assume that employees in a particular industry are expected to receive a 5 percent increase in compensation next year but health insurance premiums, which are paid by the employer and represent 10 percent of the employees' total compensation, are expected to rise by 20 percent. The employer is always concerned with the total cost of its employees; thus, cash wages in that industry would rise by only 3.3 percent. There is a trade-off between fringe benefits and cash wages.

If one firm in the industry paid its employees 5 percent higher wages plus the 20 percent increase in insurance premiums, that firm would have higher labor costs than all of the other firms in the industry. What are the consequences to the firm? To incur above-market labor costs the firm would either have to make less profit or increase the prices of the products it sells. If the firm were to make less profit, it would earn a lower return on invested capital. A lower return on invested capital will lead investors to move their capital to other firms in the industry, to other industries, or to other countries where they can earn a higher return. Capital knows no loyalties or geographic boundaries; it will move to receive the highest return (consistent with a given level of risk). Thus, higher labor costs cannot impose a permanently lower return to a firm; otherwise, the firm will shrink as it loses capital. The same would be true if labor costs among all firms in the industry increased and profits declined.

What if the firm or industry passes the higher labor costs on to consumers by raising its prices? As long as the firm's products have competitors, either from other firms in the industry or from manufacturers in other countries, and consumers are price sensitive to the firm's product, the firm will lose sales.[2] With lower sales, the firm will need fewer employees. Good substitutes to any firm's (or industry's) product are generally available, either from other products or other manufacturers. Thus, large price differences for the same or similar products cannot be maintained. The failure to keep prices in line with a competitor's prices will drastically reduce sales, with a consequent flight of capital from that firm or industry and a large reduction in the workforce.

As long as competition from other firms or from foreign competitors (or both) is possible and capital can move to other industries and

---

2. The following is an example of how global competitiveness affects a firm's sales and its labor costs. Delphi, a U.S. firm that sells automotive components, was forced into bankruptcy because of its high labor costs. It is attempting to emerge from bankruptcy by reducing its U.S. labor costs. The firm pays its U.S. unionized employees $27 an hour, but when health and retirement benefits are included, its labor costs rise to $65 an hour. Delphi's Asian operations are highly profitable. In China, it pays its workers about $3 an hour, about a third of which goes to medical and pension benefits (Sapsford and Areddy 2005).

countries, rising medical costs will not result in lower profits or higher prices but will be borne by employees in the form of lower cash wages.

Short-Term Effects

Although rising medical costs are typically carried by the employee in the form of lower cash wages, an employer could experience a short-term effect on its profits. Shifting the cost of health insurance back to employees is difficult in the short run. For example, if an employer did not anticipate how rapidly medical costs would increase and, perhaps because of a long-term labor agreement, the firm is unable to lower its employees' wages to compensate for the higher-than-expected medical costs, profitability could decline.

Few firms, however, have been unaware of how rapidly medical costs have been increasing. Thus, rising costs are built into labor agreements. However, medical costs could also rise less rapidly than anticipated, increasing profitability. In any case, unanticipated cost increases will be reflected in future wage agreements and would not affect profitability over time.

An Example

The following example illustrates why labor bears the burden of higher insurance premiums. Automobiles can be produced in Michigan or in the southern part of the United States. Unless the prices of cars produced in Michigan and in the South are the same, consumers will purchase the least-expensive cars, assuming their quality is similar. Unless labor costs and productivity were similar in both places, the automobile manufacturers would move their production facilities to the less-costly location to produce the car. Yet we observe that within certain industries, such as automobiles, employees' medical costs and insurance premiums are higher in Detroit than in the South. How can cars produced in the North compete with cars produced in the South?

Medical costs per employee could be higher in the North as long as northern employees' cash wages are lower. Unless total compensation per employee is the same in both places, the cars produced in different locations could not be sold at the same price and manufacturers would shift their production to the lower-cost site.

Effect of Unions

What if an industry was strongly unionized and the firms in that industry were not permitted to hire nonunion labor? Could the union then shift its higher medical costs to the firm or consumers? The extent to which a union can increase labor costs is always limited by the potential loss of its members' jobs. If U.S. manufacturers increase their prices relative to their competitors, foreign competition and price-sensitive consumers will cause them to suffer large declines in sales and profits. Even when foreign competitors are prevented from competing with U.S. manufacturers, consumers will demand fewer automobiles as prices rise, although the declines would be less than if greater competition were permitted. Firms facing decreased demands for their products would hire fewer employees. A powerful union that is willing to accept a certain loss of its members' jobs by forcing firms to raise its members' compensation would do so regardless of whether the increase was for medical benefits or wages. Thus, increased medical benefits to the union members are still at the expense of higher wages.

Figure 22.1 illustrates the effect of rising medical costs on employees' wages. After 1973, total employee compensation rose less rapidly than previously because of a slowdown in employee productivity. The difference between total compensation and wages increased as a greater portion of employees' total compensation went to pay for fringe benefits. Between 1973 and 1990, employers' contributions to their employees' health insurance premiums "absorbed more than half of workers' real (adjusted for inflation) gains in compensation, even though health insurance represented 5 percent or less of total compensation" (U.S. Congressional Budget Office 1992, 5).

Total employee compensation increased in the 1990s, reflecting increased productivity. However, wages and salaries remained relatively constant from the late 1980s until the mid-1990s, reflecting the increasing importance of health insurance and retirement plans in employee compensation. Until the mid-1990s, employees' wages rose very slowly because most of the increase in compensation went to pay for higher health and retirement benefits.

From the mid-1990s to 2000, both total employee compensation and wages greatly increased, again reflecting increased productivity. However, in contrast to the earlier period of the late 1980s to the mid-1990s, wages increased at a slightly faster rate than total compensation. The slowdown in the cost of health benefits occurred because of the growth of managed care. Cost-containment activities by managed care plans resulted in a slower growth in premiums and greater wage increases for employees (Figure 19.3).

The late 1990s, however, saw a backlash against restrictive managed care plans, with the consequence that between 2001 and 2005, total compensation once again increased faster than wages.

Figure 22.1: Inflation-Adjusted Compensation and Wages per Full-Time Employee, 1965–2005

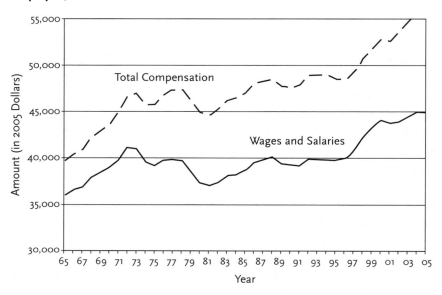

Note: Values adjusted for inflation using CPI(U).

Source: Data from the U.S. Department of Commerce, Bureau of Economic Analysis, 2006. [Online information.] http://www.bea.gov.

Rising medical costs have had a large effect on employees' take-home pay; employees have had less to spend on other goods and services. For this reason unions have been strong advocates of using government controls to limit rising health care costs.

WHO PAYS FOR RETIREE MEDICAL COSTS?

As part of their previous labor negotiations, many employers agreed to provide their employees with medical benefits when they retire in return for current wage concessions.[3] In 2005, about 21 percent of Medicare-eligible retirees in large firms (500 or more employees) were covered by

---

3. Early retirees who are not eligible for Medicare are more costly than those who are. Early-retiree health benefits cost, on average, $8,247 in 2004, whereas Medicare-eligible retirees cost firms $3,300 on average. For retirees on Medicare, the firm usually pays for the portion of the retiree's medical expenses not covered by Medicare, such as deductibles, copayments, and prescription drugs.

their employer's retiree medical plan (down from 40 percent in 1993) (Poe 2006; William M. Mercer Inc. 2005). (This survey covered employers with 500 or more employees; only about 3 percent of small firms provide their employees with retiree health benefits.)

At the time employers agreed to provide their employees with medical benefits, retiree medical costs were much lower than they are today, and employers undoubtedly underestimated how costly they could become. Instead of setting aside funds to pay these retiree obligations, as one would do with a pension obligation, firms paid their retirees' medical costs on a "pay-as-you-go" basis; that is, they paid their retirees' medical costs when they were incurred, out of current operating expenses.

Funding retiree medical costs changed as a result of a Financial Accounting Standards Board ruling that, starting in 1993, firms had to set aside funds for such benefits as they are earned. That is, retiree medical benefits must be treated similarly to pension benefits; as employees earn credit toward their retirement, the firm must set aside funds to pay for those employees' medical costs when they retire. Furthermore, the unfunded liability for current and future retirees must be accounted for on the firm's balance sheet. Firms were shocked by the size of their unfunded obligations. GM, for example, has an unfunded liability for its current and future retirees' medical costs of $77 billion (2005 data). This liability must be listed on its balance sheet, and an equivalent amount has to be deducted from the firm's net worth. GM's stockholders' equity is thereby decreased by $77 billion. In addition, GM must expense part of that liability each year. For 2005, GM's earnings had to be reduced by $5.6 billion.

How do firms like GM pay off these huge unfunded liabilities? Do they raise the prices of their products, harming U.S. competitiveness? Highly unlikely. If they raise their prices, they will lose sales to competitors, both in the United States and overseas, that did not make such commitments to their employees. Thus, U.S. competitiveness is not harmed by firms having to list unfunded retiree medical benefits on their balance sheets.

Employers also cannot reduce the wages of current employees to pay for unfunded obligations to current retirees. If they were to do so, the firm would lose its employees. The labor market is competitive. If a firm decides to reduce its employees' wages, those employees will move to firms whose retirees have not been promised medical benefits. Instead, firms are likely to use current and future profits to pay off this liability, in which case the stockholders will be the losers.

Some firms have reneged on their promises to their retirees by either reducing benefits or requiring retirees to pay part of the cost; they have tried to shift these obligations from their stockholders back to their retirees. Retirees responded by bringing lawsuits against their former employers. Court rulings, however, have generally allowed employers to reduce or eliminate the benefits for salaried, nonunion retirees, even years after they have retired. When a firm declares bankruptcy and is reorganized, it is able to reduce its obligations to its unionized employees and retirees.[4] If firms with large retiree liabilities declare bankruptcy, the stockholders, bondholders, employees, and retirees will all have to make some sacrifice for the firm to be viable again.

Rising medical costs will not directly affect U.S. competitiveness by forcing firms to increase their prices. Instead, these higher costs will be borne by the employees themselves, who will receive lower cash wages. The huge unfunded retiree medical liabilities will also not affect U.S. competitiveness, because these liabilities will not be paid off by raising prices but will be shifted to the firm's stockholders in the form of reduced equity. Do rising medical costs have any adverse effects on the economy and U.S. competitiveness?

POSSIBLE ADVERSE EFFECTS OF RISING MEDICAL COSTS ON THE U.S. ECONOMY

Rising medical costs could adversely affect the U.S. balance of trade if they were to increase the federal deficit or decrease private savings.

Increase in the Federal Deficit

The argument on the deficit is as follows. Government expenditures for Medicare and Medicaid are the fastest-increasing portion of the federal deficit. In 1970, federal spending on these two programs represented 1 percent of GDP. By 2005, spending on these programs represented 4.2 percent of GDP; this figure is expected to reach 6.2 percent by 2016. If left unchanged, these two programs will represent an increasing percentage

---

4. Another option for lowering retiree medical costs is for the firm and its union to agree to such a reduction to prevent the firm from having to declare bankruptcy, in which case the retirees, the current employees, and the firm's stockholders would likely suffer greater losses. GM's renegotiation of retiree health benefits with its union is an example of this approach (Hawkins, Boudette, and Maher 2005).

of the federal government's nonhealth spending. To fund these additional expenditures the government will have to increase its borrowing.

A higher level of government borrowing to finance a larger federal deficit will increase the value of the dollar relative to other currencies because interest rates in the United States will rise with the increased government demand for savings. In the process of moving their funds to the United States to take advantage of the higher interest rates, foreign investors will demand more dollars, which will increase their value. With a higher exchange value of the dollar, the prices of U.S.-produced goods rise and foreign goods become less expensive. As the relative prices of U.S. and foreign goods change, domestic manufacturers will sell less overseas, and imports into this country will increase as the price of foreign goods falls. American competitiveness and the trade balance will worsen.

However, the blame for the rising budget deficit need not be placed on rising medical costs. Many government programs contribute to the deficit, and many are of less value than Medicare and Medicaid. The deficit could be reduced by reducing expenditures on these other programs as well, such as farm subsidies and military projects the sole purpose of which is maintaining jobs in a community. Emphasizing medical spending as the cause of the rising federal deficit shifts attention from these other government programs and reduces the government's incentives for eliminating wasteful programs that provide less benefit than medical expenditures. Reducing expenditures on Medicare and Medicaid could also merely result in shifting these savings into expanding other or creating new government programs.

Decrease in Private Savings

The second way in which increased medical spending could adversely affect the American economy is if private savings were reduced. To finance the federal deficit the government has had to borrow, which has left less savings available for the private sector to invest in plant, equipment, and new ventures. Lower private investment eventually means lower productivity and lower real incomes. The U.S. Congressional Budget Office (1992) estimated that if federal spending on Medicare and Medicaid were limited to its 1991 share of GDP, real incomes would be 2.4 percent higher by the year 2002.

Similar to the effects of government spending, rising medical costs cause the public to spend more on medical services, decreasing the amount it has available to save. Consequently, savings in the private sector decline, as do private investments. The argument blaming the lower rate of savings on rising medical expenditures is similar to blaming the federal deficit on Medicare and Medicaid. The government could reduce the deficit by eliminating and reducing other government programs. Medicare and Medicaid are not the sole cause for large federal deficits.

It is not clear that rising medical costs decrease or increase the private savings rate. Having health insurance may reduce the need for a person to save for his medical expenses. However, medical expenses increase with age, increased out-of-pocket payments may be required, and as people live longer they will have to save for their long-term-care needs if they do not want to rely on Medicaid (and have to spend down their assets to qualify). The expectation of higher medical costs and new technology may cause people to increase their savings. The effect of rising medical expenses on savings is uncertain.

The notion that the rise in medical expenditures should be limited because it increases consumption and reduces savings for investment is also a fallacy. Some medical expenditures are in fact investments that increase productivity, such as preventive measures and certain surgical procedures that enable a person to resume normal activity. More important, if increasing the savings rate by decreasing consumption is desired, many other consumer activities—some of which are harmful, such as alcohol and cigarette consumption—should probably be reduced before limits are placed on medical spending. Many people would place a higher value on medical services than on other goods and services.

SUMMARY

It is not clear that increased medical spending has harmful effects on the economy, the budget deficit, or American competitiveness, as some have suggested. The fact that employees rather than employers bear the cost of rising health care benefits should not mean, however, that employers are absolved of the responsibility of ensuring that those funds are well-spent. As Uwe Reinhardt (1989, 20) stated:

> Even if every increase in the cost of employer-paid health care benefits could immediately be financed by the firm with commensurate reductions in the cash compensation of its employees—so that "competitiveness" in the firm's product market is not impaired—it would leave employees worse off unless the added health spending is valued at least as highly as the cash wages they would forego

[sic] to finance these benefits. Because it is the perceived value of a firm's compensation package that lures workers to the firm and away from competing opportunities, the typical business firm has every economic incentive to maximize this perceived value per dollar of health care expenditure debited to the firm's payroll expense account. Therein, and not in "competitiveness" on the product side, lies the most powerful rationale for vigorous health care cost containment on the part of the American business community.

DISCUSSION QUESTIONS

1. What determines the ratio of cash to noncash (fringe benefits) compensation that an employer will pay to its employees?

2. What are the consequences if an employer raises its prices to pay for its employees' rising medical costs?

3. How can automobile employees in Michigan receive more costly health benefits than automobile employees in the South while automobiles produced in both locations sell for the same price?

4. Even if employees bear the entire cost (in terms of lower cash wages) of rising medical costs, why should employers still be concerned with cost containment?

5. Evaluate the following statement: Rising medical costs are harmful to the economy because greater consumption expenditures on medical services result in lower savings, hence reduced private investment.

6. Evaluate the following statement: Rising Medicare and Medicaid expenditures contribute to the growing federal deficit. To finance this larger deficit the government must borrow more, which in turn increases interest rates, raises the value of the dollar, and consequently makes U.S. goods more expensive than foreign-produced goods.

REFERENCES

Mayne, E. 2004. "Ford: Health Costs Could Drive Investment Overseas." *The Detroit News*, July 20. [Online information; retrieved 12/8/06.] http://www.pnhp.org/news/2004/july/ford_health_costs_c.php.

Poe, S. L. 2006. Personal correspondence, February 23.

Reinhardt, U. E. 1989. "Health Care Spending and American Competitiveness." *Health Affairs* 8 (4): 5–21.

Sapsford, J., and J. Areddy. 2005. "Why Dephi's Asia Operations Are Booming." *The Wall Street Journal* October 17, B1.

U.S. Congressional Budget Office. 1992. *Economic Implications of Rising Health Care Costs*. Washington, DC: U.S. Congressional Budget Office.

William M. Mercer, Inc. 2005. "Health Benefit Cost Slows for a Third Year, Rising Just 6.1% in 2005." [Online information; retrieved 11/15/06.] http://www.mercerhr. com/pressrelease/details.jhtml/dynamic/idContent/1202305.

ADDITIONAL READING

Hawkins L., Jr., N. Boudette, and K. Maher. 2005. "GM, Amid Industry Overhaul, Cuts Health Benefits for Retirees." *The Wall Street Journal* October 18, A1.

Chapter 23

Why Is Getting into Medical School So Difficult?

IN 2005, ONLY 17,978 of the 37,364 students who applied to 125 medical schools in the United States were accepted, for an applicant–acceptance ratio of 2.1:1. (The number of matriculants is about 1,000 fewer because some applicants are accepted at more than one school.) The ratio, having reached a high of 2.8:1 in 1973, steadily declined to 1.58:1 in 1988, rose again in the mid-1990s, and, after declining again, has recently started increasing; in 2005 the ratio increased to 2.1:1. As shown in Figure 23.1, first-year medical school enrollments increased sharply in the early 1970s, mostly because federal legislation (the Health Manpower Training Act of 1964) gave medical schools strong financial incentives to increase their enrollments. When these federal subsidies phased out, enrollments leveled out; they have remained relatively steady since the early 1980s. However, a continual excess demand for a medical education remains.

Many qualified students are rejected each year because of the limited number of medical school spaces. Some rejected students choose to enroll in medical schools in other countries, such as Mexico. Overseas medical schools often charge higher tuition and require longer training periods than U.S. medical schools, which require four years of college before the four years of medical school. Residency training requires an additional three to seven years of graduate medical education. Unfortunately, medical education is one area in which academic excellence is not a sufficient qualification for admission to graduate or professional education. Other types of graduate-level professional education programs have experienced sharp increases in demand but not continual excess demands for admission. Although every well-qualified student who wants

Figure 23.1: Medical School Applicants and Enrollments, 1960–2005

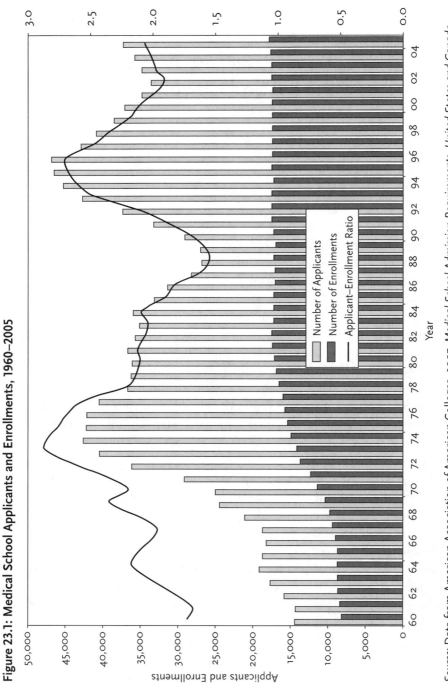

Source: Data from American Association of American Colleges. 2007. *Medical School Admission Requirements, United States and Canada,* various editions. Washington, DC: AAMC.

to become a physicist, mathematician, economist, or lawyer cannot re-alistically expect to be admitted to her first choice in graduate schools, if such students have good academic qualifications, as do most medical students, they will likely be admitted to some U.S. graduate school.[1]

MARKET FOR MEDICAL EDUCATION IN THEORY

When medicine is perceived as being relatively more attractive than other careers, demand for medical schools will increase and exceed the available number of spaces; a shortage of medical school spaces will then occur. If the market for medical education were like other markets, this shortage would only be temporary while more medical schools were built and existing schools recruited additional faculty and added physi-cal facilities to meet the increased demand. Over time, the temporary shortage would be resolved as the supply of spaces increased. Crucial in eliminating a temporary shortage is a rise in price (tuition). Increased tuition would serve to ration student demand for the existing number of spaces and provide medical schools with a financial incentive (and the funds) to invest in facilities and faculty so they could accommodate larger enrollments. Subsidies and loan programs could be made available directly to low-income students faced with higher tuition rates.

MARKET FOR MEDICAL EDUCATION IN PRACTICE

The market for medical education, however, differs from other markets. The medical education industry produces its output inefficiently (at high cost and using too many years of a student's time), and the method used to finance medical education is inequitable (large subsidies go to students from high-income families). More efficient competitors would have driven any other industry with this record out of business. How has this industry been able to survive with such poor performance?

The producers of medical education have been insulated from the marketplace. Tuition, established at an arbitrarily low level, represents less than one-third of the costs of education and approximately 10 per-cent of medical school revenues. Medical schools can maintain low tu-ition because large state subsidies and research grants offset educational costs. Tuition, being such a small fraction of educational costs and not

---

1. Medical education also differs from other graduate programs in that once accepted to medical school, a student is virtually assured of graduating. The attrition rate is approxi-mately 2 percent, compared with attrition rates of 50 percent in other graduate programs.

rising with increased demand, neither serves to ration excess demand among students nor provides an incentive to medical schools to expand their capacity. Medical schools, particularly public ones, do not depend on tuition revenue to even cover their operating expenses. Lacking a financial incentive to expand, medical schools do nothing to alleviate the temporary shortage. Instead, the shortage becomes permanent, which is a far more serious situation.

For-profit businesses respond to increased consumer demands by raising prices and increasing supplies because they want to make greater profits. New firms enter industries in which they perceive they can earn more on their investments than they can earn elsewhere. When prices are prevented from rising or barriers to new firms entering an expanding market exist, temporary shortages can become permanent. Typically, barriers to entry are legal rather than economic and protect existing firms from competition. Protected firms are able to maintain higher prices and receive above-normal profits than if new firms were permitted to enter the market.

Medical schools, being not-for-profit organizations, are motivated by more "noble" goals, such as the prestige associated with training tomorrow's medical educators. Most medical schools share the goal of having a renowned, research-oriented faculty who teach a few small classes of academically gifted students, who will be their successors as super-specialist researchers. Few, if any, medical schools seek acclaim for graduating large numbers of primary care physicians who practice in underserved areas.

Only by maintaining an excess demand for admissions can medical schools choose the type of student who will become the type of physician they prefer (who will meet their prestige goals). Both the type of student selected and the design of the educational curriculum are determined by the desires of the medical school faculty, not by what is needed to train quality physicians efficiently (in terms of both student time and cost per student). As long as a permanent shortage of medical school spaces exists, medical schools will continue to "profit" by selecting the type of student the faculty desires, establishing educational requirements the faculty deems most appropriate, and producing graduates who mirror the faculty's preferences. The current system of medical education contains inadequate incentives for medical schools to respond cost effectively to changes in the demand for medical education.

How likely is it that an organization, perhaps a health plan, could start its own self-supporting medical school, one that would admit students after only two years of undergraduate training (as is done in Great Britain), with a revised curriculum and residency requirement that would combine the last two years of medical school with the first two years of graduate medical education (reducing the graduate medical education requirement by one year, as proposed by the former dean of the Harvard Medical School), and financed either by tuition or by graduates repaying their tuition by practicing for a number of years in the organization (Ebert and Ginzberg 1988)? Such schools could satisfy the excess demands for a medical education, reduce the educational process by at least three years, and at the same time teach students to be practitioners in a managed care environment.

ACCREDITATION FOR MEDICAL SCHOOLS

Not surprisingly, starting new and innovative medical schools is very difficult. The Liaison Committee on Medical Education (LCME) accredits programs leading to the MD degree and establishes the criteria to which a school must adhere to receive accreditation (Association of American Medical Colleges and American Medical Association 1991). For example, a minimum number of weeks of instruction and calendar years (four) for the instruction to occur are specified, and an undergraduate education, usually four years, is required for admission to a medical school. Innovations in curriculum and changes in the length of time for becoming a physician (and to prepare for admission to medical school) must be approved by the LCME. The LCME further states that the cost of a medical education should be supported from diverse sources: tuition, endowment, faculty earnings, government grants and appropriations, parent universities, and gifts. Through its concern that too great a reliance should not be placed on tuition, the LCME encourages schools to pursue revenue sources and goals unrelated to educational concerns.

To be accredited medical schools must also be not-for-profit. The LCME's accreditation criteria in effect eliminate all incentives for health plans and similar organizations to invest in medical schools in hopes of earning a profit or having a steady supply of practitioners. Private organizations have no incentive to invest capital to start a new medical school.

The status quo of the current high-cost medical education system would be threatened if graduates of these new medical schools proved as qualified as those trained in more traditional schools (as evidenced by their licensure examination scores and performance in residencies offered to them) and could enter practice three years earlier.

Instead, to bring about medical education reforms, nine commissions have been set up since the 1960s to recommend changes. In a 1989 survey, medical school deans, department chairs, and faculty overwhelmingly endorsed the need for "fundamental changes" or "thorough reform" in medical student education. One examination of the lack of medical education reform indicated that faculty lack sufficient incentives to participate in reforming medical education programs because promotion and tenure are based primarily on research productivity and clinical practice expertise: "[There is] the relegation of students' education to a secondary position within the medical school . . . Faculty have tended to think of the goals of their own academic specialty and department rather than the educational goals of the school as a whole" (Enarson and Burg 1992, 1142).

RECOMMENDED CHANGES
Not surprisingly, without financial incentives a not-for-profit sector will fail to respond to increased student demands for a medical education and will not be concerned with the efficiency by which medical education is provided. Instead of relying on innumerable commissions whose proposed reforms go largely unimplemented, three changes in the current system of medical education and quality assurance should be considered: (1) ease the entry requirements for starting new medical schools, (2) reduce medical school subsidies, and (3) place more emphasis on monitoring physician practice patterns.

Ease the Entry Requirements for Starting New Medical Schools
The accreditation criteria of the LCME should be changed to permit other organizations, such as MCOs (including those that are for-profit), to start medical schools. A larger number of schools competing for students would pressure medical schools to be more innovative and efficient. With easier entry into the medical education market, the emphasis on quality will have to shift from the process of becoming a physician toward quality outcomes, namely toward examining physicians and monitoring their practice behavior. Directly monitoring physicians' practice behavior is the most effective way of protecting the public against unethical and incompetent physicians.

As more physicians participate in managed care and large medical groups associated with MCOs, physician peer review will be enhanced. These organizations have a financial incentive to evaluate the quality and appropriateness of care given by physicians under their auspices, as these organizations compete with similar organizations according to their premiums, quality of care provided, and access to services. Report cards documenting physician quality of care and patient satisfaction are increasingly being required by large employers and consumer groups. Quality assurance of physician services will increase as a result of competition among medical groups and health plans.

Reduce Medical School Subsidies

Reducing government subsidies would also cause medical schools to become more efficient by reducing the time required for a medical degree and the costs of providing it. Medical students should not be subsidized to a greater extent than students in other graduate or professional schools. A decrease in state subsidies to medical schools will force medical schools to reexamine and reduce their costs of education. Medical schools that merely raise their tuition to make up the lost revenues will find it difficult to attract a sufficient number of highly qualified applicants once more schools are competing for students. As tuition more accurately reflects the cost of education, applicants will comparison shop and evaluate schools with a range of tuition levels. To be competitive, schools with a lesser reputation will have to have correspondingly lower tuition levels. The need to reduce student educational costs most likely will result in innovative curricula, new teaching methods, and better use of the medical student's time.

To ensure that every qualified student has an equal opportunity to become a physician once subsidies are decreased, student loan and subsidy programs must be made available. Current low tuition rates in effect subsidize the medical education of all medical students, even those who come from high-income families; once these students graduate, they enter one of the highest-income professions. Providing subsidies directly to qualified students according to their family income levels would be more equitable. Furthermore, providing the subsidies directly to students in the form of a voucher (to be used only in a medical school) would be an incentive for students to select a medical school according to its reputation, total costs of education, and number of years of education required to graduate (college and medical school). Medical schools would be forced to compete for students based on these criteria.

Place More Emphasis on Monitoring Physician Practice Patterns

Currently, the process for ensuring physician quality relies wholly on graduating from an approved medical school and passing a licensing examination. Once a physician is licensed, no reexamination is required to maintain that license (although specialty boards may impose their own requirements for admission and maintenance of membership). State licensing boards are responsible for monitoring physicians' behavior and penalizing physicians whose performance is inadequate or whose conduct is unethical. Unfortunately, this approach for ensuring physician quality and competence is completely inadequate.

State licensing boards discipline very few physicians. In 1969, only 0.69 per 1,000 physicians received any disciplinary action. Between 1980 and 1982, the disciplinary rate rose slightly to 1.3 per 1,000 physicians, or one-tenth of one percent of all physicians. Recently, a change in reporting disciplinary actions increased the base number and has made comparison with previous years difficult. In 2004, however, the "total number of prejudicial acts per 1,000 practicing in-state physicians" was 6.45, or one-half of one percent of all physicians. Disciplinary actions vary greatly by state. Some states take virtually no disciplinary actions against their physicians. The number of prejudicial acts per 1,000 physicians in large states (with more than 15,000 practicing in-state physicians) varied from a low of 3.43 in Maryland to a high of 24.78 in Florida. The number of prejudicial acts per 1,000 physicians in other states was 8.14 in Arizona, 7.52 in Pennsylvania, 5.92 in California, and 11.19 in Colorado (Federation of State Medical Boards of the United States, Inc. 2006).

It is unlikely that New York, which had 7.33 prejudicial acts per 1,000 physicians, has more unethical or incompetent physicians than other states, such as Maryland, or fewer physicians requiring disciplinary action than Florida. Instead, the considerable variability among states represents the uneven efforts by the medical licensing boards of those states, which are mainly composed of physicians, to monitor and discipline physicians in their states. In fact, even when physicians lose their licenses in one state, they can move to another state and practice; some state medical boards encourage physicians to move to another state in exchange for dropping charges. As of 2003, only five states permit their licensing boards to act based solely on another state's findings. The public is not as protected from incompetent and unethical medical practitioners as it has been led to believe by the medical profession.[2]

Monitoring the care provided by physicians through the use of claims and medical records data would more directly determine the quality and competence of a physician. State licensing boards need to devote more resources to monitoring physician behavior. Requiring periodic re-examination and relicensing of all physicians would make physicians update their skills and knowledge. Rather than requiring physicians to take a minimum number of hours of continuing education, reexamination would determine the appropriate amount of continuing education on an individual basis. (Continuing education by itself is a "process" measure for ensuring quality and does not ensure that physicians actually maintain and update their skills and knowledge bases.) Reexamination is a more useful and direct measure for assessing whether a physician has achieved the objectives of continuing education.

Periodic reexamination and relicensure would determine what tasks an individual physician is proficient enough to perform. Currently, all licensed physicians are permitted to perform a wide range of tasks, although for some they may have insufficient training. Physicians may designate themselves as specialists whether or not they are certified by a specialty board. At present, any physician can legally perform surgery, provide anesthesia services, and diagnose patients. Reexamination could result in a physician's practice being limited to those tasks for which she continues to demonstrate proficiency. Instead of "all-or-nothing" licenses, physicians would be granted specific-purpose licenses. Such a licensing process would acknowledge that licensing physicians to perform a wide range of medical tasks does not serve the best interests of the public because not all physicians are qualified to perform all tasks adequately.

Specific-purpose licensure would mean that not all physicians would need to take the same educational training; training in some specialties would take much less time, whereas training to become a super-specialist

---

2. Improvements have been occurring slowly over time; as of 2003, 39 states require a new hearing if a physician has had any disciplinary actions against him in another licensing jurisdiction. All states now share formal action information with other states and report disciplinary actions to the National Practitioner Data Bank (Carlson 2006; Federation of State Medical Boards of the United States, Inc. 2006).

would of course take longer. Shorter educational requirements for family practitioners would lower the cost of their medical educations and enable them to graduate earlier and earn an income sooner. Even with higher tuition, family practitioners would incur a smaller debt and could begin paying it off at least three years earlier.[3] The number of family practitioners would increase because they would have to make a much smaller investment (fewer years of schooling and lost income) in their medical educations, which would more than compensate for not receiving as high an income as a specialist. When a physician wants an additional specific-purpose license, he could receive additional training and take the qualifying examination for that license. Training requirements for entering the medical profession would be determined not by the medical profession but by the demand for different types of physicians and the lowest-cost manner of producing them.

SUMMARY

The competition among medical schools that would result from reducing their subsidies and permitting new schools to enter would improve the performance of the market for medical education. Easing entry restrictions would make opening nontraditional schools (and innovating in existing schools) easier, allowing more qualified students to be admitted to a medical school. Qualified students would no longer have to incur the higher expense and longer training times of attending a foreign medical school. Emphasizing outcome measures and appropriateness of care will better protect the public from incompetent and unethical physicians. Reducing government subsidies to medical schools would force medical schools to be more efficient and innovative in structuring and producing a medical education. Distributing subsidies to students according to family income rather than to the medical school (which results in a subsidy to all students) would enhance equity among students receiving a medical education and force medical schools to compete for those students.

---

3. Jolly (2005) estimates that median debt levels for public medical school graduates from the class of 2007 would be $122,000. For class of 2007 graduates of private (nonprofit) medical schools the median debt level would be $158,000.

DISCUSSION QUESTIONS

1. Evaluate the performance of the current market for medical education in terms of the number of qualified students admitted and the cost (both medical education and student forgone income) of becoming a physician.

2. The current approach for subsidizing medical schools results in all medical students being subsidized. Contrast this approach with one that awards the same amount of subsidy directly to students (according to their family incomes) for use in any medical school.

3. Medical schools are typically interested in prestige. How would medical school behavior change if schools had to survive in a competitive market (with free entry) and without subsidies?

4. An important reason why there are so few family practitioners is their much lower economic returns than specialists. How would a competitive market in medical education increase the relative profitability of becoming a family practitioner?

5. Currently, the public is protected from incompetent and unethical physicians by requiring physicians to graduate from an approved medical school, pass a one-time licensing examination, and receive continuing education. What are alternative, lower-cost approaches for protecting the public's interest?

REFERENCES

Association of American Medical Colleges, and American Medical Association. 1991. *Liaison Committee on Medical Education: Functions and Structure of a Medical School.* Washington, DC: AAMC, AMA.

Carlson, D. 2006. Personal communication, February 22.

Ebert, R. H., and E. Ginzberg. 1988. "The Reform of Medical Education." *Health Affairs* 7 (2 Suppl.): 5–38.

Enarson, C., and F. Burg. 1992. "An Overview of Reform Initiatives in Medical Education: 1906 Through 1992." *Journal of the American Medical Association* 268 (9): 1141–43.

Federation of State Medical Boards of the United States, Inc. 2006. *2003 Exchange,* Table 36. Dallas: FSMB.

———. 2006. Summary of 2004 Board Actions. [Online information; retrieved 12/8/06.] http://www.fsmb.org/pdf/FPDC_Summary_BoardActions_2004.pdf.

Jolly, P. 2005. "Medical School Tuition and Young Physicians' Indebtedness." *Health Affairs* 24 (2): 527–35.

Chapter 24

The Shortage of Nurses

THROUGHOUT THE POST–World War II period, concerns over a national shortage of RNs have been recurrent. At times the shortage of nurses seemed particularly acute; at other times it appeared to be resolved, only to reassert itself several years later. Government and private commissions have attempted to quantify the magnitude of the shortage and have proposed remedies. Since 1964, the federal government has spent billions of dollars to alleviate the nursing shortage. Given the continuing concern over the shortage of nurses and the large federal subsidies that have supported nursing education, it is useful to examine why shortages of nurses have recurred and what, if anything, should be done about it.

MEASURING NURSING SHORTAGES

The measure commonly used to indicate a shortage of nurses is the nurse vacancy rate in hospitals, the percentage of unfilled nursing positions for which hospitals are recruiting. The vacancy rate was at a high of 23 percent in 1962, steadily declined throughout the 1960s, and reached single digits by the early 1970s; it rose in the late 1970s, reaching 14 percent in 1979, but by 1983 fell to approximately 4.4 percent. By the mid-1980s, the vacancy rate was climbing again; it exceeded 12 percent by 1989, after which it declined to 4.0 percent in 1998 and then rose sharply to 13.0 percent in 2001 (Figure 24.1). As of 2005, it was 8.1 percent.

Each of these periods of high or rising RN vacancy rates brought forth commissions to study the problem and make recommendations. The high vacancy rates in the early 1960s led to the start of federal support for nursing education, the Nurse Training Act of 1964, which has been renewed many times.

Figure 24.1: RN Vacancy Rates, Annual Percentage Changes in Real RN Wages, and the National Unemployment Rate, 1979–2005

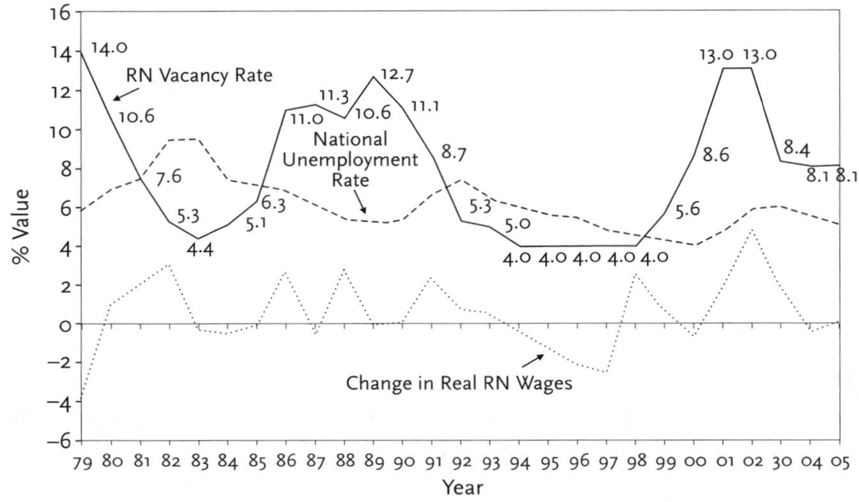

Source: Data compiled by P. I. Buerhaus, Valere Potter Professor, Vanderbilt University School of Nursing, and D. O. Staiger, Associate Professor of Economics, Dartmouth College and of Community and Family Medicine, Dartmouth Medical School, and Research Associate, National Bureau of Economic Research. 2002 and 2006. March.

NURSING SHORTAGES IN THEORY

What are the reasons for a shortage of RNs? The definition of a nurse shortage is that hospitals cannot hire all the nurses they want at the current wage. In other words, at the existing wage the demand for nurses exceeds the number of nurses willing to work at that wage. However, economic theory claims that if the demand for nurses exceeds the supply of nurses, hospitals will compete for nurses and nurses' wages will increase. As nurses' wages rise, nurses who are not working will seek employment, and part-time nurses will be willing to increase the hours they work. All those hospitals willing to pay the new, higher wage will be able to hire all the nurses they want, and hospitals will no longer have vacancies for nurses.

Thus, economic theory predicts that once shortages begin to appear, we would expect to observe rising wages for nurses followed by declining vacancy rates. Nurse employment will increase (more nurses will enter the labor force and others will work longer hours), and as nurses' wages increase, hospitals will not hire as many nurses at the higher wage as they initially wanted. Shortages could recur if the demand for nurses once again increases (more rapidly than supply). With an increase in demand the process starts over; hospitals find they cannot hire all they want at the current wage, and so on. Clearly, wages are not the only reason why nurses work or increase their hours of work. The nurse's age, whether she has young children, and overall family income are also important considerations. A change in the nurse's wage, however, will affect the benefits of working versus not working and thereby affect the nurse's choice of hours worked.

NURSING SHORTAGES IN PRACTICE

How well does economic theory that relies on increased demand for nurses explain the recurrent shortages of nurses? Nurse shortages must be separated into two periods: the period before and the period after the 1965 passage of Medicare and Medicaid.

Before the Passage of Medicare and Medicaid

Before Medicare, the vacancy rate kept rising, exceeding 20 percent by the early 1960s. Hospital demand for nurses continued to exceed the supply of nurses at a given wage. Surprisingly, however, nurses' wages did not rise as rapidly as wages in comparable occupations, which were not even subject to the same shortage pressures. Over a period of years, worsening shortages of nurses and limited increases in nurse wages could only have been the result of interference with the process by which wages were determined.

Working on the hypothesis that nurse wages were being artificially held down, economist Donald Yett (1975) found that hospitals were colluding to prevent nurses' wages from rising. The hospitals believed competing for nurses would merely result in large nurse wage increases, hence a large increase in hospital costs, without a large increase in the number of employed nurses. This collusive behavior by hospitals on the setting of nurses' wages prevented the shortage from being resolved. (For additional references on the nursing shortage and a more complete discussion of the shortage over time see Feldstein [2005].)

After the Passage of Medicare and Medicaid

Once Medicare and Medicaid were enacted, hospitals were reimbursed according to their costs for treating Medicare and Medicaid patients.

Consequently, hospitals were more willing to increase nurse wages. Nurses' wages increased rapidly in the mid to late 1960s, and the vacancy rate declined from 23 percent in 1962 to approximately 9 percent by 1971. The increase in nurses' wages brought about a large increase in the number of employed nurses, contrary to hospitals' earlier expectations. Trained nurses who were not working decided to reenter nursing. The percentage of all trained nurses who were working rose from 55 percent in 1960 to 65 percent in 1966 and 70 percent in 1972. Higher wages had an important effect on increasing nurse participation rates.

The artificial shortages created by hospitals before the mid-1960s are no longer possible. The antitrust laws make collusion by hospitals to hold down nurses' wages illegal. Therefore, the recurrent shortage of nurses since that time has been of a different type.

The lack of information in the market for nurses lengthens the time necessary to resolve shortages. For example, if a hospital experiences an increase in its admissions or a higher acuity level of its patients, it will try to hire more nurses. The hospital may, however, find that its personnel department cannot hire more nurses at the going wage. The hospital's vacancy rate increases. Other hospitals in the community may have the same experience. The hospital then has to decide whether and by how much to raise the wage of nurses to attract additional nurses. If the hospital decides to raise nurses' wages, it will have to pay the higher wage to its existing nurses as well. The hospital must then decide how many additional nurses it can afford to hire at the higher wage for new nurses and for all of its existing nurses. The cost of a new nurse is not only the higher wage a hospital must pay that new nurse but also the cost of increasing wages to all of the other nurses.

The hospital may decide that rather than increasing wages, other approaches for recruiting new nurses, such as providing child care and a more supportive environment, may be less costly. Thus, a time lag exists between the time the hospital decides to hire more nurses, raises wages, and is satisfied with the number of nurses it has.

A time lag also exists before the supply of nurses responds to changed market conditions. Once nurses' wages are increased, it takes time for this information to become widely disseminated. Nurses who are not working may decide to return to nursing at the higher wage; this would be indicated by an increase in the nurse participation rate. Other nurses who are working part time may decide to increase the number of hours they work, and with higher wages more high school graduates may decide to undertake the educational requirements to become a nurse. The most rapid response to an increase in wages will come from those who are part time followed by those who are already trained but not working as nurses. The long-run supply of nurses is determined by those who decide to enter nursing schools (and by the immigration of foreign-trained nurses). Short- and long-run supply responses to an increase in nurses' wages thus occur.

Let us now return to an examination of how well economic theory explains the recurrent shortage of nurses. Throughout the late 1960s and early 1970s, nurses' wages increased more rapidly than wages in comparable professions, such as teaching, resulting in declining vacancy rates and an increased nurse participation rate. Within several years, enrollments in nursing schools increased. A lag of several years always exists before the information on nurses' wages is transmitted to high school graduates and nursing school enrollments change. The sharp increase in nurses' wages after the passage of Medicare in the mid-1960s led to a rapid increase in nursing school enrollments (Figure 24.2).

By the late 1970s, concerns about a new shortage of nurses surfaced. The basis for this shortage began in 1971, when President Nixon imposed wage and price controls on the economy. Although these controls were removed from all other industries in 1972, they remained in effect for medical care until 1974. These wage controls, together with the increased supply of nurse graduates, began to have an effect by the late 1970s. Demand for nurses continued to increase throughout the 1970s, while the wage controls led to lower relative wages for nurses and, by the late 1970s, declining nursing school enrollments. By 1979, the vacancy rate reached 14 percent.

The shortage in 1979 and 1980, however, was short lived. As shown in Figure 24.1, nurses' wages rose sharply at the same time the economy entered a severe recession in the early 1980s. The rising unemployment rate caused more nurses to seek employment and increase their hours of work. Because 70 percent of RNs are married, the loss of a job by a spouse or even the fear of losing a job is likely to cause nurses to increase their labor force participation to maintain their family incomes (Buerhaus 1994).

Higher wages and the rising unemployment rate increased nurse participation rates from 76 percent in 1980 to 79 percent by 1984. As a consequence of these forces, vacancy rates dropped to 4.4 percent by 1983. The nursing shortage was once again resolved through a combination of rising wages, an increase in the nurse participation rate, and the

Figure 24.2: Nursing School Enrollment, 1961–2005

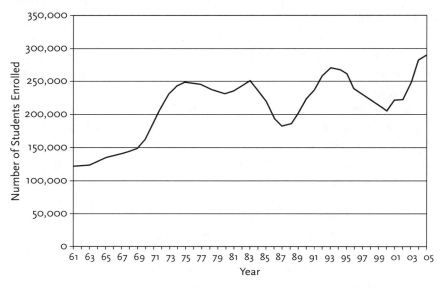

Note: 1997–1999 data are author's estimates because data are unavailable.

Sources: 1961–1996 data from American Nurses' Association. *Facts About Nursing,* various editions; 2000–2001 data compiled by P. I. Buerhaus, Valere Potter Professor, Vanderbilt University School of Nursing. March 2006; 2002–2005 data from National League for Nursing. 2006. *Nursing Data Review Academic Year 2004–2005.* New York: NLN.

national unemployment rate. As RN wages remained stable (and actually declined in real dollars) between 1983 and 1985 and the vacancy rate dropped, nursing school enrollments began a sharp decline through the late 1980s.

In the 1980s, the market for hospital services underwent drastic changes, which affected the market for nurses. The trend by government and private insurers to reduce use of the hospital resulted in shorter hospital lengths of stay. Patients required more intensive treatment for the shorter time they were in the hospital. Hospitalized patients were more severely ill, a greater number of transplants were being performed, and the number of low-birth-weight babies increased. The recovery period, which requires less-intensive care, was occurring outside the hospital. As a result, hospitals began to use a greater number of RNs per patient. The greater demand by hospitals for RNs during this period is indicated by the fact that in 1975 there were 0.65 RNs per patient; this figure increased to 0.88 by 1980, to 1.31 by 1990, to 1.63 by 1995, and to 1.95 in 2004. The percentage increase in RNs per patient exceeded the decline in patient days.

The demand for nurses also increased in outpatient and nonhospital settings. As the use of the hospital declined, use of outpatient care, nursing homes, home care, and hospices for terminally ill Medicare patients increased. From 1980 to 1991 and to 2003, annual outpatient visits (ambulatory care visits to physicians' offices, hospital outpatient departments, and emergency departments) increased from 262 million to 400 million to 1.115 billion, respectively. Use of skilled nursing homes by Medicare patients increased from 8.6 million days in 1980 to 24.1 million in 1991 and to 59 million in 2003 (MedPAC 2006). In addition to providing care in these alternative settings, cost-containment companies increased their demand for RNs to conduct utilization review and case management.

As the demand for nurses in these different settings increased faster than supply in the mid to late 1980s, nurses' wages were slow to respond to these increased demands. Nursing school enrollments had been falling, and the national unemployment rate declined as the economy began improving. Consequently, vacancy rates once again began to rise, from 5.1 percent in 1984 to 12.7 percent in 1989. By the late 1980s, concern again emerged over a shortage of nurses.

Hospitals again lobbied Congress for subsidies to increase nurse education and for an easing of immigration rules on foreign-trained nurses. The nursing shortage of the late 1980s resulted in Congress enacting the Nurse Shortage Reduction Act of 1988 and the Immigration Nurse Relief Act of 1989, which made it easier for foreign nurses to receive working visas.

Trends in the 1990s

Neither of the above legislative acts was needed, however, as economic incentives again eliminated the shortage. As the economy weakened in 1990 and the unemployment rate began to rise, nurse participation rates increased to 82 percent by 1992. Nursing school enrollment had begun increasing two years after nurse wages and the vacancy rate began to increase. With the increase in supply of new nurses and the higher participation rate, vacancy rates declined to 4 percent by 1994. The nursing shortage ended.

As the nurse shortage was over by 1994, one could have forecast that another shortage would occur by the end of the decade. As shown in

Figure 24.1, nurses' real wages (adjusted for inflation) declined starting in 1994 and did not start rising until 1998. During this time, hospitals were trying to reduce their costs to be price competitive so as to be included in managed care's provider networks. Only by 1998 did nurse wage increases finally begin to increase faster than inflation. The national unemployment rate also declined throughout the late 1990s, as the U.S. economy was doing very well.

Nursing school enrollments typically decline several years after a decline in wages and vacancy rates. As shown in Figure 24.2, nursing school enrollments peaked at 270,000 in 1994 and then declined for the remainder of the 1990s. The reduction in nurse wages during the mid to late 1990s led to a large reduction in nursing school enrollments and, consequently, in the number of nurse graduates.

In addition to declining enrollments, some concern arose that the population of nurses was aging (Buerhaus 1998). In 1980, 25 percent of RNs were under the age of 30, compared with only 8.1 percent in 2004. The percentage of nurses between 35 and 54 years of age increased from 42 percent in 1980 to 58 percent in 2004. The average age of a nurse was 37.9 in 1980, 42.4 in 2000, and 46.8 in 2004 (U.S. Department of Health and Human Services 2004). As the nurse population ages, participation rates decrease, as do the number of hours worked. (The nurse participation rate began to show a slight decline in the late 1990s.)

Current Supply and Demand for RNs

After years of declining (adjusted for inflation) nurse wages during the latter part of the 1990s, falling nursing school enrollments, and the aging of the nurse population, one would have expected to observe newspaper articles about the new shortage of nurses and hospitals once again paying bonuses to attract nurses. After years of low vacancy rates, the vacancy rate started increasing in 1999 (from 4.0 percent in 1998 to 5.6 percent) and quickly rose to 13 percent by 2001. The nurse vacancy rate has declined; however, by the end of 2005 it was still relatively high at 8.1 percent.

As a result of hospitals' recognition of the difficulty of attracting nurses, nurses' real wages increased by 4.9 percent in 2002 and 1.8 percent in 2003. (Real wages then dropped 0.5 percent in 2004 and increased 0.1 percent in 2005). With the increase in wages, RN supply started increasing faster. Part-time RNs increased their hours of work, trained RNs rejoined the workforce, and immigration of RNs from other countries increased.

Further stimulating the increase in supply of nurses was the slow-down of the economy in 2001, leading to an increase in unemployment of 5.8 percent in 2002, increasing to 6 percent in 2003. (The economy has since improved; unemployment in 2005 was only 5.1 percent.) Those states experiencing the greatest increases in unemployment saw the largest increases in married RNs reentering the workforce (Buerhaus 2004). Almost all of the increase in RNs in 2002 (94 percent) occurred among married nurses. (The low unemployment rate and lack of an increase in RN real wages in 2004 and 2005 has kept the nurse vacancy rate relatively high at 8.1 percent in 2005.)

The increased demand for RNs in the United States has led to strong financial incentives for foreign-trained RNs to immigrate to the United States. In the United States, foreign-trained RNs have increased opportunities for much higher pay (they are also able to send funds home to assist their families), improved working conditions, and greater prospects for increased learning and practice. In 2002, the median annual wage for RNs in the United States was $48,000, compared with annual salaries of $2,000 to $2,400 for RNs in the Philippines (Brush, Sochalski, and Berger 2004). (These higher wages in the United States have even led physicians in the Philippines to train as RNs to be able to immigrate to the United States.) In several countries, such as the Philippines, RNs are trained for the purpose of being able to immigrate to the United States, as they provide a major source of remittances of hard currency to these other countries (Aiken et al. 2004, 72). To facilitate the immigration of foreign-trained nurses to the United States, for-profit firms have arisen to serve as brokers between U.S. hospitals and foreign-trained RNs.[1]

The demand for RNs is expected to continue to increase, particularly by hospitals. The population is growing, and an increasing percentage

---

1. Foreign-trained RNs are limited in their entry to the United States by U.S. immigration and licensure policies. "All U.S. nurses must pass the National Council Licensure Examination (NCLEX-RN) to practice as RNs. To take the exam, foreign applicants must demonstrate that their education meets U.S. standards—most notably, that their education was at the postsecondary level. Also, nurses trained in countries in which English is not the primary language must also pass an English proficiency test (the Test of English as a Foreign Language, or TOEFL). The U.S. Commission on Graduates of Foreign Nursing Schools (CGFNS) offers an exam in many countries that is an excellent predictor of passing the NCLEX-RN. The CGFNS exam reduces the number of foreign-trained nurses who travel to the United States expecting to work as RNs who cannot pass the licensing exam" (Aiken 2004, 72).

of the population is becoming older; the baby boomers begin retiring in 2011. Medical advances will continue to stimulate the demand for expensive medical services provided by hospitals, consequently increasing the demand for hospital nurses. Government estimates are that the demand for RNs will increase by 40 percent over the next two decades (Buerhaus, Staiger, and Auerbach 2003, 196).

In addition, pressure by nursing organizations to have state-mandated minimum RN staffing ratios per hospital patient, such as occurred in California, will pressure hospitals to increase their demand for RNs. (One consequence of this conflict between nurse and hospital associations over increased RN staffing ratios has been research on whether the patient benefits of higher RN staffing ratios is worth the additional cost.[2])

With respect to the future supply of RNs to meet these expected increases in demand, several trends are emerging. The RN workforce is aging, and as these nurses retire there will be a reduced supply if efforts are not made to increase the number of younger nurses. Most of the increase in supply since 2000 came from older RNs reentering the workforce and the immigration of foreign-born RNs. (The increase in unemployment rates was important in bringing older, married RNs back to nursing.) Increased immigration of foreign-trained nurses (and older RNs) has

---

2. A recent study analyzed data from 800 hospitals in 11 states to determine whether, from the hospital's perspective, the cost-saving (or revenue-increasing) gains from expanding RN staffing ratios exceed the cost of implementing higher RN staffing ratios (Needleman et al. 2006). The authors estimated the cost of increased RN staffing compared with the improvement in patient outcomes, such as avoided deaths, fewer adverse patient outcomes, and decreased hospital lengths of stay. The authors considered three options: The first was increasing the percentage of all nurses that are RNs (the 75th percentile) without changing the total number of hours worked by all nurses; the second required increasing all nursing hours to the 75th percentile of all hospitals; and the third involved increasing both the percentage of RNs (option 1) as well as increasing all nursing hours (option 2). The increased hospital costs for each of these options are, respectively, $811 million, $7.5 billion, and $8.5 billion. According to these results, option 1 produces a net saving of $242 million. Although options 2 and 3 are expected to produce large savings, these savings are less than the costs of the additional nurse staffing, resulting in net losses of $1.7 billion and $2.8 billion, respectively.

The authors conclude that implementing option 1 would save hospitals money, whereas options 2 and 3 might require government subsidies to make it worthwhile for hospitals to undertake the additional nurse staffing required. A study of this magnitude involves a number of assumptions regarding benefits and costs and the calculation of each; in addition, the benefits and costs are considered only from a hospital's perspective, not that of the patient or his family.

offset the decline of younger people choosing a nursing career. Both have been responsive to higher RN wages. Unless there is a greater increase in younger RNs, as older RNs start retiring after 2010, the United States will have to increasingly rely on foreign-born RNs.

Men could eventually be a major source of RN supply. As a proportion of the RN workforce, male RNs have barely increased, from less than 5 percent in the early 1980s to 5.7 percent in 2004.

Expanding the supply of U.S.-trained RNs is limited by the inadequate response by nursing schools to the increased demand for a nursing education. In 2005, due to a lack of spaces, only 41 percent of student applicants were able to be admitted to nursing programs. This represents a decrease from 45 percent in recent years. The not-for-profit market for nursing education does not appear to be performing efficiently.

Since the mid-1960s, the recurrent shortages of nurses have been caused by increased demands for nurses and the failure of hospitals to immediately recognize that, at the higher demand, nurses' wages must be increased. Once hospitals realize market conditions for nurses have changed, the process that once again brings equilibrium to the market begins. The current nurse shortage, however, may take longer than usual to resolve because of the aging of the nurse population, higher state-mandated nurse staffing ratios, and capacity constraints among nursing schools.

FEDERAL SUBSIDIES TO NURSING SCHOOLS AND STUDENTS

Each time a new nursing shortage occurs, various bills are introduced in Congress to attempt to address different aspects of the nursing shortage, such as increased funding for nurse scholarships, financial support for nurses seeking advanced degrees, and funding for increasing faculty in nursing schools. Proposals for federal funding to increase the supply of nurses have been made since the enactment of the 1964 Nurse Training Act and its many renewals. These recommendations ignore the important role played by higher wages in increasing both the short- and long-run supply of nurses.

Federal subsidies to nursing schools and students cannot be directed only to those students who would otherwise have chosen a different career. Nurse education subsidies take years to affect the supply of nurses. More important, to the extent that federal programs are successful in increasing the number of nursing school graduates, nurses' wages rise more slowly. A larger supply of new graduates causes a lower rate of increase in nurses' wages, which in turn results in a smaller increase in the nurse participation rate. Nurses would be more reluctant to return to nursing or increase their hours of work if their wages did not increase.

Nursing programs complain that they cannot admit greater numbers of nursing students because of insufficient faculty. Colleges and universities attempting to expand their nursing faculties operate in a highly competitive market for RNs with graduate degrees who can receive much higher salaries from hospitals and health systems. A significant factor in the shortage of nurse faculty is salaries lower than the market wage. It is surprising that nursing schools are unable to resolve a problem of attracting new faculty, a problem that other academic programs must contend with and appear to have resolved. Given the high rate of return to students receiving their associate in arts degree and their RN training in a two-year college, such schools should be able to increase tuition levels to be able to attract the necessary resources to expand their capacity and admit a greater number of students.

Reliance on market mechanisms rather than federal subsidies is likely to bring about a quicker resolution of nurse shortages. For example, increased wages will bring about an increase in the number of hours part-time nurses work; almost 30 percent of all employed nurses work part time. Higher wages also attract qualified RNs from other countries, such as the Philippines, which trains nurses for export to the United States and whose families depend upon their remittances. Higher wages for nurses will cause hospitals and other demanders of nurses to rethink how they use their nurses. As nurses become more expensive to employ, hospitals will use nurses in higher-skilled tasks and delegate certain housekeeping and other tasks currently performed by RNs to less-trained nursing personnel such as licensed practical nurses. (Up to 50 percent of nurses' time is spent on tasks that could be delegated to others.) Higher wages and new roles for nurses would make nursing a more attractive profession, thereby increasing the demand for a nursing career. Finally, nursing is predominantly a female profession; there is no reason more men cannot be attracted to a nursing career. Higher wages and new nursing roles will increase the attractiveness of nursing to a larger segment of the population.

SUMMARY

The nursing profession faces challenges and opportunities in coming years. The major reason for recurrent RN shortages is the cyclic pattern of nurse wages. As nurse wages stagnated, the rate of return on a nursing career fell and enrollments in nursing schools declined, as did numbers of graduates. With a reduced supply of nurses and an increased acuity level of patients, hospitals eventually found that they could not attract as many nurses as they wanted at the current nurse wage rate, and RN vacancy rates increased. Each of these shortages was resolved when nurse wages increased; nursing school enrollments increased, older RNs reentered the workforce, and a greater number of foreign-trained RNs immigrated to the United States, all of which expanded the supply of nurses.

The aging of the nurse workforce is likely to result in a smaller supply of nurses over the next two decades, unless there is increased immigration of foreign-trained RNs and expanded nursing school capacity.

To forestall future shortages and make the nurse market function more smoothly, better information must be provided to the demanders and suppliers of nursing services. Information will facilitate the market's adjustment process by eliminating the time lags in wage increases and enrollments that have caused these cyclical shortages. Hospitals and other demanders of nursing services must be made more aware of approaches that increase nurses' productivity and the wages and other working conditions necessary to attract more nurses. To realize the full potential of nursing as a profession and expand the supply of nurses, potential nursing students need to be provided with timely information if they are to make informed career choices. Nurses, particularly those who are not employed or are working part time, have to be aware of opportunities in nursing, as well as wages and working conditions being offered. Efforts to increase information are more likely to eliminate shortages and lead to an increase in the supply of nurses than are policies that merely rely on large federal subsidies to nursing education.

Both public policy and private initiatives are directed at reducing the rising costs of medical care. If the outcome of public policy is to place arbitrary budget limits on hospitals and total medical expenditures, nurses' wages will not increase as rapidly as wages for comparably trained professions in the nonregulated health sector, and a permanent nurse shortage will occur. Innovation in the use of RNs and provision of new medical services will be stifled for lack of funds.

If, however, public policy reinforces what is occurring in the private sector, namely competition among MCOs on the basis of their premiums and quality of care, the demand for RNs will be determined by their productivity, the tasks they are permitted to perform, the improved patient outcomes they provide, and their wages relative to other types of nursing personnel. To the extent that RNs are able to perform more highly valued tasks, such as assuming responsibility for more primary care services, utilization management, and management of home health care, as is currently the case in many competitive organizations, they become more valuable to MCOs. In competitive markets, these organizations will be willing to increase their use of RNs and their wages to reflect the higher value of services rendered. The future roles, responsibilities, and incomes of RNs will be very much affected by the incentives created by a competitive health care system.

DISCUSSION QUESTIONS

1. Why was the demand for RNs rising faster than supply during the 1980s?

2. How have the last several shortages of nurses been resolved?

3. How does an increase in nurses' wages affect hospitals' demand for nurses and the supply of nurses?

4. Why was the shortage of nurses that occurred before Medicare different from subsequent shortages?

5. Contrast the following two approaches for eliminating the shortage of nurses:

   a. Providing federal subsidies to nursing schools

   b. Increasing information on nurse demand and supply to prospective nursing students and demanders of nursing services such as hospitals

REFERENCES

Aiken, L., J. Buchan, J. Sochalski, B. Nichols, and M. Powell. 2004. "Trends in International Nurse Migration." *Health Affairs* 23 (3): 69–77.

Brush, B., J. Sochalski, and A. Berger. 2004. "Imported Care: Recruiting Foreign Nurses to U.S. Health Care Facilities." *Health Affairs* 23 (3): 78–87.

Buerhaus, P. 1994. "Capitalizing on the Recession's Effect on Hospital RN Shortages." *Hospital and Health Services Administration* 39 (1): 47–62.

Buerhaus, P., D. Staiger, and D. Auerbach. 2003. "Is the Current Shortage of Hospital Nurses Ending?" *Health Affairs* 22 (6): 191–98.

———. 2004. "New Signs of a Strengthening U.S. Nurse Labor Market?" *Health Affairs* Web exclusive, November 17, W4-526–W4-533. [Online publication; retrieved 11/15/06.] http://content.healthaffairs.org/cgi/reprint/hlthaff.w4.526v1.

Feldstein, P. 2005. "The Market for Registered Nurses." In *Health Care Economics*, 6th ed., 392–418. Albany, NY: Delmar Publishers.

Medicare Payment Advisory Commission (MedPAC). 2006. *A Data Book: Healthcare Spending and the Medicare Program.* [Online publication; retrieved 12/8/06.] http://www.medpac.gov/publications/congressional_reports/Jun06DataBook_Entire_report.pdf.

Needleman J., P. I. Buerhaus, M. Stewart, K. Zelevinsky, and S. Mattke. 2006. "Nurse Staffing in Hospitals: Is There a Business Case for Quality?" *Health Affairs* 25 (1): 204–11.

U.S. Department of Health and Human Services, Health Resources and Services Administration. 2004. *Preliminary Findings: 2004 National Sample Survey of Registered Nurses.* [Online publication; retrieved 11/15/06.] http://bhpr.hrsa.gov/healthworkforce/reports/rnpopulation/preliminaryfindings.htm.

Yett, D. 1975. *An Economic Analysis of the Nurse Shortage.* Lexington, MA: D.C. Heath.

ADDITIONAL READING

Buerhaus, P. 1998. "Is Another RN Shortage Looming?" *Nursing Outlook* 46 (May/June): 103–08.

Chapter 25

The High Price of Prescription Drugs

SPENDING ON PRESCRIPTION drugs in the past several years has been increasing more rapidly than other medical expenditures. After reaching a peak rate of increase of 18 percent in 1999, the annual rate of increase in drug expenditures declined to 6 percent in 2005, reaching $200.7 billion (Centers for Medicare & Medicaid Services 2007). Government researchers forecast that drug expenditures will continue to increase rapidly for the rest of this decade. The new Medicare prescription drug benefit, effective 2006, will increase drug expenditures even more rapidly. (The new drug benefit is estimated to increase Medicare drug expenditures by $1 trillion in the first ten years.)

Although prescription drug expenditures represent a smaller percentage of total health expenditures (10 percent) than hospital or physician services (31 percent and 21 percent, respectively), the sharp increase in drug expenditures has become a cause for concern in both the public and private sectors. Rapidly increasing drug expenditures are a growing burden to state Medicaid programs and a major contributing factor to higher private insurance premiums. Furthermore, patients pay a higher percentage of drug expenditures out of pocket than they do for other major health expenditures. Not surprisingly, patients are more likely to complain about paying $50 for a prescription drug than about a $20,000 stay in the hospital, which is covered by insurance.

REASONS FOR THE RAPID INCREASE
IN PHARMACEUTICAL EXPENDITURES
Drug expenditures had been increasing at double-digit rates since the early 1980s. This rate of increase slowed in the early 1990s, began to

Figure 25.1: Annual Percentage Changes in the Prescription Drug Price Index and Prescription Drug Expenditures, 1980–2005

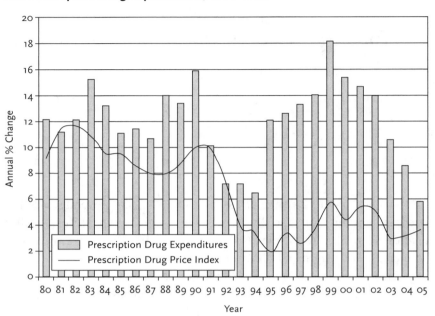

Sources: U.S. Department of Labor, Bureau of Labor Statistics. 2007. [Online information.] http://www.bls.gov/cpi/home.htm; Centers for Medicare & Medicaid Services, Office of the Actuary, National Health Statistics Group. 2007. [Online information.] http://www.cms.hhs.gov/NationalHealthExpendData.

increase sharply in the latter part of the decade, and then slowed in more recent years. The rate of increase in drug expenditures has been several times greater than the rate of increase in drug prices. The annual percentage increases in prescription drug expenditures and drug prices since 1980 are shown in Figure 25.1. Price increases (as measured by the Bureau of Labor Statistics) do not appear to be as important a contributing factor to the recent increases in drug expenditures as in the period before the mid-1990s.

Instead, increased *use* of drugs appears to be an important contributor to increased drug expenditures. As shown in Figure 25.2, the total number of prescriptions filled increased during the 1990s, reaching 3.7 billion by 2005. On a per capita basis the average number of prescriptions increased sharply, from 7.3 in 1992 to 10.4 in 2000 to 12.3 in 2005.

Figure 25.2: Total Prescriptions Dispensed and Prescriptions per Capita, 1992–2005

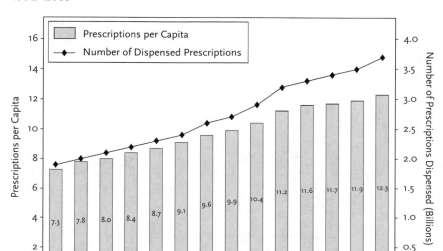

Sources: 1992–1999 data from the National Institute for Health Care Management. 2002. *Prescription Drug Expenditures in 2001: Another Year of Escalating Costs,* March 29. [Online information.] http://www.nihcm.org/finalweb/spending2001.pdf; 2001–2005 data on number of dispensed prescriptions from IMS Health. [Online information.] www.imshealth.com; 2001–2005 data on prescriptions per capita calculated using data from IMS Health at www.imshealth.com and U.S. Census Bureau, http://www.census.gov.

Two important reasons for the large increase in the number of prescriptions are an increase in the number of aged and increased insurance coverage for prescription drugs. Although population growth is about 1 percent per year, the number of aged has been increasing more rapidly, and the aged have the highest use rate of prescription drugs. Whereas those between the ages of 35 and 44 years use an average number of 2.9 prescriptions each per year, those between the ages of 55 and 64 years receive an average of about 6.5 prescriptions each. Between the ages of 65 and 74 years, the average number of prescriptions increases to more than 9 per person, and those aged 75 years and older receive more than 11 prescriptions each (Figure 25.3).

Figure 25.3: Average Number of Prescriptions Prescribed, by Age, 1997

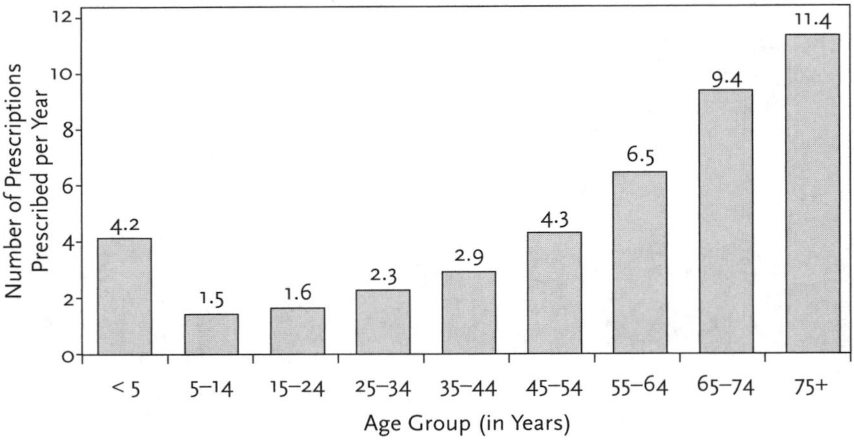

Age Group (in Years)

Note: Prescriptions prescribed at outpatient physician offices in 1997.

Sources: The Henry J. Kaiser Family Foundation. 2000. *Prescription Drug Trends: A Chartbook*; July, based on National Association of Chain Drug Stores. *The Chain Pharmacy Industry Profile, 1999*; analysis based on data from the National Ambulatory Medical Care Survey. 1997; U.S. population data from U.S. Census Bureau. [Online information.] http://www.census.gov/prod/3/98pubs/98statab/sacec.pdf.

As the aged, who are the greatest users (and beneficiaries) of prescription drugs, become an increasing proportion of the population, the volume of prescriptions should continue to increase. Starting in 2011, the first of the baby boomers will reach 65 years old. Given these trends of an increase in the number of aged and the greater number of prescriptions per aged, drug expenditures in general—and particularly among the aged—clearly will continue to increase.

The second reason for the increase in number of prescriptions per capita has been growth in insurance coverage for prescription drugs. The percentage of the population with some form of third-party payment for prescription drugs has been increasing over time. Conversely, out-of-pocket expenditures for prescription drugs have been falling. In 1970, 82 percent of drug expenditures were paid out of pocket. In each of the following ten years this percentage declined, to 70 percent in 1980, 56 percent in 1990, 28 percent in 2000, and 25 percent in 2005 (Figure 25.4). Providing a drug benefit in which the patient's copayment may be $5 per prescription represents a large price decrease, and

Figure 25.4: Share of Prescription Drug Spending, by Source of Funds, Selected Years, 1960–2005

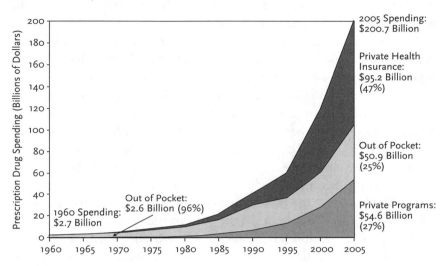

Note: Public programs cover federal, state, and local spending for prescription drugs, including Medicare, worker's compensation, temporary disability, public assistance (Medicaid and SCHIP), Department of Defense, Maternal/Child Health, Veterans Administration, and Indian Health Services.

Source: Centers for Medicare & Medicaid Services, Office of the Actuary, National Health Statistics Group. 2007. [Online information.] http://www.cms.hhs.gov/NationalHealthExpendData.

drug plans offered by MCOs led to large increases in the use of prescription drugs.

As shown in Figure 25.4, the largest share of spending on drugs comes from private health insurance and health plans, which increased from 26 percent in 1990 to 47 percent in 2005. Government payment for drugs, primarily by Medicaid and Medicare HMOs, increased from 18 percent to 27 percent over the same period. As private and government coverage of drug expenditures has increased, consumer out-of-pocket payments have decreased, from 56 percent to 25 percent over the same periods. The new Medicare drug benefit that subsidizes prescription drug use by the aged will greatly increase the government share of total drug expenditures.

Increased use of drugs and higher drug prices do not by themselves explain the rapid rise in drug expenditures since the mid-1990s. The

1990s saw a large increase in the number of innovative new drugs that cost more and have preventive and curative effects, which has resulted in greater use. These drugs can treat previously untreatable illnesses and have substituted for more costly, invasive medical treatments, leading to lower overall treatment costs. New drugs reduce nonpharmaceutical medical costs, such as new antidepressants that have reduced costly psychotherapy as well as beta-blockers and blood pressure drugs that have reduced the costs of cardiovascular-related hospital admissions and surgeries. Lichtenberg (2002) concluded that the replacement of older drugs by newer drugs has resulted in reductions in mortality, morbidity (as indicated by fewer days lost from work), and total treatment costs, particularly for inpatient care. The use of new drugs has resulted in large hospital savings because of reductions in lengths of stay and number of hospital admissions. The total reduction in nondrug medical expenses is about seven times the increase in the costs of drugs.

Some new drugs also have fewer adverse side effects. Many new lifestyle drugs, such as Viagra (treatment of male impotence), Claritin (relief from allergies), Prilosec (relief from stomach upsets), antidepressants, and pain relievers, improve quality of life. However, they may be much more expensive than older drugs. For example, new pain relievers treat severe arthritis, but they cost $150 a month, nearly 20 times more than previous pain relievers. A new biotech drug that treats rheumatoid arthritis, Enbrel, can cost $1,500 a month. Whereas drugs such as penicillin would be prescribed for a brief period to cure an infection, some modern drugs, including lifestyle drugs, can be taken for decades. The prospect of better health and a higher quality of life has led to an increase in the number of prescriptions and the price of new drugs.

To better understand the increase in drug expenditures one must account for the contribution of new drugs. Table 25.1 categorizes the increase in prescription drug expenditures into price and utilization increases based on a study examining the period 1993 to 1998. Overall utilization of prescription drugs accounted for about one-third (7.2 percent per year) of the expenditure increase, whereas price increases accounted for the remaining two-thirds of the increase (12.8 percent per year) in drug expenditures. However, when the expenditure increase over this period is classified by new drugs (introduced after 1992) versus old drugs, two-thirds of the expenditure increase (13.0 percent per year) is due to new drugs (8.4 percent per year increase in prices and 4.6 percent per year increased use). Older drugs accounted for only one-third of the

Table 25.1: Percentage Contribution of Changes in Price and Utilization to 1993–1998 Increase in Prescription Drug Spending

	Average Annual Increase in Price Effect	Average Annual Increase in Utilization Effect	Total Average Annual Increase
New drugs (1992 and later)	8.4%	4.6%	13.0%
Older drugs	4.4	2.6	7.0
Total	12.8	7.2	20.0

Source: National Institute for Health Care Management Research and Educational Foundation. 1999. *Factors Affecting the Growth of Prescription Drug Expenditures.* July. [Online information.] http://www.nihcm.org/FinalText3.pdf.

total expenditure increase over this period (4.4 percent per year increase in price and 2.6 percent per year increase in use).

These findings imply that *the replacement of old drugs by new drugs is the most important reason for rising drug expenditures.* Prescription drug expenditures are likely to continue their rapid rise, driven by new drug discoveries and greater use of drugs, particularly among an increasingly older population. Rising drug expenditures should be viewed with favor, as they often indicate new and improved drugs. A greater number of prescriptions per person, particularly for the aged, may indicate that chronic diseases can be better managed, the aged can live longer, and their quality of life can be improved.

PRICING PRACTICES OF U.S. PHARMACEUTICAL COMPANIES

Drug manufacturers sell their drugs to different purchasers (intermediaries), who in turn sell them to patients. Retail (independent and chain) pharmacies sell about 49 percent of all prescription drugs; health care organizations such as HMOs, hospitals, long-term-care facilities, home health care, federal facilities, and clinics sell 27 percent; mail-order pharmacies sell 15 percent; and food stores sell 9 percent (Figure 25.5). (HMO and insurance company patients rely on mail-order and retail pharmacies that are in their insurers' networks for their drugs.)

Figure 25.5: Prescription Sales by Outlet, U.S. Market, 2005

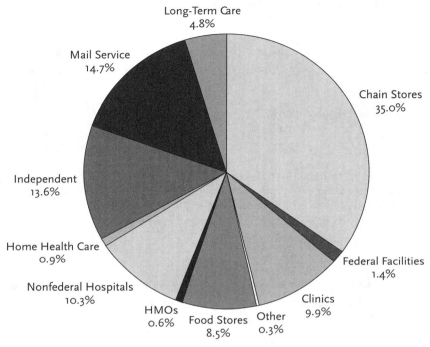

Long-Term Care
4.8%

Mail Service
14.7%

Chain Stores
35.0%

Independent
13.6%

Home Health Care
0.9%

Federal Facilities
1.4%

Nonfederal Hospitals
10.3%

HMOs
0.6%

Food Stores
8.5%

Other
0.3%

Clinics
9.9%

Total U.S. Sales in 2005 = $251.8 Billion

Source: IMS Health. 2005. *U.S. Top-Line Industry Data.* [Online information.] http://www.imshealth.com.

Drug manufacturers sell the same prescription drug to different purchasers at different prices. An HMO pays less for its drugs than an independent retail pharmacy, although the latter sells a much greater volume of drugs. Similarly, patients without any prescription drug coverage (often the poor and sick) pay more for the same drug at a retail pharmacy than those who are part of a managed care plan.

Two aspects of the pricing practices of pharmaceutical companies have been criticized as being unfair and have led to proposals for government intervention. First, different purchasers are charged different prices for the same drug, and second, prescription drugs have a high price markup.

Pricing According to Cost

A new prescription drug is priced many times higher than its actual costs of production. This high markup of price over cost has generated a great deal of criticism. If the drug were priced closer to its production cost, it would be less of a financial burden on those with low incomes, those without prescription drug coverage, and state Medicaid budgets.

Drug manufacturers often claim that their drug prices are determined by the high costs of developing those drugs. High research and development (R&D) costs, however, are not the reason for high or rising drug prices. Large fixed, or "sunk," costs are costs that have already been incurred; hence, they are not relevant for setting a drug's price. Fixed costs must eventually be recovered or the drug company will lose money; however, a new drug that is no different than drugs already on the market could not sell for more than these competitive drugs regardless of how much that drug cost to develop.

Pricing According to Demand

When price differences for the same drug cannot be entirely explained by cost differences, according to economic theory the reason for price differences must be related to differences in the purchaser's price sensitivity or willingness to pay. Purchasers who are not price sensitive will be charged higher prices than those who are. *A purchaser who is willing to buy less or switch to other drugs when the price increases is more price sensitive than one who will not.*

The higher price charged to one purchaser is not meant to make up for the lower price charged to another purchaser. Instead, the reason for different prices is that the seller can simply make more money by charging according to each purchaser's willingness to pay.

The ability to shift market share rather than just the volume purchased drives discounts. Not all large-volume purchasers receive price discounts. Retail pharmacies in total sell a large volume of drugs, but they do not receive the same price discounts as do managed care plans. When an HMO negotiates with a drug company on one of several competing brand-name drugs within a therapeutic class, the HMO's willingness to place the drug on its formulary while excluding a competitor's drugs can result in substantial discounts for the HMO.[1] Similarly, pharmacy benefit managers (PBMs), who manage health plans' drug benefits for

---

1. As HMOs and health plans seek volume discounts from drug companies, they are willing to limit their subscribers' choice of drugs in return for negotiating lower drug prices. Drug formulary committees focus on drugs for which therapeutic substitutes exist and evaluate different drugs according to their therapeutic value and price; higher-priced drugs are used only when justified by greater therapeutic benefits. Restrictions are then placed

drugs sold through retail pharmacies, can promote brand-name substitution and thereby receive large discounts.[2]

Retail pharmacies pay the highest prices for their prescription drugs because they must carry all branded drugs. Furthermore, the pharmacy cannot promote substitution between branded drugs because the physician may be prescribing according to a health plan's formulary. Because pharmacies cannot shift volume, drug manufacturers see no need to give them a price discount.[3] (To receive price discounts government entities

---

on their physicians' prescribing behavior. These organizations are also using computer technology to conduct drug utilization review; each physician's prescription is instantly checked against the formulary, and data are gathered on the performance of each physician as well as on the health plan's use of specific drugs.

2. PBMs are firms that provide administrative services and process outpatient prescription drug claims for health insurers' prescription drug plans. To control growth in prescription drug expenditures, PBMs will also contract with a network of pharmacies, negotiate pharmacy payments, negotiate with drug manufacturers for drug discounts and rebates, develop a drug formulary listing preferred drugs for treating an illness, encourage use of generic drugs instead of high-priced brand-name drugs, operate a mail-order pharmacy, and analyze and monitor patient compliance programs. Some PBMs have been very aggressive in switching physicians' prescriptions; they may call a physician and tell him that a less-expensive drug is available for the same medical condition and suggest that the physician switch drugs to one on which the PBM receives a large price discount or rebate.

3. In 1993, an antitrust suit was filed by 31,000 retail pharmacies against 24 pharmaceutical manufacturers, claiming that the drug companies conspired to charge HMOs, PBMs, and hospitals lower prices while denying price discounts to retail pharmacies. Most of the drug companies settled by paying a relatively small average amount per retail pharmacy and said they would give the same discounts to retail pharmacies *if they could demonstrate that they were able to shift market share of their drugs*. Five drug companies refused to settle. The retail pharmacies had to prove that price discrimination harmed competition and that the discounts were not a competitive response to another drug firm's lower prices. At the trial in 1998, the judge dismissed the lawsuit, which was upheld on appeal.

According to a study by The Boston Consulting Group (1993), as of 1992, mail-order pharmacies received an average drug price discount of 30 percent, managed care companies received a 35 percent discount, hospitals and nursing homes each received a 5 percent discount, and retail pharmacies received no discount. The drug companies claimed they did not offer a price discount to retail pharmacies because the discounts would not increase the drug company's market share. Retail pharmacies had to carry a wide selection of drugs because they merely filled orders of prescribing physicians. The greater the ability of the buyer to switch market share away from one drug manufacturer to a competitor's drug, the greater was the discount. The drug companies claimed that retail pharmacies were unable to switch volume from one drug company to another; therefore, there was no reason to give them a discount.

have resorted to price regulation; see Chapter 28.) For a pharmacy to be included in a health plan or a PBM network it must charge lower dispensing fees, which also results in lower prices to the PBM and to health plan enrollees.

Price discrimination, whereby a seller charges different prices to different purchasers, occurs in many other areas of the economy. For example, seniors and students pay lower prices at the movies and other events. Prices may differ by time of day, such as early-bird dinner specials and drinks, and airlines charge business travelers more than vacationers because they book flights on short notice. Those who are less likely to switch are less price sensitive and are charged more for the same service.

Price discrimination actually promotes price competition between drug manufacturers for more price-sensitive purchasers, which results in lower prices for purchasers and consumers. To price discriminate a seller must prevent low-price buyers from reselling the product to those who are charged more. A 1987 federal law prevented resale of prescription drugs on the basis of preserving the safety and integrity of those drugs.

Pricing Innovative Drugs

Pharmaceutical manufacturers are strategic in how they mark up the price of their drugs (price–cost ratio) and negotiate price discounts. A drug's price markup is determined by demand. New drugs are priced according to their therapeutic value and the availability of good substitutes. When a new drug for which there is no close substitute comes on the market and is clearly therapeutically superior to existing drugs, it will have a higher price markup. Sometimes a drug is priced according to some concept of value, such as comparing the drug's price to the surgical procedure it replaces. Approving an existing drug for a new use also increases its value, as its therapeutic effects for that new use are greater than existing drugs; the drug company is thus able to increase its price.

The greater the price markup over costs, the more innovative the drug and the fewer the close substitutes to it. Innovative drugs command higher price markups than imitative drugs. The price of a new drug is determined by a purchaser's willingness to pay for its greater therapeutic benefits. A new breakthrough drug that is the first to treat a disease is priced much higher than any other drug in its therapeutic class (typically more than three times the price) because no good substitutes are available. New drugs with modest therapeutic gains are priced about two times the average for available drug substitutes. New drugs with little or no gain over existing drugs are priced at about the same level as existing substitutes. Once the patent has expired on a branded drug, generic drugs are introduced and are typically priced at about 30 percent to 70 percent of the branded drug's price before the patent expired. As more generic versions become available, the prices of generic drugs fall.

New, higher-priced drugs will fail commercially if their therapeutic benefits are similar to those of existing drugs. As MCOs evaluate drugs for inclusion in their formularies based on therapeutic benefits and price, differences in drug prices will reflect differences in therapeutic benefits. Knowledgeable purchasers evaluating a higher-priced new drug will pay a higher price only if its therapeutic benefits were greater than the older drug.

A new drug that is similar to an existing drug (a "me-too" drug) cannot be priced much higher than the existing drug because purchasers will switch to a good substitute (the existing drug) at a lower price. Although drug companies have been criticized for producing me-too types of drugs, their availability contributes to price competition.

Once competitors enter the market originally served by an innovative drug, prices decline. Interestingly, when generic versions enter the market after the patent on a branded drug has expired, the branded drug loses market share to the generic drug but the price of the branded product actually increases; the price-sensitive customers switch to the generic drug, and those who do not switch are not price sensitive. Therefore, the seller of the branded drug is able to raise its price. Some physicians (and consumers) have strong preferences for the branded drug and do not want to substitute the generic version; they are willing to pay more for the security of the brand-name drug.[4] Drug manufacturers have determined that serving a smaller market at a higher price is more profitable

---

4. The Bureau of Labor Statistics drug price index overstates drug price increases when a generic equivalent of a branded drug comes on the market. The lower-priced generic drug rapidly expands its market share at the expense of the branded drug for which it is a substitute. As the branded drug loses market share to the generic drug, its price is increased to the remaining patients who are less price sensitive and reluctant to use the generic version of the drug. The drug price index picks up the price increase of the branded drug but does not measure the price decline experienced by the large proportion of consumers who switch to the generic version. Thus, the drug price index fails to reflect the sharp price decline with the introduction of the generic drug.

than reducing the price of the branded drug to compete with generic versions.[5]

Thus, the pricing strategy of pharmaceutical companies is based on two principles. The first is the price sensitivity of the purchaser. The greater the price sensitivity of the purchaser, such as an HMO that is willing to shift its drug purchases to a competitor's drug, the lower the price. Second, the more innovative the drug, such as a drug that does not have a close substitute, the higher the price markup will be. These pricing strategies are designed to maximize drug firm profits.

Drug Companies' Marketing Response to Managed Care Plans

Purchaser decision making with respect to pharmaceuticals has changed. Previously, physicians chose a patient's prescription drug. As a result, drug manufacturers spent a great deal of money marketing directly to physicians. With the growth of managed care and its use of closed formularies, drug companies began to develop new marketing strategies. As the purchasing decision over prescription drugs shifted from the individual physician to the committee overseeing the organization's formulary, sending sales representatives to individual physicians caring for an HMO's patients was less useful than marketing to the HMO itself. Drug companies have had to demonstrate that their drugs are not only therapeutically superior to competitive drugs but that they are also cost effective, namely that the additional benefits of their drug are worth a higher price. Physicians continue to be important in prescribing drugs to their patients, but PBMs and health plans determine which brand-name drugs the physician is able to prescribe and the prices paid for those drugs.

To counteract the closed formularies, drug manufacturers started direct-to-consumer television and newspaper advertising to generate consumer demand for certain drugs from their physicians. Direct-to-consumer advertising, the cost of which increased from about $600

---

5. When the patent on a branded drug expires, the first generic version of that drug has a six-month period of exclusivity over other generics; the first generic can capture up to 90 percent of the market from the branded drug. Typically, the branded drug manufacturer does not produce the generic version when its patent expires. Recently, however, Pfizer has decided to do so to gain the six-month period of exclusivity. The FTC has decided to examine whether Pfizer's practice serves as a disincentive for generic manufacturers to compete when the market for that drug is not very large, thereby lessening competition (Hensley 2006).

million in 1997 (the first year it was permitted by the U.S. Food and Drug Administration [FDA]) to $2.5 billion by 2000, to $4 billion by 2004, has proved very effective in increasing sales of advertised prescription drugs (Henry J. Kaiser Family Foundation 2005). Previously, physicians almost never wrote prescriptions for drugs requested by patients because most patients did not know enough to demand drugs by name or therapeutic class. As more medical information has become available to patients, they have begun demanding more input into the therapeutic decisions that affect their lives. Drug companies claim that ads are meant to inform the patient and stimulate a discussion between the patient and her physician. Critics claim that the ads do not inform patients about who is most likely to benefit from that drug, its possible side effects, or other treatment options.

Drug costs have become the fastest-increasing expense for health plans. In response to rising costs, health plans have provided patients with incentives to use less-expensive drugs. A three-tiered copayment system is used. Patients pay a small copayment for generic drugs, a higher copayment for prescription drugs on the health plan's formulary (for which the manufacturer gives a large discount), and a much higher copayment for branded drugs not on the health plan's formulary.

SUMMARY

Prescription drug expenditures will continue to increase because of increased use of drugs and the introduction of newer, higher-priced drugs. Prices of new drugs have a very high markup in relation to their cost of production. To those without drug coverage and to large purchasers of drugs, such as health plans and state Medicaid agencies, these facts are a cause for concern.

However, the public should view rising drug expenditures and even high price markups favorably. Rising drug prices are often an indication that new drugs are more effective than existing drugs or alternative treatments. (When new drugs are of higher quality, that is, when they provide greater benefits than the drugs they replace, the "quality-adjusted" price of these drugs may well be lower than the price of older drugs. Thus, counting the higher prices of new drugs as mere price increases is misleading.) Furthermore, when new drugs replace older drugs, purchasers value the greater therapeutic benefits of the newer drugs more and are willing to pay higher prices for their increased value. Consumers are clearly better off. The replacement of older drugs by newer drugs is the most important reason for the increase in drug expenditures. Also contributing to greater use of newer drugs has been increased demand resulting from the increase in third-party payment for prescription drugs, population growth, and the aging of the population. All of these factors will likely cause drug expenditures to continue to increase in the future.

Drug manufacturers charge different prices to different buyers for the same drug (price discrimination) to give price discounts to purchasers who are willing to switch their drug purchases and charge higher prices to those who are less price sensitive. The cost-containment strategies of health plans and PBMs have caused drug firms to compete on price to have their drugs included in the formularies of large purchasers and to emphasize the cost effectiveness of their drugs. Drug firms have also started direct-to-consumer advertising to develop consumer pressure to demand the drug from their physicians. To limit the effect of such tactics health plans have instituted three-tiered copayment systems that give consumers incentives to use drugs on the health plan's formulary.

DISCUSSION QUESTIONS

1. Which factors have contributed most to the sharp increase in drug expenditures?

2. Are rising drug expenditures necessarily bad?

3. Is the high price of drugs determined by the high cost of developing a new drug?

4. Why do drug manufacturers charge different purchasers different prices for the same prescription drug?

5. What methods have managed care plans used to limit their enrollees' drug costs?

REFERENCES

Centers for Medicare & Medicaid Services, Office of the Actuary, National Health Statistics Group. 2007. *National Health Expenditure Data: Overview.* [Online information; retrieved 1/10/07.] http://www.cms.hhs.gov/NationalHealthExpendData.

Henry J. Kaiser Family Foundation. 2005. *Prescription Drug Trends*, November. [Online information; retrieved 11/15/06.] http://www.kff.org/insurance/upload/3057-04.pdf.

Hensley, S. 2006. "Pfizer to Make Generic Version of Its Zoloft." *The Wall Street Journal* June 29, B1.

Lichtenberg, F. R. 2002. *The Benefits and Costs of Newer Drugs: An Update.* NBER Working Paper No. 8996. Cambridge, MA: National Bureau of Economic Research.

The Boston Consulting Group, Inc. 1993. *The Changing Environment for U.S. Pharmaceuticals: The Role of Pharmaceutical Companies in a Systems Approach to Health Care.* New York: The Boston Consulting Group, Inc.

ADDITIONAL READINGS

Frank, R. G. 2001. "Prescription Drug Prices: Why Do Some Pay More than Others Do?" *Health Affairs* 20 (2): 115–28.

Scherer, F. M. 2000. "The Pharmaceutical Industry." In *Handbook of Health Economics*, vol. 1, edited by A. J. Culyer and J. P. Newhouse, 1297–336. New York: Elsevier Science.

Chapter 26

Ensuring Safety and Efficacy of New Drugs: Too Much of a Good Thing?

INNOVATIVE NEW DRUGS have decreased mortality, increased life expectancy, and improved the quality of life for many millions of people. New drugs have also reduced the cost of medical care, substituting medicines for more costly surgeries and long hospital stays. At the time of discovery, however, the effects of new drugs are not fully known. Powerful drugs that have the potential for curing cancer may also have harmful side effects. Some drugs may cause illness or even death for some people, while providing beneficial effects to others. New drugs offer a trade-off: improvements in the quality and length of life versus possible serious adverse consequences.

The FDA's approval is required before any new drug may be marketed in the United States. The FDA's objective should be to achieve a balance between the concerns of drug safety and the prospective benefits of pharmaceutical innovation. Ensuring that a new drug does not harm anyone delays the introduction of a beneficial drug that may save many lives. This delay may result in the deaths of thousands of people whose lives could have been saved had the new drug been approved earlier. Similarly, introducing potential breakthrough drugs immediately may cause the deaths of many, as the full effects of the new drug are not completely understood.

How should this trade-off in lives be evaluated? Is each type of life—those potentially saved by early introduction of a new drug versus those who might die from early approval—valued equally? Regulatory delay increases the time and cost of bringing a new drug to market. Thus, excessive caution or expediency incurs risks. Either may cause a loss of lives. This chapter discusses the FDA and its history and performance with regard to the drug-approval process.

HISTORY OF REGULATION OF PRESCRIPTION DRUGS

The Pure Food and Drug Act of 1906 was the federal government's first major effort at regulating the pharmaceutical industry. The supporters of this act, however, were primarily concerned with the quality of food rather than drugs. Pure food acts had been submitted to Congress at least ten years before one was finally passed. Media publicity on the ingredients of food and drugs generated popular support for legislative action. A great deal of publicity was generated by newspapers, magazine articles, and Upton Sinclair's 1906 book *The Jungle*, with its graphic descriptions of what was being included in the foods the public was eating. The result was public outrage, to which Congress responded by passing the Pure Food and Drug Act.

The act required drug companies to provide accurate labeling information, including whether the drug was addictive. (A number of medicines contained alcohol, opium, heroin, and cocaine, which were legal at that time.) The government could verify the accuracy of the drug's contents. Subsequent court cases resolved that therapeutic claims made by the sellers of a drug would not be considered fraudulent if the sellers believed their therapeutic claims. Thus, the drug-related portion of the act was quite limited and was modeled by the public's concern with the contents of food.

In the 1930s, the modern drug era began with the development of sulfa drugs. As drugs were introduced, a tragedy provided the impetus for new legislation. A company seeking to make a liquid form of elixir sulfanilamide for children dissolved it in ethylene glycol (antifreeze), unaware of the toxic effects. As a result, more than 100 children died before the drug was recalled. Responding to the public outcry, Congress passed the Food, Drug, and Cosmetic Act in 1938. This law, which created the FDA, was intended to protect the public from unsafe, potentially harmful drugs. A company had to seek approval from the FDA before it could market a new drug. Drug companies were left to determine the necessary amount and type of premarket testing to prove to the government that the drug was safe for its intended use.

A 1950 amendment to the 1938 act authorized the FDA to distinguish prescription from nonprescription drugs by stating that some types of drugs could only be sold by prescription, as they could be harmful to the individual if bought on their own.

In 1959, Senator Estes Kefauver held hearings on the drug industry. (He was running for the Democratic nomination for president at that time.) Critics of the industry were concerned that drug prices were too high, that drug companies undertook unnecessary and wasteful advertising expenditures, and that the drug industry earned excessive profits.

In the late 1950s, a new drug was introduced in Europe to treat morning sickness for pregnant women. After the introduction of thalidomide in Europe, an FDA staff member expressed doubts about the safety of the drug because of reported side effects and delayed its approval. An American drug company, however, was able to introduce it into the United States on an experimental basis. (The 1938 FDA amendments permitted such limited distribution to qualified experts so long as the drug was labeled as being under investigation.) As soon as reports began to appear in Europe that deformed babies were born to mothers who had taken the drug during pregnancy, the American company withdrew the drug.

The resulting media attention given to thalidomide and its effects in Europe shifted Congress's concern about high drug prices, wasteful expenditures, and excessive profits to concern with public safety. Congress responded to the public's fears about drug safety and passed the 1962 amendments to the Food, Drug, and Cosmetic Act. (Richard Harris [1964] provides a history of the 1962 FDA amendments.)

The 1962 amendments resulted in a major change in the regulation of pharmaceuticals. Drug companies were now required to prove the safety of their new drugs and their efficacy (beyond a "placebo" effect) for the indications claimed for them in treating a particular disease or condition. (Effectiveness must be determined by a controlled study in which some patients are given the new drug and others are given a placebo, an inactive substance such as a salt or sugar pill.) Once the FDA approves a new drug for marketing, the drug is approved only for specific claims. If the drug company wants to broaden those claims, it must file a new application with the FDA and provide evidence to support the new uses of that drug. (Physicians may, however, prescribe a drug for a use for which the FDA has not approved it.)

The steps that a drug company must take to meet the FDA's safety and efficacy standards are costly and time consuming. The FDA specifies the type of premarketing tests that are required. Before undertaking clinical trials using humans, animal trials are used to determine whether the drug is sufficiently safe and promising to justify human trials. Based on this evidence the FDA will approve clinical trials using humans. Each of the three different stages of clinical trials uses a greater number of subjects so that more dangerous drugs are identified before they can affect larger numbers of patients. Stage one introduces the drug to a small number of healthy individuals, and stage two uses a small number of persons with the disease to be treated. The third stage uses a large number of patients, half of whom take a placebo, and is designed to demonstrate efficacy and provide additional evidence of safety. Clinical trials take, on average, six years to complete. Once completed, the drug firm must receive FDA approval, which can take an additional several years.[1] Once approved by the FDA, the new drug must be manufactured according to specified standards.

After the 1962 amendments were enacted, generic and patented drugs were treated in the same manner. Both had to meet the same stringent FDA requirements as a new drug seeking a patent. Manufacturers of generic drugs had to independently prove the safety and efficacy of their products to receive FDA approval. Because the research of generic drugs had to be undertaken in the same process as the patented drug, the cost and time for developing generic drugs increased. Once a new drug received its patent and was approved by the FDA, the drug had no competition for a longer period and the price could be kept high for a longer time. Consumers continued to face high prices for prescription drugs for which the patents had expired because of FDA requirements that delayed the entry of generic substitutes.

The 1984 Drug Price Competition and Patent Term Restoration (Hatch-Waxman) Act simplified and streamlined the process for FDA approval of generic drugs in exchange for granting patent extensions to innovative drugs. Generic drugs no longer had to replicate many of the clinical trials performed by the original manufacturer to prove safety and efficacy. Instead, the generic drug manufacturer was only required to demonstrate that the generic drug was "bioequivalent" to the already approved patented drug, which was much less costly than proving safety and efficacy. (Bioequivalence means the active ingredient is absorbed at the same rate and to the same extent for the generic drug as for the patented drug.) The effect of this act was to reduce the delay between patent expiration and generic entry from more than three years to less than three months. Generic substitutes for branded drugs with expired

---

1. Once the FDA approves a new drug as being safe and efficacious for its intended use, the new drug must also pass the health plan's review process to show that it is also cost effective. Unless the drug can pass this review, the new drug may not be added to the health plan's drug formulary.

patents are now quickly available at much-reduced prices. The market share of the generic substitute rapidly increases after patent expiration. Previously, only 35 percent of top-selling drugs whose patents expired had generic copies; currently, almost all do.[2]

Although the 1984 act made generic drug entry easier and less costly once a patent expired, it also extended the patent life of branded drugs to compensate for patent life lost during the long FDA approval process. (Effective patent life is measured from the time the FDA approves a new drug to the end of the patent.) The act permitted drugs that contain a new chemical entity to qualify for a patent life extension. These patent extensions postpone generic entry by an average of about 2.8 years. The 1984 act was a compromise between the generic drug manufacturers, which wanted easier entry, and the brand-name drug manufacturers, which wanted a longer patent life.[3]

State legislation in the 1970s and 1980s also enabled generic drugs to rapidly increase their market share once a drug patent expired. Through the early 1970s, pharmacists in many states could not legally dispense a generic drug when a prescription specified a brand-name drug. By 1984, all states had enacted drug substitution legislation that permitted a pharmacist to substitute a generic drug even when a brand-name drug was specified, *as long as the physician had not indicated otherwise on the prescription.*

During the 1980s and 1990s, AIDS activists were very critical of the FDA's approval process. AIDS patients were dying from the disease and wanted promising new drugs to be immediately available. Approval would be too late for many if these drugs were delayed for years because of research protocols required by the FDA. To provide half of terminally

---

2. The FTC has been investigating anticompetitive behavior in the drug industry. Drug companies that hold patents on brand-name drugs have been accused of making special deals with generic drug manufacturers to keep the generic drugs off the market, thereby not competing with the branded drug, for longer than the 1984 Hatch-Waxman Act intended. Drug manufacturers have been alleged to pay generic drug companies to delay introducing their products. Congress and the FDA are also examining whether changes to the 1984 act are required to close loopholes in the law. Industry critics claim that another tactic drug companies use to delay the entry of generic drugs is to sue the generic manufacturers, allowing the branded drugs months more of lucrative, exclusive sales.

3. Olson (1994) describes why, after several years of failure, the 1984 drug legislation was ultimately enacted. Her analysis includes the proposals of different interest groups, turnover in key Senate committees, and a change in the majority party.

ill AIDS patients with a placebo was believed to be immoral; they would be denied a possible life-saving drug. Terminally ill AIDS patients were willing to bear the risk of taking drugs that might prove to be unsafe or have adverse side effects.

AIDS activists pressured Congress and the FDA for an accelerated approval process. As a result, new laws and regulations were enacted between 1987 and 1992 that enabled seriously ill patients to have access to experimental drugs. These types of drugs were provided with a "fast-track" approval process. For other serious or life-threatening diseases, drugs in the clinical trial stages that were shown to have meaningful therapeutic benefit compared with existing treatments were also given an expedited review. In return for early approval of these new drugs, the drug firm had to periodically notify the FDA about any adverse reactions to the drug that were not detected during the clinical trial periods.

In 1992, Congress enacted the Prescription Drug User Fee Act (renewable every five years), which authorized the FDA to collect fees from drug manufacturers seeking a drug approval. The revenues from these fees were to be used to increase the number of FDA staff reviewing drug approvals. As a result the approval process took less time and the number of new drugs approved increased compared with previous years.[4]

Both the fast-tracking approval process and the funds from user fees reduced the time for FDA approvals of new drugs. As shown in Figure 26.1, in the late 1980s the FDA took about 32 months to approve a new drug. By 1998, the average approval time was less than 12 months. Unfortunately, in recent years the average FDA approval time has been increasing, rising to 19.1 months in 2004.

FDA'S STRINGENT GUIDELINES FOR SAFETY AND EFFICACY

It is difficult to be opposed to increased drug safety. As a consequence of FDA regulatory requirements, physicians and the public are better

---

4. In 1994, new federal legislation (the Uruguay Round Agreements Act) changed the patent life of prescription drugs (and all types of inventions) from 17 years from the date a patent is granted to 20 years from the date the application is filed. Between two and three years elapse from the time an application is filed until a patent is granted. The average period for which a new drug can be marketed under patent protection has risen from about 9 years to about 11.5 years.

Figure 26.1: Number of and Mean Approval Times for New Molecular Entities* in the United States, 1984–2004

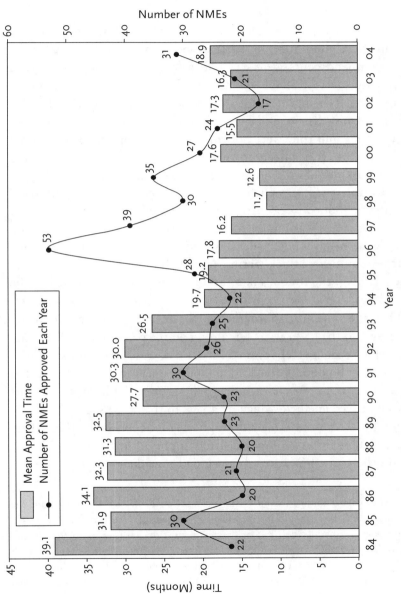

*New molecular entities (NMEs) are new medicines that have never been marketed before, including diagnostic and nondiagnostic drugs.

Sources: 1984–2004 data on the number of NMEs approved each year and 1984–1999 data on the mean approval time from U.S. FDA, Center for Drug Evaluation and Research. [Online information.] http://www.fda.gov/cder; 2000–2004 data on the mean approval time from Tufts Center for the Study of Drug Development Approved New Molecular Entities Data Set.

informed about approved drug uses and possible side effects. However, FDA regulation has had some adverse consequences.

The U.S. Drug Lag

One measure of the FDA's performance is how long it takes to approve a drug in the United States compared with other countries. After the 1962 drug amendments were enacted, a long lag developed between the time drugs were available for use in other countries and when they could be used in the United States. For example, drugs proven effective for treating heart disease and hypertension were used in Great Britain as early as 1965, but they were not fully approved for use in the United States until 1976. It has been estimated that between 7,500 and 15,000 people died in 1988 alone from gastric ulcers while waiting for the FDA to approve misoprostol, which was already available in 43 countries. Furthermore, about 20,000 people are estimated to have died between 1985 and 1987 while waiting for approval of streptokinase, the first drug that could be intravenously administered to reopen the blocked coronary arteries of heart attack victims (Gottlieb 2004).

The drug lag, the time it takes for a new drug to be approved in the United States after it has been approved in another country, has two effects. First, the longer the approval time, the greater the cost of producing a new drug and the fewer years remaining on the patent life of that drug, both of which reduce R&D profitability and decrease the number of new drugs likely to be developed. Second, and perhaps most important, the longer it takes to approve a new drug, the greater the harm to patients who would have benefited by having access to that drug sooner.[5]

Early studies looking at data through the 1970s concluded that a drug lag existed. Researchers compared drugs approved in the United Kingdom and the United States and concluded that drugs approved in the

---

5. One analyst who examined the 1962 drug amendments concluded that they made the public worse off. Sam Peltzman (1974) attempted to quantify the benefits of the 1962 amendments by estimating the effect of the new regulations on keeping ineffective and dangerous drugs (of which there were very few before 1962) off the market compared with the lost benefits of having fewer new drugs, higher prices for existing drugs (because of less competition from new drugs), and reduced availability of drugs because of the time lag. The decline in the development of new drugs was the greatest disadvantage of the amendments; this factor alone, according to Peltzman, made the costs of the new amendments greatly exceed the potential benefits.

United States lagged behind those approved in the United Kingdom by about two years. However, in more recent years the U.S. drug lag appears to have disappeared. As shown in Figure 26.1, the approval rate of new drugs by the FDA was 50 percent faster in the mid-1990s compared with the previous decade. Understanding changes in the FDA's drug approval rate requires an understanding of the FDA's decision process.

FDA's Incentives

The two main criticisms of FDA regulation are the long delays before new drugs are approved (currently about 19 months) and the increasing R&D cost imposed on drug companies for bringing a new drug to market. The FDA makes a choice when it decides how much emphasis to place on drug safety and efficacy versus approval delays and increased R&D cost. It is important to understand the political incentives that the FDA faces in making this trade-off.

Politically, a large difference exists between statistical (or invisible) persons who could have been saved and identifiable persons who died as a result of a new drug. When the FDA approves a drug that subsequently results in the deaths of a number of individuals, these deaths will be publicized in the media. Congress is likely to become involved as the publicity increases. The congressional committee that has oversight of the FDA will have hearings at which the relatives of the deceased patients testify. The FDA staff will have to explain why they approved an unsafe drug. As FDA Commissioner Schmidt stated in 1974:

> In all of the FDA's history, I am unable to find a single instance where a Congressional Committee investigated the failure of the FDA to approve a new drug. But, the times when hearings have been held to criticize our approval of new drugs have been so frequent that we aren't able to count them . . . The message to FDA staff could not be clearer. Whenever a controversy over a new drug is resolved by its approval, the Agency and the individual involved likely will be investigated. Whenever such a drug is disapproved, no inquiry will be made (p. 76).

Deaths caused by a drug are "visible" or "identifiable" deaths because the individuals affected can be readily identified. Minimizing identifiable deaths, however, delays the FDA approval process. Each day a life-saving drug is unavailable is a day someone may die for lack of that drug. Persons who may die because a life-saving drug is unavailable are referred to as statistical deaths.[6]

People who die because a life-saving drug has not yet received FDA approval, although it may be available in Europe, are difficult to identify and are not as visible. The media do not publicize all the nameless people who may have died because a new drug was too costly to be developed or was slow in receiving FDA approval. No media attention is given to the thousands of individuals in need of the drug and their families. Deaths that can be attributed to drug lag, particularly with the early beta-blockers to prevent heart attacks, number in the tens of thousands. The large number of these statistical deaths has greatly outweighed the number of victims of all drug tragedies before the 1962 amendments (including those deaths caused by elixir sulfanilamide in the 1930s).

Statistical lives and identifiable lives are not politically equal. The media and members of Congress place a great deal more pressure on the FDA when a loss of identifiable lives results from a prematurely approved drug than if a much greater loss of statistical lives occurred as a result of the FDA delaying approval of a new drug. The FDA's incentives are clearly to minimize the loss of identifiable lives at the expense of a greater loss of statistical lives. The FDA can make one of two types of errors, as shown in Table 26.1. Type I error occurs when the FDA approves a drug that is found to have harmful effects; Type II error occurs when the FDA either delays or does not approve a beneficial drug. Both types of errors are not weighted equally by the FDA. The FDA places greater emphasis on preventing type I errors.

Although a human life is a human life, the decision maker's calculation of the costs and benefits of early versus delayed approval is on the side of delayed approval. The political pressure on FDA staff to justify

---

6. Statistical deaths are calculated as follows. Assume that a new drug is introduced in Europe and two years elapse before that same drug receives FDA approval to be marketed in the United States. Further assume that the new drug is more effective than the drug currently on the market to treat that same disease, such that it is able to decrease mortality from 5 percent to 1 percent. Suppose 100,000 persons each year are affected by that illness. The number of lives that would have been saved by earlier FDA approval is 8,000. The percentage difference in mortality rate (0.05 − 0.01 = 0.04), multiplied by the two-year lag when the drug could have been on the market (0.04 × 2 = 0.08), multiplied by the number of people at risk each year (0.08 × 100,000) equals 8,000 statistical deaths because of the two-year delay.

Table 26.1: FDA and Type I and Type II Errors

	Drug Is Beneficial	Drug Is Harmful
FDA allows the drug	Correct decision	Type I error
		Allows a harmful drug; victims are identifiable, and FDA staff must explain to Congress
FDA does not allow the drug	Type II error	Correct decision
	Disallows a beneficial drug; victims are not identifiable	

their decisions will cause them to be overly cautious in approving new drugs until they can be sure no loss of life will occur.

The cost-benefit decision to the FDA of when it approves a drug has undergone a change in recent years (Carpenter 2004). Previously, the FDA bore little cost of delaying approval of a drug (from those who would have benefited from the drug), while it benefited by gathering more and more information as to the drug's safety; the FDA minimized the chances that Congress would criticize it for endangering the public's safety. Under these cost-benefit calculations, it was in the FDA's interest to delay approval until it was much more certain as to the drug's safety. In recent years, the cost to the FDA of delaying approval has increased. Patient advocacy groups, at times allied with the drug company whose drug is being reviewed, have pressured the FDA for accelerated approval of drugs. Advocacy groups for AIDS patients were among the first such groups to publicize the cost of delays in drug approval. (Pharmaceutical firms supported these patient advocacy groups because they wanted to start earning revenues sooner.)

The effect of patient advocacy groups and media publicity on drug approval times is illustrated by data on approval times for different types of cancer drugs (Carpenter 2004). Although lung cancer has a higher mortality rate and is more costly to treat (requiring a greater number of hospitalizations and a longer length of hospital stay) than breast cancer, breast cancer has more advocacy groups who were able to generate greater media attention; consequently, breast cancer drugs were more quickly approved than drugs for lung cancer patients. The same relationship between media publicity and drug approval times exists for other drugs as well.

Patient advocacy groups that are able to generate a great deal of media attention have increased the visibility of the consequences of delay. In doing so, they have raised the political cost to the FDA of drug approval delays (type II errors). However, whenever an approved drug is shown to be less safe than originally believed, as occurred with Vioxx, which was traced to a small but higher risk of heart attacks among patients who use it (type I error), the FDA staff will come under a great deal of criticism and revert toward excessive caution in approving new drugs.

Increased Cost of Drug Development

Stringent FDA guidelines and long approval times have greatly increased the cost of developing new drugs. After the 1962 drug amendments required more rigorous clinical testing, proof of efficacy, and safety criteria for FDA approval, the cost and time for bringing a new drug to market increased sharply. Before the 1962 amendments, the cost of a new drug, including the cost of failed drugs, was $6.6 million in 2005 dollars. The median time in which a new drug proceeds from starting clinical testing to receiving FDA approval has been increasing over time, from 4.7 years on average during the 1960s (after the 1962 drug amendments) to 6.7 years in the 1970s, to 8.5 years in the 1980s, and to 9.1 years in the mid-1990s. As of 2003, it took, on average, about 16.5 years from a research idea until a drug was marketed.

The cost of developing a new drug has increased dramatically. In 1987, drug companies spent about $231 million to develop a new drug; if the costs had increased at the same rate as inflation, this would have been $397 million in 2005. However, a study conducted by DiMasi, Hansen, and Grabowski (2003) estimated that the cost has soared to $802 million. (Adams and Brantner [2006] estimate the cost to be from $500 million to more than $2 trillion.) An important reason for the rapidly increasing cost of drug development is the cost of human trials. The typical clinical trial currently involves 4,000 people, compared with 1,300 in the 1980s. Managed care companies are demanding that drug companies prove the value of their drugs in larger and longer clinical trials.

Included in the costs of drug development are actual expenditures as well as the opportunity cost of the interest forgone on these investment costs. For example, only $403 million of the estimated $802 million represents actual out-of-pocket costs. The rest is the estimated cost of capital, or the amount that investing the money at an 11 percent rate of return would have earned over time. This opportunity cost of capital is significant, as long time lags exist between investment expenditures and revenues generated by new drugs.

These investment costs include expenditures on many drugs that will never make it to market (failures). Of every 5,000 potential new drugs tested in animals, only five are likely to reach human clinical trials; of those five, only one will eventually be marketed.

Also important to a drug firm's profitability is the fact that the longer it takes to achieve the FDA's stringent research guidelines and receive FDA approval, the shorter the remaining patent life on the drug and the period in which to make profits. Profit is the principal motivating factor behind drug companies' willingness to assume risk and invest large amounts in R&D. *The pharmaceutical manufacturers' profitability over time is determined by their investment in R&D.* As shown in Figure 26.2, R&D expenditures as a percentage of U.S. sales are about 19 percent of revenue. This rate of investment is one of the highest of any industry.

Profitability over time (as a percentage of revenue) for pharmaceutical firms has also been higher than for any other industry. Although profits are high, so are the risks, as the costs of developing a new drug and bringing it to market are as high as $800 million. Furthermore, drug development is a very risky business; only a small percentage of drugs will make it through all of the clinical phases and become financially viable. *The high rates of profit earned by drug manufacturers to finance R&D result from the few breakthrough drugs discovered.* Even those that are marketed may not be financially successful; about three of ten drugs marketed make a profit, and about 10 percent of all drugs marketed provide 52 percent of the industry's profits.

Figure 26.3 describes the percentage of drugs the profits of which exceed average R&D costs. As can be seen, the distribution of profits is skewed. Very few drugs offer a profitable return, but for the 10 percent of drugs considered to be "blockbuster" drugs the profits are substantial. Thus, a drug company needs a few "winners," especially blockbusters, to repay the costs on the majority of drugs that do not even repay their R&D investments.

Patent protection is essential for protecting a drug manufacturer's investments in R&D. Once a new drug is discovered, it can be reproduced

Figure 26.2: Domestic R&D Expenditures as a Percentage of U.S. Domestic Sales, Pharmaceutical Companies, 1970–2005

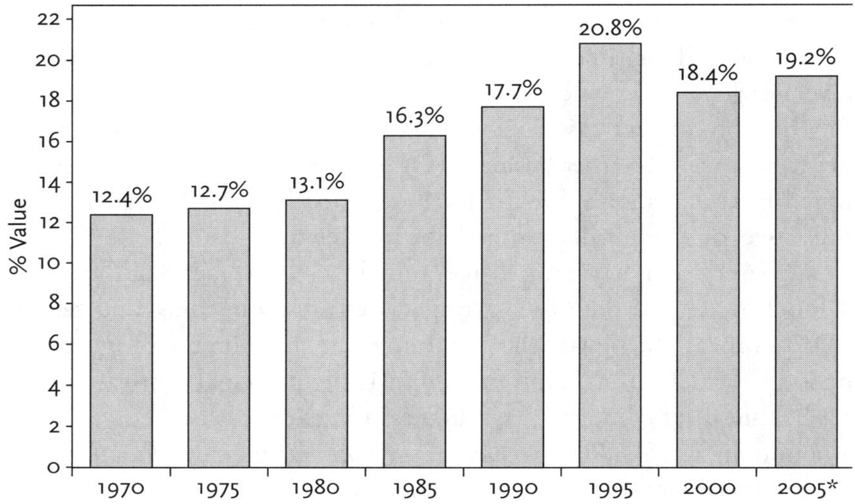

*Estimated data.

Source: Pharmaceutical Research and Manufacturers of America. 2006. *PhRMA Annual Membership Survey.* [Online information.] http://www.phrma.org/files/2006%20Industry%20Profile.pdf.

relatively easily. Without the period of market exclusivity that patents provide, drug manufacturers could not recover their R&D investments. Patents provide a drug manufacturer with market power, the ability to price above costs of production. Breakthrough drugs have a great deal more market power than a "me-too" drug. Although a new breakthrough drug (the first drug to treat an illness) may initially have a great deal of market power, other companies can eventually patent drugs that use the same mechanism to treat the illness. Once patent protection expires, generic versions priced much below the branded drug quickly increase their share of the market. For example, in 1997, the patent on Zantac expired, and the generic version captured 90 percent of the market served by Zantac within two years. Currently, about half of all prescription drugs dispensed are off-patent generic drugs.

Public policy with respect to the drug industry must deal with the following trade-off. To increase R&D investments, drug manufacturers

Figure 26.3: Decile Distribution of Present Values of Postlaunch Returns for the Sample of 1990–1994 New Chemical Entities

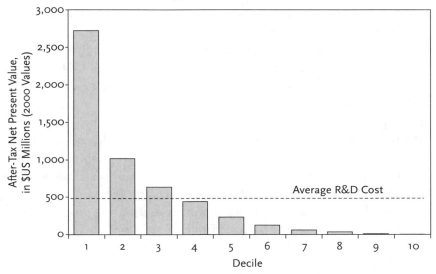

Source: Grabowski, H. G., et al. 2002. "Returns to Research and Development for 1990s New Drug Introductions." *Pharmacoeconomics* 20 (15, Suppl. 3): 11–29, Figure 7.

must earn high profits on innovative drugs that provide significant increases in therapeutic value. However, the cost of producing these drugs is but a small fraction of their selling price. If prices on these breakthrough drugs were made more affordable (closer to their production costs) to alleviate the large burden on those with low incomes, the high profits that provide the incentive to invest in R&D would disappear. *Lower drug prices that benefit today's patients mean fewer innovative drugs in the future.*

Orphan Drugs

As R&D costs and the time for drug approval have increased, long and costly clinical trials to develop "orphan" drugs, those that would benefit small population groups, became unprofitable. The potential revenue for a new drug may be small because few people are afflicted with a particular disease or a small percentage of those afflicted do not respond to the standard treatment. Rising R&D costs make targeting these small therapeutic markets unprofitable. Market size (potential revenue) is an important determinant of drug development. Congress enacted the Orphan Drug Act in 1984 to provide drug companies with a financial incentive (tax incentives or exclusive marketing rights) to develop drugs that provide therapeutic benefits for fewer than 200,000 patients.

Similar to the orphan drug issue is the concern that drug development is targeted toward people living in wealthy countries. Only 5 percent of global R&D is directed at health problems unique to developing nations, although 90 percent of the global disease burden is in the developing world. Private-sector R&D is determined by prospective demand conditions. For example, malaria is a parasitic disease that has a global incidence of 200 to 300 million cases annually. About 1 million deaths are caused by malaria each year, and the majority of these deaths are children under the age of five years living in sub-Saharan Africa. Drug development aimed at health problems confronting people in poor countries will need to be subsidized from government sources.

SUMMARY

The rationale for FDA regulation of drugs is presumably to provide a remedy for the lack of information that exists among physicians and consumers when buying drugs. Lack of information on a drug's safety could cause serious harm to patients. Given this serious information problem, what should FDA's role be? Should the FDA continue to be the sole decision maker on the availability of new drugs? Or should the FDA play a more passive role by merely providing information on the safety and efficacy of new drugs and leave the decision about whether to use a new drug to the physician and the patient?

What is the optimum trade-off between statistical and identifiable deaths? Who should make that decision? Decreased identifiable deaths means increased testing, increased R&D costs, delays in FDA approval, and a consequent increase in statistical deaths. Clearly, for saving lives and treating serious illnesses the choice should be less concern with drug safety and efficacy and quicker approval to minimize the number of statistical deaths. The costs of delay vary depending on the seriousness of the illness. Even two patients with the same disease will differ on the types of risks they are willing to accept. Under the current system the FDA is determining the level of risk acceptable to society, while some patients would be willing to go above that level.

Proponents of strengthening the FDA's current role (rather than changing it to be merely a provider of information) are concerned that physicians and patients would still have incomplete information to make appropriate decisions on new drugs. Physicians may be too busy or unwilling to invest the time to fully understand the safety and efficacy information on new drugs and may even be influenced by drug company advertising. Changing the FDA's role from that of a decision maker to simply a provider of information does not appear to have much public support. Instead, public policy is more concerned with speeding up the FDA's approval process. The time for approving a new drug has declined but is beginning to rise again. Various proposals have been made to speed up the FDA's review process for drug approval, such as having the FDA also rely on evidence gathered from other countries that have high approval standards, dropping the proof-of-efficacy requirement, and requiring less evidence of a drug's safety for life-saving drugs that have no alternative therapy.

Speeding up the FDA's approval process will require greater post-marketing surveillance of drug interactions and safety. Evidence of the effects of a new drug may not be known for several years. The long preapproval process continues to miss dangerous drugs. For example, Trovan, an antibiotic drug, had to be withdrawn because of unforeseen liver injuries. Only after a drug has been on the market and used by large numbers of people can its safety and efficacy be truly evaluated.

In addition to speeding up the FDA's approval process and expanding postmarket surveillance of new drugs, concerns exist about the time and cost required to bring a new drug to market. High R&D costs (like longer times for approval that shorten patent life) decrease the profitability of an investment in new drugs. Decreased profitability leads to a lower investment and results in fewer new drugs being discovered. As the costs of drug discovery are increased, drug companies are less likely to develop drugs that have small market potential. An additional consequence of the high cost and long time requirements to introduce a new drug is that, with fewer new drugs being introduced, drug prices are higher than if more competition existed.

High R&D costs also have a greater effect on small drug firms. Large drug firms have many new drugs in the discovery pipeline and on the market. Small firms invest their capital in the particular drug that is going through the R&D and approval process. The longer the delay in being able to market their drug, the greater is their capital requirement. To minimize their chance of running out of money, small drug firms with a promising new drug will merge or partner with larger firms that have greater capital resources and experience with the drug approval process. The longer and more costly the FDA's research and approval process, the greater is the burden on small drug firms.

Economics is concerned with trade-offs. Choosing one policy, namely increased drug safety and efficacy, has a "cost," namely fewer new drugs being developed. A greater number of statistical deaths will occur, the drug industry will become more consolidated, and drug prices will be higher because fewer new drugs will compete with existing drugs. Thus, merely favoring increased drug safety and efficacy is not a simple choice without consequences. The issue is how to strike an appropriate balance between these choices.

DISCUSSION QUESTIONS

1. How have the 1962 drug amendments affected the profitability of new drugs?

2. What is the consequence of the FDA providing the public with greater assurance that a new drug is safe?

3. What is the difference between identifiable and statistical deaths?

4. What are orphan drugs, and why are drug firms less likely to develop such drugs today?

5. Why has the FDA's drug approval process sped up in recent years?

6. What are the advantages and disadvantages of greater reliance on premarket testing versus postmarket surveillance?

REFERENCES

Adams, C., and V. Brantner. 2006. "Estimating the Cost of New Drug Development: Is it Really $802 Million?" *Health Affairs* 25 (2): 420–28.

Carpenter, D. 2004. "The Political Economy of FDA Drug Review: Processing, Politics, and Lessons for Policy." *Health Affairs* 23 (1): 52–63.

DiMasi, J., R. Hansen, and H. Grabowski. 2003. "The Price of Innovation: New Estimates of Drug Development Costs." *Journal of Health Economics* 22 (2): 151–85.

Gottlieb, S. 2004. "The Price of Too Much Caution." *New York Sun* December 22. [Online information; retrieved 11/15/06.] http://www.aei.org/news/newsID.21746, filter./news_detail.asp.

Harris, R. 1964. *The Real Voice*. New York: MacMillan.

Olson, M. K. 1994. "Political Influence and Regulatory Policy: The 1984 Drug Legislation." *Economic Inquiry* 32 (3): 363–82.

Peltzman, S. 1974. *Regulation of Pharmaceutical Innovation*. Washington, DC: American Enterprise Institute.

Schmidt, A. 1974. "The FDA Today: Critics, Congress, and Consumerism." Speech given at the National Press Club, Washington, DC, October 29. Quoted in Grabowski, H. 1976. *Drug Regulation and Innovation*. Washington, DC: AEI Press.

ADDITIONAL READINGS

Temin, P. 1980. *Taking Your Medicine: Drug Regulation in the United States,* 27–31. Cambridge, MA: Harvard University Press.

U.S. Congress, Office of Technology Assessment. 1993. *Pharmaceutical R&D: Costs, Risks and Rewards,* OTA-H-522. Washington, DC: U.S. Government Printing Office.

U.S. Congressional Budget Office. 1998. *How Increased Competition from Generic Drugs Has Affected Prices and Returns in the Pharmaceutical Industry*. Washington, DC: U.S. Government Printing Office.

Chapter 27

Why Are Prescription Drugs Less Expensive Overseas?

ANECDOTES ABOUND ABOUT people traveling to Canada or Mexico to buy a prescription drug at a much lower price than offered by retail pharmacies in this country. In addition to anecdotal evidence, studies by the U.S. General Accounting Office (1992, 1994) have shown that branded prescription drugs are more expensive in the United States than in other countries. The studies concluded that U.S. prices were 32 percent higher than prices in Canada and 60 percent higher than prices in the United Kingdom. Another study (U.S. House of Representatives, Committee on Government Reform and Oversight 1998) found that senior citizens in Maine paid an average retail price of $116.01 for Prilosec, whereas consumers in Canada and Mexico paid $53.05 and $29.46, respectively (Figure 27.1).

Cross-national comparison studies of branded (prescription) drug prices generally conclude that lower drug prices in other countries are a result of regulatory price controls, implying that the United States can similarly lower drug prices by using price controls. The following sections discuss the accuracy of cross-national drug price studies, why higher prices for prescription drugs in the United States are not surprising, and the implications of requiring U.S. drug manufacturers to charge a single uniform price overseas and in the United States.

ACCURACY OF STUDIES ON INTERNATIONAL VARIATIONS IN DRUG PRICES

The methodology used in the General Accounting Office studies and similar studies that concluded that prescription drug prices are higher in the United States than in other countries has been widely criticized.

Figure 27.1: Prices for Prilosec, Selected Countries, 2001

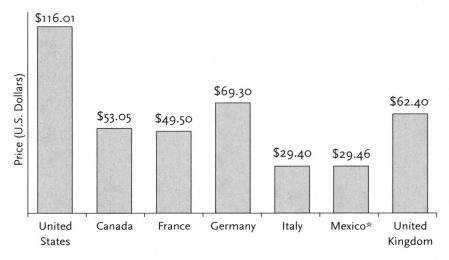

*1998 data.

Sources: U.S. House of Representatives, Committee on Government Reform. 2001. Minority Staff, Special Investigation Division. Prepared for Rep. Thomas A. Allen. *Rx Drugs More Expensive in Maine than in Canada, Europe, and Japan.* Washington, DC: U.S. Government Printing Office; U.S. House of Representatives, Committee on Government Reform and Oversight. 1998. Minority Staff Report. Prepared for Rep. Thomas A. Allen. *Prescription Drug Pricing in the 1st Congressional District in Maine: An International Price Comparison.* Washington, DC: U.S. Government Printing Office.

What these studies purport to analyze and the methods used should be subject to greater examination before their implications for the United States are accepted.

Retail Price Comparisons

Typically, cross-national studies compare the retail prices of selected prescription drugs that are bought by cash-paying patients in the United States to the retail prices of those same drugs in another country. (The General Accounting Office studies used listed wholesale prices in the United States, which were intended to approximate prices charged to retail pharmacies.) These comparisons greatly overstate U.S. drug prices because they assume that all purchasers of the prescription drug in the United States pay the same price. Using retail (or even wholesale) prices as the prescription drug price in the United States does not account for the large discounts and rebates received by large U.S. purchasers such as MCOs, PBMs, mail-order drug firms, and federal government programs, including Medicaid. (Patients in these organizations merely pay a copayment that is a small fraction of the price the organizations pay for the drug.) Discounts and rebates lower the average selling price to these large purchasers compared with the retail or wholesale prices used in these comparison studies. Not only do these large purchasers comprise the majority of the U.S. prescription drug market, but they also represent a larger percentage of the purchasers in the United States than in comparison countries.

These large purchasers pay substantially less for prescription drugs than cash-paying U.S. patients who do not have prescription drug insurance and buy directly from a retail pharmacy. Cash-paying patients represent a small segment of the prescription drug buyers in the United States, so comparisons using these patients greatly overstate prices.

Rather than assuming a single U.S. retail price, comparing prices paid on average by all those purchasing drugs in the United States to the prices paid by overseas patients would be more appropriate.[1]

Cost of Drug Therapy

Given the public policy implications of cross-national studies, the purpose of these comparisons must be clarified so that an appropriate study design can be determined. One objective of such studies might be to estimate the cost of drug therapy (by disease) to patients in different countries, not just the differences in prices for specific prescription products. To accurately examine differences in drug therapy cost across countries such studies should adjust for the use of generic substitutes and weighting of the different drugs used in a country's drug price index.

Cross-national studies have excluded generic drugs, which are priced between 40 and 80 percent lower than branded drugs. Furthermore, U.S. purchasers rely much more on generic drugs than do patients in other countries. (Generics accounted for 46 percent of prescriptions in the United States in 1998, whereas use of generics in countries with strict drug price regulation, such as France and Italy, is very low.) If generic

---

1. A number of other issues are involved in examining retail drug prices, such as dosage form; strength; and pack size, for example, price per gram of active ingredient or price per dose (standard unit), which may be one tablet, one capsule, or 10 mL of a liquid. Differences in prescription drug prices also occur because of differences in dosage form, strength, and pack size used in the comparison countries.

drugs are more frequently substituted for expensive branded drugs in the United States than in other countries, a comparison based solely on branded drugs overstates the cost of a prescription for U.S. patients.

Another important issue in cross-national comparisons is the mix or consumption pattern of drugs used in different countries. Comparisons of drug prices between countries rely on a simple average of the prices paid for several leading brand-name drugs. For example, the General Accounting Office study (1992) comparing branded drug prices in the United States and Canada merely compared U.S. prices to Canadian prices for a number of branded drugs. (These prices were then added up and compared to the sum of the U.S. retail prices for those same drugs. Dividing the sum of the prices of one country by the sum of prices in the other country resulted in a ratio of prices between the two countries.) In doing so, the study gave an equal weight to each branded drug being compared. Whether some branded drugs were widely or infrequently used did not matter; each received an equal weight.

Because the United States and other countries have different drug consumption patterns, any price index should reflect these differences by weighting the volume of use of different branded drugs. Some branded drugs represent a greater percentage of purchased branded drugs than others; these percentages differ by country.

Cross-national comparisons should use a weighted average of the prices of branded drugs. The index should also include the use of generic drugs as well as the average prices paid for all drugs, including the discounted prices paid by MCOs and other large purchasers in the United States and the volume they purchase. This would result in a much lower weighted average price than simply observing the price of the branded drug (and its volume) sold to retail customers. Furthermore, for some branded drugs a great deal of substitution of the generic version, which is sold at a lower price, occurs. A weighted average price of that drug would include the branded and generic versions, which would result in a much lower price than simply using the branded version. Each drug should also be given a weight in the index according to its use in that country.

A Drug Price Index

Research conducted by Danzon and Chao (2000) determined that when a drug price index is constructed for each country using average prices paid by different purchasers, including generic drugs, and weighting drug prices by their frequency of use, the index may be no higher in the

United States than in other countries. *Although individual prescription drugs may be more expensive in the United States, the costs of drug therapy across countries (based on an accurately constructed drug price index) are not much different.* (For a detailed discussion of cross-national comparisons, including additional limitations such as the unit of measurement and the availability of branded drugs, as well as appropriate methodologies and results, see Danzon and Furukawa [2003].)

WHY PRESCRIPTION DRUGS ARE EXPECTED TO BE PRICED LOWER OVERSEAS

Numerous examples can be found of prescription drugs that are less expensive in other countries than in the United States. Why would a manufacturer of a patented prescription drug be willing to sell the same drug at greatly reduced prices overseas? This pricing behavior is based on two characteristics of the drug industry, its cost structure and differences in each country's bargaining power.

The costs of developing and bringing to market an innovative new drug are very high (DiMasi, Hansen, and Grabowski 2003). The R&D costs for a prescription drug can go as high as $800 million dollars. Experimental trials must be conducted, and the FDA's approval is required. It may take seven to ten years to develop a new drug and receive FDA approval. The R&D costs, as well as the costs involved in receiving FDA approval, are termed *fixed costs*. These development costs are the same regardless of how much of the patented new drug is produced and sold. The actual costs of producing the new drug, once its chemical entities have been determined through the R&D process and it has received FDA approval, are relatively small. Thus, patented drugs are characterized by very large fixed costs and relatively small variable costs (the actual costs of producing the drug).

The drug manufacturer would like to receive the highest possible price for that new drug. For some purchasers, however, the manufacturer would be willing to accept any price that exceeds its variable costs. A price in excess of variable costs makes a contribution to covering those large fixed costs and to profit. The manufacturer is better off receiving $5 even if it costs $4 to produce that drug; the $1 revenue from some purchasers is better than nothing.

The drug industry is very sophisticated in its pricing of the same medicine across different countries. A drug manufacturer would like to add new users (sell the drug in different countries) because the variable

Figure 27.2: World Pharmaceutical Market, 2005

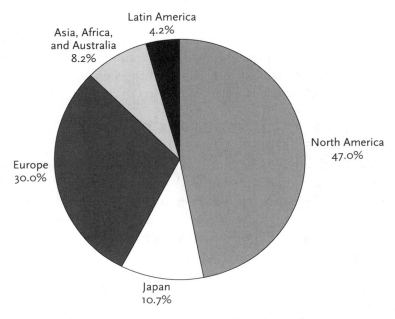

Total World Pharmaceutical Market = $566 Billion

Source: IMS Health. 2006. [Online information.] http://www.imshealth.com.

costs of producing the drug are so low, but it is not willing to add new users if it has to reduce the price and revenues it earns in higher-priced markets. The single largest market for new innovative drugs is in the United States, which accounts for 43 percent of the world pharmaceutical market (North America, comprising the United States and Canada, represents 47 percent [Figure 27.2]). People in the United States are on average wealthier than those in other countries and want access to innovative drugs as soon as possible; they are therefore less price sensitive to high drug prices (about two-thirds of the U.S. population has insurance to pay for prescription drugs). Not surprisingly, drug manufacturers charge higher prices when consumers are less price sensitive.

In countries that regulate the price of drugs, the same manufacturer is willing to sell the same drug at a lower price as long as the regulated price exceeds the manufacturer's variable cost of producing that drug.

The drug manufacturer would be very concerned if purchasers in the lower-priced countries were to resell the drug in the higher-priced markets. If resale from the lower-price countries to the higher-priced countries were possible, a differential pricing system could not persist.

As long as the manufacturer is able to prevent resale of the same drug from low- to high-priced markets, this system of differential pricing allows markets that would otherwise be neglected to be served. Differential pricing, whereby a drug manufacturer charges different prices to different countries for the same medicine, results in the greatest number of people gaining access to a drug. The manufacturer is willing to reduce its price to countries that regulate drugs and to poor countries that cannot afford to pay much for drugs not because the manufacturer has a social conscience, but because any sales at a price that exceeds the drug's variable cost contribute to profits. By trying to increase profits, however, the drug manufacturer also provides the greatest number of people with access to its drug.

Canadian and European governments, which pay for most of their populations' health expenditures, keep drug prices down because they have limited budgets for health care. These tight budgets for drug expenditures have had unintended side effects. The introduction of cost-effective drugs has been delayed because the budget for drugs would be exceeded. Consequently, surgical and hospital expenditures have been greater than if costly new innovative drugs had been used, and delays have occurred in approving life-saving drugs for citizens of these countries.

For example, "Herceptin, which was considered to be a breakthrough drug for about a third of all breast cancer patients . . . was approved two years ago by regulators in the U.S., where it benefited from an accelerated review offered to novel cancer therapies. It is still awaiting regulatory approval in most of Europe" (Moore 2000). Furthermore,

> Many European countries also attempt to restrict demand after new medicines reach pharmacy shelves. European . . . countries with tight pharmaceutical budgets have made it difficult for cancer patients to have access to older cancer drugs (Taxol) that were top selling anti-cancer drugs. One study (industry funded) examining prescribing patterns between 1996 and 1998 finds the following: while 99.9% of patients with advanced breast cancer in the U.S. received treatment with taxane, the comparable [rate] was 48% for the Netherlands and only 25% for Britain (Moore 2000).

Figure 27.3: Pharmaceutical Expenditures as a Percentage of Total Health Expenditures, Selected Countries, 2003

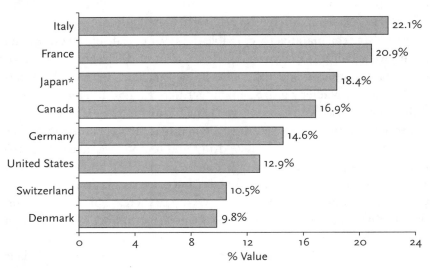

*Data for 2002.

Note: Pharmaceuticals include prescription and nonprescription drugs.

Source: Data from Organisation for Economic Cooperation and Development. 2005. *OECD Health at a Glance, 2005.* Paris: OECD.

Another consequence of regulated lower drug prices overseas is that total drug expenditures represent a higher portion of total medical expenditures in those countries than in the United States (Figure 27.3) because the prices for drugs in those countries are quite low (generally for older molecules), and neither patients nor their physicians have any incentive to use fewer drugs. For example, to reduce drug expenditures the German government in recent years imposed financial penalties on physicians to limit their prescribing too many drugs. The United States spends a smaller portion on drugs (12.9 percent of total health expenditures) than Italy (22.1 percent), France (20.9 percent), Japan (18.4 percent), Canada (16.9 percent), or Germany (14.6 percent).

PUBLIC POLICY ISSUES

Cross-national studies that have found that the United States has higher prescription drug prices imply that the United States should institute a price-control system similar to those of countries that have lower drug prices. By publicizing these study findings, along with examples of aged persons who cannot afford to pay high retail drug prices, advocates of price controls hope to build political support for imposing controls on U.S. prescription drugs.

Two methods for equalizing U.S. and overseas prices on prescription drugs are favored by proponents of a regulatory approach. The first is having the U.S. government require that the retail price of prescription drugs sold in the United States be no different from the price at which those same drugs are sold in other countries, such as Canada and Mexico. The second approach is to allow pharmacists to import FDA-approved U.S. prescription drugs to the United States from other countries where they sell for substantially less. Each of these proposals has short-term effects as well as indirect, or unintended, longer-term consequences.

A Single Price for Prescription Drugs Across Countries

What would happen to prescription drug prices in both the United States and overseas if U.S. drug manufacturers were required to price U.S.-branded drugs at the same price at which they are sold to other countries? Proponents of a single price for the same medicine assume that the uniform price will be the lowest of the different prices charged for that same drug. Assume that a prescription drug, ABC, sells for $10 in the United States and $5 in Canada. Further assume that the United States enacts a law stating that the manufacturer of drug ABC must charge the same price regardless of the country in which the drug is sold. Would the price of drug ABC be reduced to $5 and U.S. consumers receive a $5 benefit?

The answer is no.

The manufacturer of drug ABC would have to determine which single price would result in the greatest amount of profit. Because the United States is the largest single market for innovative branded drugs, and its consumers are less price sensitive, greatly reducing the drug's price in the U.S. market would not result in a large increase in the number of users of that drug. Consequently, a large decrease in price (without a corresponding large increase in volume) would cause a large decrease in revenue.[2] Given the large profits earned in the United States (the price markup over variable cost in the United States multiplied by the large

---

2. When consumers are less price sensitive, changes in price cause smaller proportionate changes in volume. By increasing price, total revenue increases because the percentage change in price is greater than the percentage change in volume. Similarly, lowering price when

number of users), the uniform price of the drug will likely be closer to the U.S. price than to the lower prices paid in other countries. The drug company will lose less money if it raises the prices in other countries by a greater amount than it lowers the U.S. price.

Keeping the uniform price closer to the U.S. price for a drug means the new uniform price of the drug will be increased in other countries. Raising the price in these countries is likely to cause a decrease in use. These countries typically have limited government budgets for health care, and a large increase in the price of drugs would cause the government to restrict their use. Whether total revenue to the U.S. manufacturer from sales of the drug in other countries increases or decreases depends on whether the percentage increase in price exceeds the percentage decrease in use in those countries.

In either case, requiring a uniform price for drug ABC in the United States and other countries means overseas patients who need the drug will be worse off. Whereas formerly they (or the government on their behalf) paid $5, they would now have to pay a higher price. Some patients would no longer have access to the drug. If close substitute drugs are available, patients will buy these other drugs (assuming the price of these other drugs has not also been similarly increased). If close substitutes are not available for innovative drugs, patients/government will have to spend more of their income on the drug. If patients cannot afford to buy the drug or their government restricts its use because of its higher price, adverse health consequences will result. Requiring a uniform pricing policy in the United States and other countries will likely lead to a small reduction in the U.S. price of a drug and an increase in the drug's overseas price so that it is equal to the new U.S. price. This policy would inflict a tragic loss on patients in other countries, who would have to go without innovative drugs.

Reimportation

The second regulatory approach to reducing U.S. retail prices for prescription drugs is to allow U.S. pharmacists and drug wholesalers to buy lower-priced supplies of FDA-approved medicines in Canada and other

---

consumers are not price sensitive will result in a decrease in total revenue. Conversely, when consumers are price sensitive, the percentage change in price is less than the percentage change in volume. With price-sensitive consumers, total revenue increases when prices are reduced.

nations for resale in the United States. Drugs reimported into the United States from Canada would likely be less expensive than the same drugs sold in the United States because of Canadian price controls on those drugs. The presumed effect of this policy would be to reduce the U.S. retail price of drugs to prices comparable to those in the countries from which they are reimported.

A federal law permitting reimportation was enacted in October 2000. This law overturned a 1988 law that permitted only pharmaceutical manufacturers to reimport prescription drugs based on the concern that drugs were being improperly stored and repackaged overseas. Although reimportation was vigorously opposed by the pharmaceutical industry, senators and congressional candidates from both political parties running for reelection during fall 2000 voted for the bill, which was then signed into law by President Clinton. As both political parties could not agree on a Medicare prescription drug benefit, legislators running for reelection believed voting for reimportation would be viewed by the public as being in favor of helping the aged with their prescription drug costs.

In December 2000, Donna Shalala, Secretary of the Department of Health and Human Services, refused to implement the new law, claiming that it was unworkable and would not lower drug costs (Kaufman 2000). At the time of the debate the FDA said it could oversee the drug reimportation system, but only at considerable cost. Unless funding was provided ($93 million a year), the safety of the reimported drugs could not be monitored; full funding was not included in the legislation. Furthermore, the administration believed the bill had several fatal flaws that would deter reimportation, namely that the drug companies would retaliate against reimporters and would not provide the reimporters with the necessary package labeling inserts.

A U.S. manufacturer of a branded prescription drug would be unlikely to increase its sales to a country that resells that drug in the United States. Drug manufacturers could easily monitor drug sales to each country to determine whether sales of a particular drug had suddenly increased. (If the drug importer in a country resells the country's limited supply of that drug back to the United States, patients in that country are harmed by not having access to that drug.)

Thus, to be able to reimport drugs into the United States, U.S. pharmacists and wholesalers would have to buy those chemical entities from a foreign producer of those drugs. When a drug is manufactured in the United States, the manufacturer must adhere to strict FDA guidelines to ensure that the drug is produced with certain quality standards. If a drug is manufactured in another country without extensive monitoring of the reimported drug by the FDA, no guarantee can be given that the drug will meet the same quality standards. The concern over drug safety resulted in 11 former FDA commissioners opposing the reimportation bill.

Thousands of illegal shipments of prescription drugs have been entering the United States each month through the postal service. This growth in overseas sales to U.S. patients has dramatically increased because of the Internet. The sheer volume of such overseas drug shipments has overwhelmed the ability of the FDA and customs officials to verify the safety of the imported drugs. Finally, on June 7, 2001, the FDA proposed stopping overseas drug products from being mailed to individuals unless they met certain strict conditions. The FDA claimed that these drug products could be counterfeit or even dangerous and that the volume is so large that it no longer has the ability to inspect them.

Reimportation is unlikely to be effective in reducing U.S. prescription drug prices, first because U.S. drug manufacturers will be unwilling to sell large quantities of their drugs at greatly reduced prices to other countries so that these countries can sell the same drugs back to U.S. pharmacists at lower prices.[3] Second, if foreign drug manufacturers are permitted to produce a drug patented by a U.S. manufacturer and sell that drug to customers in the United States, those foreign producers would be violating U.S. patent laws and the imports would be prohibited. Third, if other countries are unable to receive sufficient supplies of U.S.-produced drugs to sell back to the U.S., counterfeit drugs are likely to be produced and sold to U.S. patients, resulting in significant safety issues, which will eventually halt mail-order drug sales from overseas.

SUMMARY

Cross-national comparison studies that claim drug prices are less expensive in other countries have been seriously misleading. Although the retail prices of certain prescription drugs may be lower overseas than in the

---

3. In an effort to eliminate drug shipments to Canadian Internet pharmacies that sell lower-cost U.S.-produced drugs to U.S. consumers, Pfizer notified all Canadian drug retailers of its policy to halt all sales of Pfizer drugs to them if they sell Pfizer drugs to U.S. consumers. Pfizer receives information on all drug orders from individual drug stores from its distributors (Carlisle 2004).

United States, the more relevant comparison is the cost of drug therapy in different countries. Only a small percentage of the U.S. population pays retail prices for drugs. The majority of the U.S. population has some form of third-party payment for drugs, and these large purchasers buy their drugs at discounted prices. Generic drugs are also much more widely used in the United States than in other countries. Absent from these cross-national comparisons is any discussion of the availability of innovative drugs overseas.

Public policy affecting prescription drugs should be evaluated on its effect on R&D expenditures. The incentive for drug manufacturers to invest large sums in R&D and develop breakthrough drugs is based on the prospect of earning large profits. Once a drug has been discovered and approved by the FDA for marketing, the actual cost of producing that drug is very low. Not surprisingly, therefore, countries can regulate the price of drugs and still have access to U.S. drugs. (Evidence exists that other countries' regulation of drug prices resulted in a decline in R&D by drug firms in those countries.) These countries can receive a "free ride" on the large R&D expenditures by U.S. drug firms. However, if the United States were to regulate its drug prices as do other countries or permit reimportation by foreign drug producers, R&D investment would decline, as would the supply of innovative drugs. Without government enforcement of patent rights and pricing freedom, the drug industry will decrease its investment in R&D; drugs are easy to copy but expensive to develop. Consumers in both the United States and other countries benefit from differential pricing policies. In other countries more consumers benefit by having access to lower-priced drugs, whereas in the United States the higher prices generate greater profits for the drug companies and provide them with an incentive to invest more in R&D.

If the objective of cross-national studies is to lower the retail prices of drugs so that cash-paying seniors can buy them at lower prices, a better alternative than mandating uniform prices across all countries or permitting reimportation is available. Now that seniors have been provided with a prescription drug benefit as part of the 2003 Medicare Modernization Act, their health plan or a PBM can negotiate lower drug prices from the drug manufacturer, substitute generic drugs when appropriate, and manage the drug benefit to reduce the total cost of drug therapy. Seniors can have access to needed drugs, and competition will reduce prescription drug prices.

DISCUSSION QUESTIONS

1. What are some criticisms of cross-national studies of drug prices?

2. Although some prescription drugs are priced lower in other countries, is the cost of a drug treatment also lower in those countries?

3. Why would a drug manufacturer be willing to sell a drug that is priced high (in relation to its variable costs) in the United States at a low price overseas?

4. What would be the consequences, in terms of drug prices and drug users, if prices of prescription drugs sold in the United States had to equal the price at which those same drugs are sold in other countries?

5. Why would a policy of reimportation of prescription drugs be ineffective?

REFERENCES

Carlisle, T. 2004. "Pfizer Pressures Canadian Sellers of Drugs to U.S." *The Wall Street Journal* January 14, A6.

Danzon, P. M., and L. W. Chao. 2000. "Cross-National Price Differences for Pharmaceuticals: How Large, and Why?" *Journal of Health Economics* 19 (2): 159–95.

Danzon, P., and M. Furukawa. 2003. "Prices and Availability of Pharmaceuticals: Evidence from Nine Countries." *Health Affairs* Web exclusive, October 29, W3-521–W3-536. [Online publication; retrieved 11/15/06.] http://content.healthaffairs.org/cgi/reprint/hlthaff.w3.521v1.

DiMasi, J., R. Hansen, and H. Grabowski. 2003. "The Price of Innovation: New Estimates of Drug Development Cost." *Journal of Health Economics* 22 (2): 151–85.

Kaufman, M. 2000. "Shalala Halts Bid to Lower Drug Costs." *The Washington Post* December 27, A1.

Moore, S. D. 2000. "In Drug-Cost Debate Europe Offers U.S. a Telling Side Effect." *The Wall Street Journal* July 21, 1.

U.S. General Accounting Office. 1992. *Prescription Drugs: Companies Typically Charge More in the United States than in Canada,* GAO/HRD 92–110. Washington, DC: U.S. Government Printing Office.

———. 1994. *Prescription Drugs: Companies Typically Charge More in the United States than in the United Kingdom,* GAO/HEHS 94–29. Washington, DC: U.S. Government Printing Office.

U.S. House of Representatives, Committee on Government Reform and Oversight. 1998. *Prescription Drug Pricing in the 1st Congressional District in Maine: An International Price Comparison.* Minority Staff Report Prepared for Rep. Thomas A. Allen. Washington, DC: U.S. Government Printing Office.

ADDITIONAL READINGS

U.S. Congressional Budget Office. 2004. *Would Prescription Drug Importation Reduce U.S. Drug Spending?* Economic and Budget Issue Brief, April 29. [Online publication; retrieved 11/15/06.] http://www.cbo.gov/showdoc.cfm?index=5406&sequence=0#F4.

U.S. House of Representatives, Committee on Government Reform. 2001. *Rx Drugs More Expensive in Maine than in Canada, Europe, and Japan.* Minority Staff, Special Investigation Division Report Prepared for Rep. Thomas A. Allen. Washington, DC: U.S. Government Printing Office.

Chapter 28

The Pharmaceutical Industry: A Public Policy Dilemma

THE PHARMACEUTICAL INDUSTRY is subject to a great deal of criticism regarding the high prices charged for its drugs, its large (some would say "wasteful") marketing expenditures, and its emphasis on "lifestyle" and "me-too" drugs rather than investing more on drugs to cure infectious diseases and chronic conditions. Yet the industry has developed important drugs that have saved lives, reduced pain, and improved the lives of many. Public policy that attempts to respond to industry critics may at the same time change the industry's incentives for R&D and thereby reduce the number of potential blockbuster drugs.

To evaluate the criticisms of this profitable industry and the consequences of public policy directed toward it, an understanding of the structure of this industry is important.

The pharmaceutical industry comprises two distinct types of drug manufacturers: pharmaceutical manufacturers, who engage in R&D and market brand-name drugs, and generic manufacturers. Pharmaceutical manufacturers invest large sums in R&D, whereas generic manufacturers do not. Consequently, the former group develops innovative branded drugs for new therapeutic uses, while generic firms sell copies of branded drugs (when their patents expire) at greatly reduced prices. These two industries differ in their economic performance and in the public policies directed toward them. Most public policy is directed at pharmaceutical manufacturers.

Understanding the distribution channel for prescription drugs is also important for understanding the structure of the industry. Manufacturers produce the drugs and, for the most part, sell them to wholesalers, who then sell them to pharmacies where they are purchased by patients.

Pharmacies can be chain drug stores such as Rite-Aid, mass merchandis-ers such as Wal-Mart, food store pharmacies such as Safeway, mail-order or retail pharmacies, and, more recently, Internet pharmacy web sites. Over time, the number of independent retail pharmacies has been declin-ing. Wholesalers and retail pharmacies are each competitive industries.

PUBLIC POLICY DILEMMA

An important characteristic of the drug industry is the low cost of actu-ally producing a drug once it has been discovered. Very large costs are incurred by the pharmaceutical manufacturer in the research and drug-development phase and in marketing the new drug once it has been approved by the FDA. A new drug's price is not determined by its R&D costs, however, because these costs have already been incurred. Instead, the price is based on the demand for that drug, namely its therapeutic value and whether it has close substitutes. Because the production costs of a drug (marginal costs) are very low, a drug with great therapeutic value and few, if any, substitutes will command a high price. The result-ing markup of price over production costs will therefore be very high, leading to criticism of the drug company that the drug is priced too high for those who need it.

The public policy dilemma is that if the high price markups over cost are reduced so that more people can buy the drug, profits for R&D will also be reduced, thereby reducing future R&D investment and the dis-covery of new drugs with great therapeutic value.

STRUCTURE OF THE PHARMACEUTICAL INDUSTRY

The structure of the pharmaceutical industry, together with regulatory restraints and government payment policies, affects drug prices and the rate of investment in new, innovative drugs. Industry performance is gen-erally measured by the number of "blockbuster" drugs produced. High price markups over cost for innovative, high-value drugs with no existing substitutes have greater justification than high price markups on older drugs, an indication of lack of price competition, because the industry is unable (or lacks the incentive) to produce new, innovative drugs to take their place. Industry performance is also affected by regulations that in-crease the cost of developing new drugs, the time it takes for a new drug to receive FDA approval, and whether the government establishes the prices it will pay for new drugs; each of these government policies affect the profitability of new drugs, hence incentives for R&D investment.

The pharmaceutical industry has undergone major changes since the mid-1970s. Previously, most pharmaceutical firms were very large, were able to take advantage of economies of scale, and were vertically integrated, that is, most activities were performed "in house," from drug discovery, clinical trials, and regulatory approval process, to marketing. The firm's investments in R&D were financed by internally generated funds (Cockburn 2004).

Revolutionary discoveries in biologic sciences changed the structure of the industry. New biotechnology firms were started. Venture capital funded many of these startups, which were not expected to be profitable for a number of years. Although the risk was high, the profit potential from new drug discoveries was believed to be so large that investors were willing to risk substantial sums in these new firms. The biotechnology industry has become a major source of drug innovation.

Most of the small, new biotechnology firms, however, do not have the capabilities of large drug firms to bring a new product to market. Similarly, large drug firms recognize the profit potential of the drug research being undertaken by these small firms. As a result, advantages accrued to both types of firms from developing relationships to capitalize on each of their strengths. Large drug firms developed contractual relationships and bought smaller biotechnology companies. Thus far, few biotechnology firms have made a profit, although their products offer tremendous profit potential. These small firms face large risks and huge investment costs before their products can be marketed. The process of discovery, clinical trials, and drug approval is lengthy and costs hundreds of millions of dollars. Larger firms are able to bear these costs and have the expertise to navigate the drug-approval process. Greater risk pooling also occurs when many different drugs are in the discovery and development phase, as only a few of the many drugs developed will be successful. Only a large firm can afford to undertake these large research efforts. Small firms may not have the financial resources to complete the long drug-approval process or the expertise to perform all of the steps required.

Mergers and Acquisitions

During the past decade, a large number of mergers have occurred among pharmaceutical companies. These mergers have been of two types. The first were vertical mergers, whereby a firm diversifies into another product line. The growth of managed care and the growing importance of PBMs led several large drug manufacturers to spend many billions of dollars to buy PBMs in the early 1990s. (Merck, for example, paid $6.6 billion for the PBM Medco in 1993.) These drug firms believed that by buying PBMs they could gain greater control over the market for their drugs; the PBMs would presumably substitute their drugs for those of their competitors, increasing their market share and drug sales. PBMs, however, were unable to merely include their owner's drugs to the exclusion of others because their credibility in serving health plans would have been adversely affected. The drug firms' PBM strategy does not appear to have been worthwhile. Pharmaceutical companies that did not buy PBMs were also able to increase their drug sales, and some companies that bought PBMs sold them. The growth of managed care turned out to be a benefit rather than a threat to drug manufacturers. As more people enrolled in managed care, they received prescription drug coverage, use of prescription drugs increased, and sales at all drug firms sharply increased.

The second type of merger that has been occurring is horizontal, where one drug manufacturer purchases another. There are several reasons for horizontal mergers. First, by becoming larger, firms expect that economies of scale will increase efficiency and decrease costs. Merging two companies can result in decreased administrative costs and increased efficiency of the two companies' sales forces, which is critical to the success of any drug firm. Consolidating research units can eliminate competing efforts.

For some large firms mergers are a response to patent expirations and gaps in a firm's product pipeline (Danzon, Epstein, and Nicholson 2004). A wider array of prescription drugs diversifies the financial risk of a firm that has just a few best-selling drugs. For small pharmaceutical firms, mergers are primarily an exit strategy, an indication of financial trouble. Horizontal mergers can improve the combined drug firms' market power. However, few mergers have occurred between firms with drugs in the same therapeutic category. Instead, the types of drugs offered by the combined drug firms are in different therapeutic categories, offering a broader range of prescription drugs across many therapeutic categories to large purchasers.

Industry Competitiveness

The pharmaceutical industry appears to be relatively competitive, as measured by the degree of market concentration. Concentration, which is measured by the combined market share of the top four firms, is only about 22 percent. However, when therapeutic categories are used, the degree of market concentration is much higher, in some cases 100 percent, as a therapeutic category may include only one drug. Thus, the competitiveness of the pharmaceutical industry depends on the definition of the market.

Markets that are less concentrated (i.e., have more competitors) are typically more price competitive. The higher the degree of market concentration, the fewer substitutes that are available for a particular drug and firms generally have greater market power, that is, the ability to raise price without losing sales. Thus, the manufacturer of the first breakthrough drug in a therapeutic category has a great deal of market power. As additional branded drugs are developed in that therapeutic category ("me-too" drugs), better substitutes become available and price competition increases. When the patents on those drugs expire and generic versions are introduced, a great deal of price competition occurs. At each of these stages purchasers are able to buy the prescription drug at a lower price.

DEVELOPMENT OF NEW DRUGS BY THE U.S. PHARMACEUTICAL INDUSTRY

Several measures are used to indicate the productivity of the U.S. pharmaceutical industry. "Global" NCEs are drugs that are marketed to a majority of the world's leading purchasers of drugs; it is preferred, compared to total NCEs, as an indicator of a drug's commercial and therapeutic importance. "First in (a therapeutic) class" is another measure of how innovative a drug is. In addition, the introduction of biotechnology and orphan drugs is examined, as both are major sources of industry growth and innovation.

Grabowski and Wang (2006) analyzed all NCEs introduced worldwide between 1982 and 2003. During that period, 919 NCEs were introduced: 42 percent were global NCEs, 13 percent were first-in-class NCEs, 10 percent were biotechnology drugs, and 8 percent were orphan drugs. Over this period, the total number of NCEs introduced each year showed a downward trend. However, when the measures of a drug's importance are examined (global NCEs, first-in-class, biotechnology, and orphan drugs), the trend has increased over time. The authors conclude that although the trend in total NCEs declined, the relative quality of new drugs has been increasing, and most of the biotechnology and orphan drugs were introduced from 1993 to 2003. The number of

NCEs considered global or first in class varied by therapeutic category, the highest number being oncology drugs, an emphasis of the biotech industry with the U.S. as the dominant source of biotech drugs.

When the introduction of drugs was analyzed by country, the United States was found to be a leader in the development of innovative drugs, particularly in the period from 1993 to 2003; U.S. manufacturers accounted for 48 percent of first-in-class drugs, 52 percent of biotechnology products, and 55 percent of orphan drugs. (These data are shown in Table 28.1.) Furthermore, when the country in which important new drugs are first introduced was examined, the United States was again a strong leader compared with the rest of the world in the most recent, 1993 to 2003, period. Both foreign and domestic drug firms prefer to introduce their important new drugs first in the U.S. market. U.S. patients benefit from having earlier access to important new drugs (although there is also an associated risk with being the first users of such drugs).

The decline in the total number of NCEs appears to indicate that the productivity of the U.S. drug industry has been declining. However, when measures of the importance of new drugs are used, productivity in the U.S. drug industry has increased. Biotechnology drugs, in which the United States is a leader, have been a source of important new drugs and industry productivity growth.

The U.S. market provides greater incentives to drug firms than other countries for development of important new drugs and for the first introduction of innovative new drugs. Whether the U.S. predominance in drug innovation and first choice of introduction will continue depends on government payment policies to reduce the costs of new drugs.

THE MEDICARE PRESCRIPTION DRUG BENEFIT

In coming years industry demand, pricing, and profitability, hence performance, are likely to be greatly affected by a new Medicare drug benefit. The Medicare Modernization Act (which was enacted in 2003 and took effect in 2006) provided the aged with a new outpatient prescription drug benefit.

The design of the prescription drug benefit was the result of a political compromise. Given the size of the federal budget deficit, President Bush proposed a drug benefit for the aged that would cost the federal government $400 billion for the first ten years. The Democrats proposed a drug benefit that would cost $800 billion over the same period. Large prescription drug costs can be a catastrophic financial expense to the

Table 28.1: Country-Level Output of NCEs by Category and Time Period, 1982–1992 and 1993–2003

Country	All NCEs 82–92	All NCEs 93–03	Global NCEs 82–92	Global NCEs 93–03	First-in-Class NCEs 82–92	First-in-Class NCEs 93–03	Biotech NCEs 82–92	Biotech NCEs 93–03	Orphan NCEs 82–92	Orphan NCEs 93–03
European Union total	230	183	99	112	23	27	6	23	9	20
France	35	18	9	11	2	3	0	3	0	4
Germany	53	42	21	27	5	5	2	6	2	5
Italy	29	14	4	1	1	0	0	0	0	0
Switzerland	42	41	26	30	8	11	3	8	1	8
United Kingdom	34	36	23	27	6	7	0	3	5	2
Others	38	33	17	16	2	2	1	3	1	2
Japan	125	88	12	12	5	3	5	9	1	0
United States	120	152	66	81	24	30	9	37	10	27
Rest of world	7	13	3	1	0	2	0	2	0	2
Total	482	437	179	206	53	62	19	71	20	49

Source: Reprinted with permission from Grabowski, H. G., and Y. R. Wang. 2006. "The Quantity and Quality of Worldwide New Drug Introductions, 1982–2003." *Health Affairs* 25 (2): 425–460, Exhibit 4. © 2006 Project HOPE-The-People-to-People Health Foundation, Inc.

small percentage of the aged who incur such costs. If the drug benefit only covered those prescription drug costs that exceeded several thousand dollars a year for an aged person, only about 20 percent of the aged would receive any subsidy from the new drug benefit. To enable more of the aged to receive some benefit (and thereby express their gratitude to legislators at election time), smaller drug expenses were also covered. The resulting design, which includes very large as well as some small drug expenses while not exceeding the $400 billion allocated for the new drug benefit, is shown in Figure 8.3.

After a small ($250) deductible is paid by the aged, they are then liable for 25 percent of the next $2,000 in drug expenses. A gap in coverage then occurs, and the aged are responsible for the next $2,850 in drug expenses (referred to as the "doughnut hole"). After incurring the additional $2,850 of expenses out of pocket, the aged person and her third-party insurer would have already incurred a total expenditure of $5,100 in drug expenses; the aged person would then be responsible for only 5 percent of any remaining drug expenses.

The new drug benefit is expected to greatly increase the demand for prescription drugs by the aged, who are the highest users of prescription drugs, and pharmaceutical manufacturers' revenues are expected to sharply increase. However, increased revenues to the pharmaceutical companies mean higher federal expenditures for the aged's prescription drugs. The Medicare Modernization Act prohibits the federal government from negotiating drug prices with pharmaceutical firms. The aged enroll in a private drug plan, which then negotiates drug prices with the drug manufacturer.

As the cost of the drug benefit to the federal government continues to increase, however, Congress is likely to change the law and have the government regulate drug prices. (A number of legislators have already proposed changing the law to allow the government to negotiate directly with pharmaceutical companies.) The new drug benefit creates a huge unfunded federal liability at a time when the federal government's budget deficit is already very large. As long as the government is ultimately responsible for paying for the elderly's drug expenses, regardless of who administers the benefit, drug expenditures will eventually be regulated, as the government currently regulates payment for each type of provider participating in Medicare.

Proponents of government regulation of drug prices claim that in addition to reducing federal expenditures, the aged would also benefit by lowering their high out-of-pocket drug expenses. As evidence of the benefits of price controls, proponents claim that prices on branded drugs are as much as 30 percent higher in the United States than in Canada, which uses price controls.

Price controls on new breakthrough drugs are politically attractive. Politicians try to provide their constituents with short-term visible benefits at seemingly no cost. In the short run, drug prices will be reduced and there would be no decrease in access to drugs currently on the market. Because the costs of R&D have already been incurred, the only cost of producing an existing drug is its relatively small variable costs. As long as the regulated drug price is greater than the drug's variable costs, the firm will continue selling the drug. Profits from that drug will be lower, but the drug firm will make more money by continuing to sell the drug, even at the regulated price, than by not selling it.

CONSEQUENCES OF PRICE CONTROLS ON PRESCRIPTION DRUGS

Price controls would not decrease access to innovative drugs currently on the market or even to those currently in the drug-approval process. Imposing price controls seemingly has no adverse effects. Those who would benefit include patients who cannot afford expensive drugs, states with rapidly increasing Medicaid expenditures, and the federal government, which is responsible for bearing 75 percent of the cost of the prescription drug benefit. The aged, who have the highest voting-participation rate, state Medicaid programs, and legislators interested in decreasing federal drug expenditures are likely to favor legislation to reduce drug prices. The only apparent loser would be drug companies.

The real concern with price controls is not their effects on current drugs but on R&D for future drugs. Although there is a short-term visible benefit, price controls impose a long-term cost on patients. This long-term cost is not obvious because it occurs in the future, and the public is unaware of breakthrough drugs that would have been developed but are not. Price controls reduce profitability of new drugs. With lower expected profits, drug companies would be less willing to risk hundreds of millions of dollars on R&D. Most new drugs (about 70 percent to 80 percent) are not therapeutic breakthroughs and, although their price may exceed their variable costs, the drugs do not generate sufficient profit to cover their R&D investments. Thus, the drug company loses money on these drugs. (See Figure 26.3.) The small percentage that are

Figure 28.1: Life Cycle of a New Drug

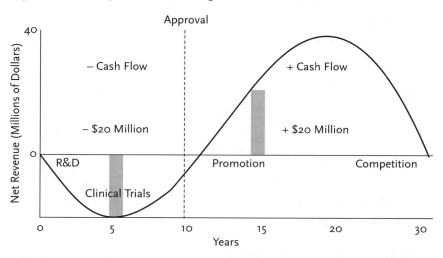

Solid line = expected net returns on a new drug.

Source: Helms, R. B. 2004. "The Economics of Price Regulation and Innovation." *Supplement to Managed Care* 13 (6): 10–12.

considered to be blockbuster drugs have high price markups over their variable costs. The large profits generated by these blockbuster drugs generate the funding used for the drugs that lose money.

These blockbuster drugs, with their high price markups, would be targeted by price controls. With price controls, profit would be insufficient to provide R&D funding for new drugs. Fewer breakthrough drugs would mean treating a disease will be more costly; these drugs might make surgical intervention unnecessary or might even prevent the disease from occurring. Through R&D and the development of new drugs the total cost of medical treatment is lowered. With price controls, R&D investments would decline. Drug companies would also reallocate their R&D efforts away from diseases affecting the elderly, where price controls limit profits, toward diseases affecting other population groups where profits would not be limited.

Figures 28.1 and 28.2 illustrate the effects of imposing price controls on the product life cycle of a blockbuster drug (Helms 2004). During the beginning phases of R&D, including clinical trials, the company incurs a negative cash flow. Once the FDA approves the drug and the drug

Figure 28.2: Effect of Price Controls on Drug Returns

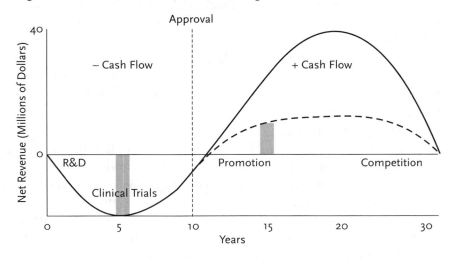

Solid line = expected net returns on a new drug.

Dashed line = expected net returns on a new drug if price controls are imposed.

Source: Helms, R. B. 2004. "The Economics of Price Regulation and Innovation." *Supplement to Managed Care* 13 (6): 10–12.

company markets the drug, the cash flow is positive, until other branded drugs (substitutes) enter the market, and eventually the patent expires and generics enter the market.

If price controls are imposed on a drug after it is approved by the FDA and marketed, the positive cash flow from the new drug is greatly diminished, as shown by the dashed line in Figure 28.2. To illustrate the financial effects of imposing price controls in the previous example, one would have to examine the present value of both the cash outlay and the positive cash return.

Money received in the future is worth less than if the same amount of money were received today. These money outflows (before the drug is being sold) and money inflows occur at different times. The cost of developing a new drug includes all of the costs of bringing it to market, such as research expenditures, the cost of clinical trials, the cost of having the drug approved by the FDA, and marketing costs once it is approved. A company would calculate what it could have earned on that investment if the funds were instead invested in a corporate bond and gained interest. For example, if $10 were invested today and earned 6 percent interest per year, in 5 years that initial investment would grow to $13.38. Thus, in calculating the cost of developing a new drug, the firm calculates both its cash outlay and what it could have earned on that money ("opportunity cost"). Similarly, in calculating the return received from that new drug, which generates a positive cash flow in the future, it is necessary to discount (using the same interest rate) the positive cash flow and determine what money received in the future is worth in to-day's dollars ("present value").

Using the Helms example, if a firm invests $20 million in year five, the present value of that investment equals $14.95 million. (In other words, $14.95 million invested today would be worth $20 million in five years.) If, after 15 years, a new drug earns $20 million, the present value of that return is only $8.35 million. Clearly the $20 million spent and the $20 million earned are not equal. In this example, the drug firm would lose money on its investment, $6.6 million. Thus, the longer it takes to bring a drug to market, the longer the negative cash flow and the smaller the present value of the positive cash flow once the drug is marketed.

If price controls are imposed on a drug once it is marketed, as shown by the dashed line in Figure 28.2, the lower will be both its positive cash flow and the present value of that reduced cash flow. Thus, if the firm earns only $10 million in year 15, the present value equals only $4.17 million. The present value of the cash outflow remains at $14.95 million (Helms 2004).

In the previous example of price controls reducing future returns, a drug firm would change its investment strategy: It would reduce its overall investment in R&D; invest in drugs with a quicker pay-off; seek drugs with less-risky profitability outcomes; and invest in drugs whose market potential is very large and profitable, thereby abandoning re-search on drugs for diseases affecting fewer people.

Examples of Price Controls on U.S. Prescription Drugs

The debate over President Clinton's health plan, introduced in the fall of 1993, provides an indication of the likely effect of price controls on prescription drugs. Included in the plan was an Advisory Council on Breakthrough Drugs, whose purpose was to review prices of new drugs. If the proposed council believed a new drug's price was "excessive," it would try to have it reduced and, failing that, to have the drug excluded from health insurance payment. The targeted drugs were those that were

Figure 28.3: Annual Percentage Change, U.S. R&D, Pharmaceutical Companies, 1971–2005

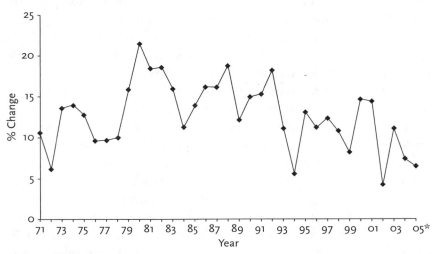

*Estimated data.

Note: Domestic U.S. R&D includes expenditures within the United States by all PhRMA member companies. R&D abroad includes expenditures by U.S.-owned PhRMA companies outside the United States and R&D conducted abroad by the U.S. divisions of foreign-owned PhRMA member companies. R&D performed abroad by the foreign divisions of foreign-owned PhRMA member companies is excluded. Data for 1995 R&D affected by merger and acquisition activity.

Source: Pharmaceutical Research and Manufacturers of America. 2006. *PhRMA Annual Membership Survey.* [Online information.] http:/www.phrma.org/files/2006%20Industry%20Profile.pdf.

the most profitable and had high price markups, namely breakthrough drugs. The pharmaceutical industry was concerned that if the plan was enacted, price controls would be imposed on prescription drugs and profitability of new drugs would be decreased. As a result, the annual rate of increase in R&D expenditures decreased sharply, falling from 18.2 percent in 1992 to 5.6 percent by 1994, the smallest annual rate of increase in 30 years (Figure 28.3). Once it became clear that the Clinton health plan would be defeated and price controls would not be imposed on new drugs, the annual rate of increase in pharmaceutical R&D spending increased again.

History does not offer much hope for drug manufacturers evading price controls. Governments in other countries have used various approaches to lower their drug expenditures. Eleven European countries use some form of price control on prescription drugs (U.S. Department of Commerce, Office of Trade Administration 2004). The types of controls used by these countries include fixing the price of drugs, delaying approval for expensive new drugs for several years, restricting the use of a drug once it has been approved, and setting the price of all drugs within a specific therapeutic category at the cost of the lowest-price drug (Bandow 2005).

Several approaches have already been used in the United States to reduce government expenditures for prescription drugs. State Medicaid programs, because of their tight budgets, have more restrictive formularies than managed care plans. Newer drugs that are more expensive but also more effective are more likely to be excluded in favor of less-expensive generics. Furthermore, Medicaid programs delay inclusion of expensive new innovative drugs in their formularies for several years.

A price-control approach used by the federal government requires the drug manufacturer to sell the drug to the government at its "best" price. In the 1980s, as a result of price competition among drug companies to have HMOs and group purchasing organizations (GPOs) include their drugs in HMO and GPO drug formularies, drug manufacturers gave large price discounts to certain HMOs and GPOs. In 1990, the federal government, in an attempt to reduce Medicaid expenditures, enacted a law that required drug manufacturers to give state Medicaid programs the same discounts they gave their best customers. Consequently, the drug companies gave smaller discounts to HMOs and GPOs. A study by the Congressional Budget Office (1996) found that the best (largest) price discount given to HMOs and GPOs declined from 24 percent and 28 percent, respectively, in 1991 to 14 percent and 15 percent, respectively, the minimum amount required by the government, by 1994. The study concluded that drug companies were much less willing to give steep discounts to large purchasers when they had to give the same discounts to Medicaid. Drug prices and expenditures consequently increased for many private buyers.

Some states are trying to use their Medicaid programs' buying power to reduce drug prices for residents who do not qualify for Medicaid. Maine, for example, enacted a law in May 2000, called Maine Rx, requiring drug manufacturers to give the 325,000 state residents without prescription drug coverage the same discounts they provide to the state's Medicaid program (Mello, Studdert, and Brennan 2004). If the drug manufacturer does not agree to offer the same discount, the drug firm will find that its drugs are excluded from the state Medicaid program, thereby sharply limiting its drug sales. (The drug could be prescribed only with prior authorization from the state.) The state does not appear to be willing to shift volume to only one drug in a therapeutic class, which is the way HMOs and GPOs negotiated price discounts for their drug formularies. Instead, the state wants all prescription drugs to be discounted. Drug companies that have branded drugs with no close substitutes will be less willing to give deep discounts. If the state limits access to that drug, adverse health consequences to those patients who need it will likely occur, or patients would have to buy it on their own. Government-enforced discounts provide short-term financial benefits, but over time Medicaid patients will bear a greater health cost.

SUMMARY

Two important characteristics of the pharmaceutical industry are, first, the very low costs of actually producing a drug pill and, second, the very high cost of developing a new drug. The price at which a new drug is sold is determined not by its cost of production or the R&D investment in that drug, but instead by its value to purchasers and whether there are any close substitutes to that drug. Very valuable drugs that have no close substitutes (blockbuster drugs) will be priced very high relative to their costs of production. Lowering the price of these blockbuster drugs to make them more affordable will decrease pharmaceutical companies' incentive to invest hundreds of millions of dollars in drugs that may have great value to society. That is the public policy dilemma.

The pharmaceutical industry has been changing over time from large vertically integrated organizations to an industry that still has large firms but also many small biotechnology firms, funded by venture capital, that are also engaged in developing new blockbuster drugs. A great deal of private money is invested in these highly risky ventures in the hope of developing a valuable (and profitable) new drug.

The U.S. drug industry, compared with the rest of the world, has been a leader in developing important new drugs and is the country of first choice for introducing innovative new drugs. Government payment policies to reduce drug expenditures threaten both the U.S. industry's leadership and patients' access to innovative drugs.

A growing concern is that federal government, which has become a large, indirect purchaser of prescription drugs as a result of the Medicare Modernization Act, will attempt to lower its drug expenses by controlling the price of prescription drugs. Direct government negotiations with drug companies over the price of their drugs will be tantamount to the government fixing the price of drugs.

Implementing price controls will not have any immediate effect on access to drugs by the aged. However, over time drug companies will invest less in R&D and redirect their R&D toward population groups and diseases where profitability is greater.

In coming years, enormous scientific progress is likely. The mapping of the human genome and advances in molecular biology are expected to lead to drug solutions for many diseases. Drug prices and expenditures will also likely be higher to reflect the increased willingness of people to pay for these new discoveries. It would be unfortunate if the desire to reduce the cost of drugs through price controls decreased the availability of breakthrough drugs.

Any public policy must deal with trade-offs: reducing the high price markup of breakthrough drugs versus maintaining incentives for investing in R&D. It is important to distinguish between the short- and long-term effects of public policy. Using price controls to lower drug prices results in a visible short-term benefit but comes at a less-visible longer-term cost of fewer breakthrough drugs. Future patients would be willing to pay for life-saving breakthrough drugs that were not developed because the government removed the incentives to do so. Given the trade-off between instituting regulation to reduce the cost of drugs or having innovative drugs to cure disease, reduce mortality, and reduce the cost of medical treatment, society would likely choose the full benefits scientific discovery will offer.

An alternative approach to the problem of high drug prices and rising drug expenditures is a policy that subsidizes the purchase of drugs for people with low incomes.

DISCUSSION QUESTIONS

1. How has the structure of the pharmaceutical industry changed over time?

2. What are alternative ways of judging whether the pharmaceutical industry is competitive?

3. Why are price controls on prescription drugs politically attractive?

4. Why would price controls not limit access to blockbuster drugs that are either currently on the market or have almost completed the FDA approval process?

5. What are the expected long-term consequences of price controls on R&D investments, quality of life, mortality rates, and the cost of medical care?

REFERENCES

Bandow, D. 2005. *Avoiding Medicare's Pharmaceutical Trap*, Policy Analysis No. 556. Washington, DC: Cato Institute.

Cockburn, I. 2004. "The Changing Structure of the Pharmaceutical Industry." *Health Affairs* 23 (1): 10–22.

Danzon, P., A. Epstein, and S. Nicholson. 2004. *Mergers and Acquisitions in the Pharmaceutical and Biotech Industries*, NBER Working Paper 10536. Cambridge, MA: National Bureau of Economic Research.

Grabowski, H., and Y. Wang. 2006. "The Quantity and Quality of Worldwide New Drug Introductions, 1982–2003." *Health Affairs* 25 (2): 452–60.

Helms, R. 2004. "The Economics of Price Regulation and Innovation." *Supplement to Managed Care* 13 (6): 10–12.

Mello, M., D. Studdert, and T. Brennan. 2004. "The Pharmaceutical Industry Versus Medicaid—Limits on State Initiatives to Control Prescription-Drug Costs." *New England Journal of Medicine* 350 (6): 608–13.

U.S. Congressional Budget Office. 1996. *CBO Papers: How the Medicaid Rebate on Prescription Drugs Affects Pricing in the Pharmaceutical Industry*. Washington, DC: U.S. Government Printing Office.

U.S. Department of Commerce, Office of Trade Administration. 2004. *Pharmaceutical Price Controls in OECD Countries: Implications for U.S. Consumers, Pricing, Research and Development, and Innovation*. Washington, DC: U.S. DOC.

Chapter 29

Should Kidneys and Other Organs Be Bought and Sold?

BETWEEN 1995 AND 2005, 62,367 people on the waiting list for an organ died. During this period, the number of people waiting for a transplant rose 121 percent, from 43,937 to 97,081, while the number of organs donated increased by just 45 percent, from 23,247 in 1995 to 33,736 in 2005 (Figure 29.1). More than 70 percent of those waiting for organ transplants are waiting for kidneys; the remainder are waiting for a heart, liver, lung, or pancreas. The number of people who die each year while waiting for an organ transplant is increasing. In 2005, 6,439 people died waiting for an organ transplant.

Although the total number of transplants is increasing each year (Figure 29.2), the gap between those waiting for organ transplants and the supply of organs has also been growing rapidly as more patients are being recommended for such transplants. The discovery of immunosuppressive drugs to reduce the risk of rejection has greatly increased the success rate of organ transplants; success rates for kidney transplants have increased from approximately 60 percent to 96 percent. Unfortunately, the number of organs is insufficient to keep up with the growing demand. Consequently, many of those waiting for a transplant will die before an organ becomes available.

Patients waiting for a kidney transplant (the most common organ transplant) must rely on kidney dialysis, which is costly. Kidney transplantation is a lower-cost form of treatment than dialysis. Thus, if all of the patients on dialysis who are waiting for a transplant could be given a kidney, the federal government, which pays for kidney dialysis and kidney transplants under Medicare, could save approximately $1 billion over a five-year period. In addition to being higher cost, dialysis takes

Figure 29.1: Demand for Organs and Total Number of Organs Donated, 1995–2005

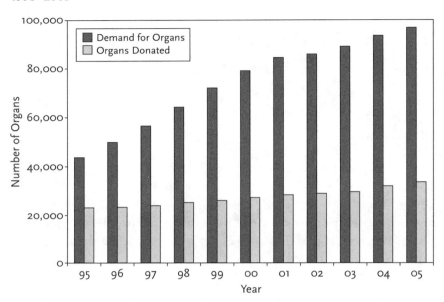

Sources: Data for the number of organs demanded is based on UNOS Organ Procurement and Transplantation Network (OPTN) Waiting List on the last day of each year; data for the number of organs donated is based on OPTN data as of March 17, 2006. [Online information.] http://www.unos.org.

time, up to seven hours per day for several days a week. Kidney dialysis patients have a reduced quality of life as well as lower productivity.[1]

SOURCES OF ORGANS FOR TRANSPLANT

Two sources of supply for organ transplants exist, living donors, such as family members who donate one of their kidneys, and cadavers. Approximately 71 percent of kidneys, as well as other organs used for transplants (96 percent of livers, 98 percent of lungs, and 100 percent of pancreas and hearts), come from victims who have just been killed in an accident. A total of 82 percent of all organs come from accident victims.

The motivating force on which transplant patients have long depended is altruism. According to the National Organ Transplant Act

---

1. The discussion in this chapter is based on Hansmann (1989) and Kaserman and Barnett (2002).

Figure 29.2: Number of Organ Transplants, Selected Years 1981–2005

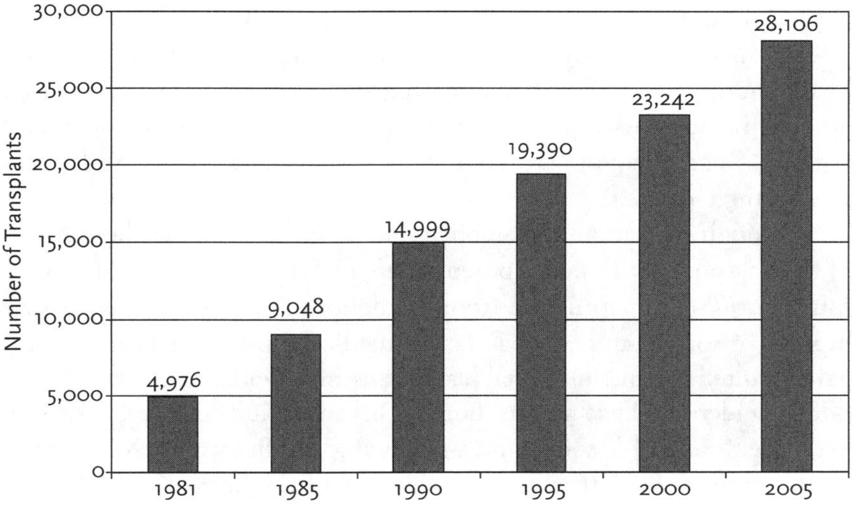

Source: Based on UNOS OPTN data as of March 3, 2006. [Online information.] http://www.unos.org.

of 1984, purchase or sale of human organs is illegal. Current efforts to increase the supply of organs rely on approaches to stimulate voluntary organ donations by the family members of those who die in accidents.

Currently, shortly after they have been notified of the death of a family member, medical personnel ask the family of the deceased to donate their loved one's body organs. Physicians are often reluctant to make such a request to a grieving family, and the grieving family is reluctant to agree while still shocked by the death of a loved one. For some families the sorrow might be somewhat offset by the belief that another person's life might be saved. However, only a small fraction of families are willing to give permission for their deceased family member's organs to be used for transplant patients. For psychologic reasons, such as the thought of dismemberment of a loved one, and religious reasons families of the deceased are often reluctant to donate the deceased's organs. The period in which such a request can be made is short; otherwise, the organ will deteriorate. The family must be located, permission must be received, a recipient must be located through the national organ network, and a tissue match must be made between the recipient and the deceased.

Various approaches have been proposed to increase voluntary organ donations. One is to use improved "marketing" techniques on how to approach (and who should talk to) grieving families, whose sorrow, as already mentioned, may be lessened by the knowledge that they have saved another person's life by donating the deceased's organs. Another approach is to provide greater publicity and education to the public on the use of signed donor cards, which make a person's organs available to potential recipients.

Although education and publicity are likely to increase the number of signed donor cards, hence potential organs, the organ transplant community *still* seeks permission from the donor's family before harvesting organs. In some states, such as Texas, medical authorities have been legally granted permission to harvest organs from bodies if the family has not been identified within four hours. This authority, however, has rarely been used. Fear of lawsuits and unfavorable publicity and the desire to maintain the public's trust prevent physicians from immediately harvesting a deceased donor's organs.

Presumed consent laws have been proposed that would make the deceased's organs available unless the deceased or their family had previously opposed it. These laws, which are in force in many European countries, have not increased organ donation rates over those in the United States, likely for the same reasons permission is still sought with signed donor cards.

Waiting for permission from the deceased's family often results in the organs being lost. Although about 20,000 people who die each year have organs suitable for harvesting, such as those who die in accidents, only a small percentage of those organs are actually donated. Under the current system of altruism, the supply of donors has increased very slowly, from 5,902 in 1988 to 9,206 in 1996 and 14,492 in 2005.

DONOR COMPENSATION PROPOSALS

The growing imbalance between supply and demand for organs has led some persons to advocate compensating donors to increase the supply of donated organs. Compensating donors (or their families) is highly controversial and would require a change in current legislation prohibiting the purchase or sale of body organs. Organ payment proposals cover the spectrum from "mild"—paying family members for organs of their deceased kin—to "strong"—paying a living donor for his second kidney. The following discussion covers three such proposals.

Compensating Families After Death of the Donor

One approach proposes that the burial costs of the deceased be paid if the family permits harvesting of the deceased's organs. Similarly, the family of the deceased could be paid an amount varying between $1,000 and $5,000. A potential problem with these proposals is that negotiating a financial transaction with families traumatized by the death of a loved one may be awkward at the time of death. Another possible problem is that organ purchases of the deceased, which would presumably be directed toward those with low incomes, might offend low-income minority families, who may feel that they are being exploited to benefit wealthy white people.

Compensating Donors Before Death

Allowing people to sell their organs in advance of their death has the advantage that family members would not be subject to the psychologic and social pressure to make a quick decision at the time they suffer the loss of a loved one. Thus, a second approach is to allow people to sell the rights to their organs in return for reducing their health or auto insurance premiums. Health or automobile insurance companies might offer annually a choice of lower premiums to those who are willing to donate their organs if they die during the coming year. The insurance company would then have the right to harvest (sell) the deceased's organs during the period of the insurance contract. Each of the potential donors would be listed in a central computer registry, which a hospital would check when a patient died. Transplant recipients would also be listed in a national registry, and their health insurer or the government would reimburse the insurer a previously stated price for the organ.

For example, if the value of all of a deceased's organs is $100,000 at time of death and the probability of dying during the year is 10,000:1 (the current average chance of dying during a year), the annual premium reduction would be $10. If the value of all of the organs is greater than $100,000 or the probability of death is lower than 10,000:1, the premium reduction would be greater. Young drivers and motorcyclists would presumably be offered large automobile insurance reductions.

The price of organs could either be established competitively or by the government, for example, $10,000 for a kidney. These prices would be used by insurance companies, together with the probability that a subscriber will die during the next year, to establish the annual premium reduction for a potential donor. If too few insurance subscribers are willing to accept the premium reduction, the price of the organ (if established by the government) could be increased until the likely supply is large enough to satisfy the estimated demand for transplants. The greater the shortage of organs, the larger would be the reductions in insurance premiums for organ donors.

Paying Living Kidney Donors

The most controversial approach for increasing the supply of organs is to pay living donors a sufficiently high price for them to part with one of their kidneys. Paying a market price to bring forth an increase in supply is already occurring in other highly sensitive areas of human behavior, such as with the use of sperm banks and surrogate mothers, who are willing to be impregnated with another couple's fertilized egg in return for a fee.

Market transactions consist of a voluntary exchange of assets between two parties. *People engage in voluntary exchange because they differ in their valuation of the asset and both parties expect to benefit from the transaction.* If sales of kidneys were permitted, the person selling the kidney would receive a fee that she believes would compensate her for the loss of a kidney. The purchaser believes the kidney is worth at least what he is willing to pay for it. The purchaser is likely to be the government rather than an individual, as kidney transplants are covered under Medicare; in this case, paying for the kidney would be similar to paying the surgeon for the operation. No one is made worse off by voluntary trade. Thus, the first major advantage of legalizing the sale of kidneys is that no one is worse off and both parties are likely better off with the voluntary exchange than when it is prohibited.

Permitting a commercial market for kidneys has other important advantages. Organs that would save the lives of all those waiting for a kidney could be purchased. No longer would they have to endure the suffering that occurs while waiting for a kidney donation, possibly dying before one becomes available. Furthermore, the government would save a great deal of money by substituting kidney transplants for kidney dialysis, as a transplant is a lower-cost method of treatment than dialysis, the current form of treatment for those awaiting transplants. Lastly, the quality of donated kidneys would increase, increasing the success rate of transplants. Currently, donated kidneys that do not have good tissue matches are used because of the severe shortage of kidneys. Paying living donors for their kidneys would result in greater choice of donors, enabling tissue matches between recipient and donor to be made in advance.

OPPOSITION TO FINANCIAL INCENTIVES TO ORGAN DONATION

Opposition to using financial incentives for increasing the supply of organs is based on several reasons. First, some believe using financial incentives would discourage voluntary donations of organs, resulting in a smaller supply of organs. Evidence that may be indicative of what is likely to happen to the overall supply of organs when financial incentives are offered is what happened when financial incentives were used to increase the supply of blood. Voluntary donations of blood declined, but the decline was more than offset by an increase in the supply of paid donations.

Second, some claim that paying living donors for their organs would exploit the poor to benefit the wealthy; the poor are likely to be the sellers of organs, whereas those with higher incomes would be the beneficiaries. The poor, it is claimed, would be forced to sell their organs to provide for their families. However, if the poor have inadequate funds, it is because society is unwilling to provide them with sufficient subsidies to increase their incomes or provide them with education that would increase their productivity and incomes. Prohibiting the poor from selling one of their assets would leave them worse off, and they would be prevented from doing something they believe will improve their situation.

Although little risk is involved in selling one's kidney, a donor will be accepting a slightly higher risk of dying in return for increased financial rewards. Many people seek additional compensation by choosing to work in higher-risk occupations. Working in a coal mine, on a skyscraper, or on an offshore drilling platform carries occupational risks, yet society does not interfere with these voluntary transactions. Someone willing to make the trade-off between greater compensation and the loss of a kidney is not "forced" to sell her organs.

Third, some are concerned that those selling their kidneys might be subject to fraud and then regret selling their kidneys. Various protections could be included in legislation legalizing the sale of kidneys. A waiting period, such as six months, could be used in case the person decides to change his mind. The donor could also be required to be of a minimum age. The donor could also be approved by a panel that includes a psychiatrist or social worker to assess her ability to make rational choices.

When demand exceeds supply in a market, prices rise. When prices are not permitted to rise or sales are illegal, the potential for a black market exists. Although the sale of kidneys in the United States is illegal, a wealthy patient has access to an international black market, particularly from donors from less-developed countries such as India and China. Demand for kidney organs is lower when the activity is illegal than if sales were legal. Finding an organ donor on the black market incurs higher search costs, purchasers are less certain of the organ's quality, no legal remedies are available if fraud occurs, and the purchaser would have to pay the hospital's and surgeon's costs out of pocket. However, again, this option is available to the wealthy. Therefore, prohibiting the sale of organs discriminates against the poor, who do not have access to the international black market in kidneys.

If a legal market in organs were permitted, would only the wealthy be able to afford kidney transplants once the price of a kidney is included in the already-high price of a transplant? The answer is no. Kidney transplants are currently paid for by the federal government; the higher cost would not be a deterrent to any recipient needing a transplant. Most of the costs for a transplant are for hospital and physician services; including the price of the organ would not be a large addition to those costs. Currently, everyone associated with the transplant benefits—the recipient receives a new kidney, and the physician and hospital receive payment for their services. Why should the donor not also benefit?

What if a low-income person desperate for money sells his kidney and subsequently suffers from kidney disease? Because the government currently pays for all kidney transplants as part of Medicare, that donor would become eligible for a free transplant. A new donor would be paid for a kidney to be used for the previous donor's transplant.

Would the opponents of a compensation system who are concerned with its effects on the poor be more positively inclined to using financial incentives if the poor (defined, for example, as those with incomes below the federal poverty level) were prohibited from selling their organs? Would the poor be better off if they were denied the right to sell one of their assets? A belief that society helps the poor when those with higher incomes limit their choices is paternalistic.

ADDITIONAL CONSIDERATIONS

The poor and minority groups are placed at a disadvantage by the present altruistic system for securing and allocating organs. Many of those waiting for transplants have low incomes. Furthermore, although African Americans are statistically more likely to suffer from kidney disease than whites, they are less likely to receive an organ transplant. African Americans make up 35 percent of the waiting list for kidney transplants.

The reason for the higher proportion of African Americans on the waiting list is that African American kidney patients have a low tissue match with whites and, although the rate is increasing over time, African Americans donate proportionately fewer kidneys (10 percent) than whites. The refusal rate for organ donations among African American families is 60 percent, compared with 29 percent for white families (General Accounting Office 1997).

The growing demand for transplants, together with their profitability to both the hospital and the surgeon, has resulted in more hospitals becoming "transplant centers." A federal rule that requires organs to be allocated first to those living in the area before they can be sent to another territory has resulted in vastly different waiting times for an organ depending on the area in which one lives. The waiting time for a liver transplant could be three months in New Jersey and 15 months in New York. The federal government is in the process of changing this rule to create one national waiting list for organs; those who are most in need and have been waiting the longest would have first priority. Although the proposed new rule of a national waiting list would appear to be fairer, local physicians and hospitals would have a decreased incentive to solicit and encourage donations because they would not be able to keep donated organs for their own patients. Furthermore, people would be more inclined to donate their own or a family member's organ to benefit persons in their community. Although the new rule is likely to improve the allocation of organs to those most in need, it will likely decrease voluntary donations.

SUMMARY

As the feasibility of transplants increases and more hospitals and physicians find status and profit in performing transplants, the demand for transplantation will continue to grow. However, without any incentives on the part of donors or physicians and hospitals to recruit donors, the shortage of organs will become more severe. As Cohen (2005) says, "If the benefits of an organs market are so clear, then why do we still . . . condemn people to death and suffering while the organs that could restore them to health are instead fed to worms?"

Perhaps the strongest objection to compensating donors for their organs is some people's ideologic and moral beliefs.[2] Financial incentives

---

2. The only ideology inherent in market proposals is the belief that supply is responsive to price.

governed by greed would substitute for altruism as the motivating force for donating one's (cadaveric) organs, an idea that is deeply offensive to many persons. However, a trade-off must be considered. Although the thought of having people sell their (cadaveric) organs is offensive, thousands of people die each year for lack of a kidney donor, and this number will increase. Which choice is more offensive—violating the strongly held beliefs of some persons regarding the repugnance of a market for human organs or the suffering and loss of life of thousands of people needing an organ transplant?

DISCUSSION QUESTIONS

1. Why have voluntary methods for increasing the supply of body organs been unsuccessful?

2. Evaluate the following proposal: People would be permitted to sell the rights to their organs (in the form of reduced health or auto insurance premiums) if they die in an accident in the coming year.

3. Would government expenditures for kidney disease (currently covered as part of Medicare for all persons) be higher or lower under a free-market system for kidneys?

4. Would the poor be disadvantaged to the benefit of those who are wealthy under a free-market system for selling kidneys?

5. Would it be more equitable to prohibit the poor from selling their kidneys in a free market that permitted the sale of kidneys?

REFERENCES

Cohen, I. 2005. "Directions for the Disposition of My (and Your) Vital Organs." *Regulation* 28 (3): 32–38.

Hansmann, H. 1989. "The Economics and Ethics of Markets for Human Organs." *Journal of Health Politics, Policy and Law* 14 (1): 57–85.

Kaserman, D., and A. Barnett. 2002. *The U.S. Organ Procurement System: A Prescription for Reform*. Washington, DC: American Enterprise Institute.

U.S. General Accounting Office. 1997. *Organ Procurement Organizations*, GAO/HEHS-98-26, 8. Washington, DC: U.S. Government Printing Office.

Chapter 30

The Role of Government in Medical Care

GOVERNMENT INTERVENTION IN the financing and delivery of medical services is pervasive. On the financing side, hospital and physician services for the aged are subsidized (Medicare), and a separate payroll tax pays for those subsidies; Medicaid, a federal/state matching program, pays for medical services for the poor; a large network of state and county hospitals is in place; health professional schools are subsidized; loan programs for students in the health professions are guaranteed by the government; employer-paid health insurance is excluded from taxable income; veterans have access to a separate medical program; the Civilian Health and Medical Program of the Uniformed Services (CHAMPUS) finances health benefits for military dependents; and medical research is subsidized. These programs and others make government a 45 percent partner in total health expenditures.

In addition to these financing programs, extensive government regulations influence the financing and delivery of medical services. For example, state licensing boards determine the criteria for entry into the different professions, and practice regulations determine which tasks can be performed by various professional groups. In some states hospital investment is subject to state review, hospital and physician prices under Medicare are regulated, health insurance companies are regulated by the states, each state mandates what benefits (e.g., hair transplants in Minnesota) and which providers (e.g., naturopaths in California) should be included in health insurance sold in that state, and some states have required employers to provide health insurance benefits to their employees.

The role of government in the financing and delivery of medical services, as well as through federal and state regulation, is extensive. To

understand the reasons for these different types of government intervention and at times seemingly contradictory policies, it is necessary to have
a view of what the government is attempting to achieve.

PUBLIC-INTEREST VIEW OF GOVERNMENT

The traditional, or public-interest, role of government can be classified
according to its policy objectives and the policy instruments to achieve
those objectives. The policy objectives of government in the health field
are twofold: (1) to redistribute medical resources to those least able to
purchase medical services and (2) to improve the economic efficiency by
which medical services are purchased and delivered. These traditional
objectives of government, redistribution and efficiency, can be achieved
by using one or more of the following policy instruments: expenditures,
taxation, and regulation. (Government provision of services, such as Veterans Administration hospitals, is rarely proposed as a policy instrument
in the United States.) These policy instruments—expenditures, taxation,
and regulation—can be applied to either the purchaser (demand) side or
the supplier side of the market. These policy objectives and instruments,
which can be used to classify each type of government health policy
according to policy objectives, the type of policy instrument used, and
whether the policy instrument is directed toward the demand or supply
side of the market, are shown in Figure 30.1.

Redistribution

Redistribution causes a change in wealth. According to the public-
interest view of government, society makes a value judgment that medical services should be provided to those with low incomes and financed
by taxing those with higher incomes. Redistributive programs typically
lower the cost of services to a particular group by enabling members of
that group to purchase those services at below-market prices. These benefits are financed by imposing a "cost" on some other group. Two large
redistributive programs are Medicare for the aged and Medicaid for the
medically indigent. The benefits and costs of a redistributive medical
program, such as Medicaid, are shown in Figure 30.2.

Efficiency

The second traditional objective of government is to improve the efficiency with which society allocates resources. Inefficiency in resource allocation can occur, for example, when firms in a market have monopoly

Figure 30.1: Health Policy Objectives and Interventions

Government Policy Instrument		Government Objective	
		Redistribution	Improved Efficiency
Expenditures	Demand side		
	Supply side		
Taxation (±)	Demand side		
	Supply side		
Regulation	Demand side		
	Supply side		

Figure 30.2: Determining the Redistributive Effects of Government Programs

	Low Income	High Income
Benefits	X	
Costs		X

power or when externalities exist. A firm has monopoly power when it is able to charge a price that exceeds its cost by more than a normal profit. Monopoly is inefficient because it produces too small a level of service (output). The additional benefit to purchasers from consuming a service (as indicated by its price) is greater than the cost of producing that benefit; therefore, more resources should flow into that industry until the additional benefit of consuming that service equals the additional cost of producing it.

The bases of monopoly power are several: There may be only one firm in a market, as with a natural monopoly like an electric company; there may be barriers to entry in a market; firms may collude on raising their prices; or a lack of information means consumers are unable to judge price, quality, and service differences among different suppliers. In each of these situations, the prices charged will exceed the costs of producing the product (which includes a normal profit). The appropriate government remedy for decreasing monopoly power is to eliminate barriers to entry into a market, prevent price collusion, and improve information among consumers.

The second situation in which the allocation of resources can be improved is when "externalities" occur, that is, when someone undertakes an action and in so doing affects others who are not part of that transaction. The effects on others could be positive or negative. For example, a utility using high-sulfur coal to produce electricity also produces air pollution. As a result of the air pollution residents in surrounding communities may have a higher incidence of respiratory illness. Resources are misallocated because the cost of producing electricity excludes the costs imposed on others. As a result, too much electricity is being produced. If the costs of producing electricity also included the costs imposed on others, the price of electricity would be higher and its demand lower. The allocation of resources would be improved if the utility's cost included production costs and external costs.

The appropriate role of government in such a situation is to determine the costs imposed on others and to tax the utility an equivalent amount. (This subject is discussed more completely in Chapter 31.)

ECONOMIC THEORY OF REGULATION

Dissatisfaction with the public-interest theory occurred for several reasons. Instead of simply regulating natural monopolies, government has also regulated competitive industries, such as airlines, trucks, and taxicabs, as well as various professions. Furthermore, unregulated firms always want to enter regulated markets. To prevent entry into regulated industries the government establishes entry barriers. If the government supposedly reduces prices in regulated markets, hence the firm's profitability, why should firms seek to enter a regulated industry?

To reconcile these apparent contradictions with the public-interest view of government, an alternative theory of government behavior, the economic theory of regulation, was developed (Stigler 1971). (For a more complete discussion of this theory and its applicability to the health field see Feldstein [2006].) The basic assumption underlying the economic theory is that political markets are no different from economic markets; individuals and firms seek to further their self-interest. Firms undertake investments in private markets to achieve a high rate of return. Why would the same firms not invest in legislation if it also offered a high rate of return? Organized groups are willing to pay a price for legislative benefits. This price is political support, which brings together the demanders and suppliers of legislative benefits.

The Suppliers: Legislators

The suppliers of legislative benefits are legislators, and their goal is assumed to be to maximize their chances for reelection. As the late Senator Everett Dirksen said, "The first law of politics is to get elected; the second law is to be reelected." To be reelected requires political support, which consists of campaign contributions, votes, and volunteer time. Legislators are assumed to be rational and to make cost-benefit calculations when faced with demands for legislation. However, the legislator's cost-benefit calculations are not the costs and benefits to society of enacting particular legislation. Instead, *the benefits are the additional political support* the legislator would receive from supporting the legislation, and *the costs are the lost political support* she would incur as a result of her actions. When the benefits to the legislators exceed their costs, they will support the legislation.

The Demanders: Those with a Concentrated Interest

Those who have a "concentrated" interest—that is, the legislation will have a large effect on their profitability by affecting their revenues or costs—are more likely to be successful in the legislative marketplace. It becomes worthwhile for the group to organize, represent its interests before legislators, and raise political support to achieve the profits favorable legislation can provide. For this reason only those with a concentrated interest will demand legislative benefits.

Diffuse Costs

When legislative benefits are provided to one group, others must bear those costs. When only one group has a concentrated interest in the legislation, that group is more likely to be successful if the costs to finance those benefits are not obvious and can be spread over a large number of people. When this occurs, the costs are said to be "diffuse." For example, assume that there are ten firms in an industry, and if they can have legislation enacted that would limit imports that compete with their products, they will be able to raise their prices and thereby receive $280 million in legislative benefits. These firms have a concentrated interest ($280 million) in trying to enact such legislation. The costs of these legislative benefits are financed by a small increase in the price of the product amounting to $1 per person.

Often the fact that legislation increases their costs is not obvious to consumers. Furthermore, even if consumers were aware of the legislation's effect, it would not be worthwhile for them to organize and represent their interests to forestall a price increase that will decrease their incomes by $1 a year. The costs of trying to prevent the cost increase would exceed their potential savings.

It is easier (less costly) for providers than for consumers to organize, provide political support, and impose a diffuse cost on others. For this reason so much legislation has affected entry into the health professions, which tasks are reserved to certain professions, how (and which) providers are paid under public medical programs, why subsidies for medical education are given to schools and not students (otherwise schools would have to compete for students), and so on. Most health issues have been relatively technical, such as the training of health professionals, certification of their quality, methods of payment, controls on hospital capital investment, and so on. The higher medical prices resulting from regulations that benefit providers have been diffuse and not visible to consumers.

Entry Barriers to Regulated Markets

The economic theory of legislation provides an explanation for these dissatisfactions with the public-interest theory. Firms in competitive markets seek regulation to earn higher profits than are available in competitive markets. Prices in regulated markets, such as interstate airline travel, were always higher than in unregulated markets, such as intrastate air travel, enabling regulated firms to earn greater profits. These higher prices provided unregulated firms with an incentive to try to enter regulated markets. Government, on behalf of the regulated industry, imposed entry barriers to keep out low-priced competitors. Otherwise the regulated firms could not earn more than a competitive rate of return. Through legislation, firms try to receive the monopoly profits they are unable to achieve through market competition.

Opposing Concentrated Interests

When only one group has a concentrated interest in the outcome of legislation and the costs are diffuse, legislators will respond to the political support the group is willing to pay to have favorable legislation enacted. When there are opposing groups, each with a concentrated interest in the outcome, legislators are likely to reach a compromise between the competing demanders of legislative benefits. Rather than balancing the gain in political support from one group against the loss from the other, legislators prefer to receive political support from both groups and impose diffuse costs on those offering little political support.

Visible Redistributive Effects

When the beneficiaries are specific population groups, such as the aged, the redistributive effects of legislation are meant to be very visible. An example of this is Medicare. By making clear which population groups will benefit, legislators hope to receive their political support. The costs of financing such visible redistributive programs, however, are still designed to be diffuse so as not to generate political opposition from others. *A small, diffuse tax imposed on many people, such as a sales or a payroll tax, is the only way large sums of money can be raised, with little opposition, to finance visible redistributive programs.* These taxes are regressive—the tax represents a greater portion of income from low-income employees and consumers. Economists have determined that payroll taxes, even when imposed on the employer, are borne mostly by the employee. (The employer is only interested in the total cost of an employee; thus, the employee eventually receives a lower wage than if those costs were not imposed.) By imposing part of the tax on the employer, however, employees appear to be paying a smaller portion of it than they really are. The remainder of the tax is shifted forward to consumers in the form of higher prices for the goods and services they purchase, which is also regressive.

Medicaid and Medicare

Differences in the sources of political support are important for understanding the two main redistributive programs in the United States. Medicaid is a means-tested program for the poor funded from general tax revenues. Because the poor (who have low voting-participation rates) are unable to provide legislators with political support, the support for Medicaid comes from the middle class, who must agree to higher taxes to provide the poor with medical benefits. The inadequacy of Medicaid in every state, the conditions necessary for achieving Medicaid eligibility, the low levels of eligibility, and beneficiaries' lack of access to medical providers are related to the generosity (or lack thereof) of the middle class. The beneficiaries of Medicare, on the other hand, are the aged themselves, who (together with their adult children) provide the political support for the program. As the cost of Medicare has risen, government has raised the Medicare payroll tax and reduced payments to providers rather than reducing benefits or beneficiaries from this politically powerful group.[1]

The political necessity of keeping costs diffuse explains why Medicare and producer regulation are financed using regressive taxes, either payroll taxes or higher prices for medical services. Spreading the costs over large populations keeps those costs diffuse, with the net effect that low-income persons pay the costs and higher-income persons, such as physicians or high-income aged, receive the benefits. Those receiving the benefits and those bearing the costs, according to the economic theory, are not based on income (see Figure 30.2), but instead according to which groups are able to offer political support (the beneficiaries) and which groups are unable to do so (they bear the costs). Regressive taxes are typically used to finance producer regulation and to provide benefits to specific population groups.

Changes in Health Policies

Health policies change over time because groups who previously bore a diffuse cost develop a concentrated interest. Until the 1960s, medical societies were the main group with a concentrated interest in the financing and delivery of medical services. Thus, the delivery system was structured to benefit physicians. The physician–population ratio remained constant for 15 years (until the mid-1960s) at 141 per 100,000, state restrictions

---

1. The political support offered by providers, such as hospitals and physicians, is important in determining how such redistributive legislation is designed. Providers benefit because such programs increase demand by those with low incomes. However, medical societies have opposed government coverage of entire population groups, such as the aged, regardless of income level, because government payment would merely substitute for private payment for those who are not poor. Physicians were concerned that if government covered everyone or all of the aged, regardless of income, the cost of such programs would increase, and the government would eventually control their fees. This was the American Medical Association's basic reason for opposing Medicare. To gain the political support of physicians Congress acceded to physicians' preferences when Medicare was established by permitting physicians to decide whether or not to accept the government payment for treating Medicare patients. Medicaid was not controversial because it covered those with low incomes, and hospitals and physicians were paid according to their preferences. As the federal and state governments experienced large expenditure increases under each of these programs, government developed a concentrated interest in controlling hospital and medical expenditures.

were imposed on HMOs to limit their development, advertising was prohibited, and restrictions were placed on other health professionals to limit their ability to compete with physicians. Financing mechanisms also benefited physicians; until the 1980s, capitation payment for HMOs was prohibited under Medicare and Medicaid, and competitors to physicians were excluded from reimbursement under public and private insurance systems.

As the costs of medical care continued to increase rapidly to government and employers, their previously diffuse costs became concentrated. Under Medicare the government was faced with the choice of raising taxes or reducing benefits to the aged, both of which would have cost the administration political support. Successive administrations developed a concentrated interest in lowering the rate of increase in medical expenditures. Similarly, large employers were concerned that rising medical costs were making them less competitive internationally. The pressures for cost containment increased as the costs of an inefficient delivery and payment system grew larger. Rising medical expenditures are no longer a diffuse cost to large purchasers of medical services.

Other professional organizations, such as those for psychologists, chiropractors, and podiatrists, saw the potentially greater revenues their members could receive if they were better able to compete with physicians. These groups developed a concentrated interest in securing payment for their members under public and private insurance systems and expanding their scope of practice. The increase in opposing concentrated interests weakened the political influence of organized medicine.

SUMMARY

The public-interest and economic theories of government provide opposing predictions of the redistributive and efficiency effects of government legislation, as shown in Table 30.1. To determine which of these contrasting theories is a more accurate description of government, we must match the actual outcomes of legislation to each theory's predictions. Do the benefits of redistributive programs go to those with low incomes, and are they financed by taxes that impose a larger burden on those with higher incomes? Does the government try to improve the allocation of resources by reducing barriers to entry and, in markets where information is limited, by monitoring the quality of physicians and other medical services and making this information available?

Table 30.1: Health Policy Objectives Under Different Theories of Government

	Objective of Government	
Theory of Government	Redistribution	Improved Efficiency
Public-interest theory	Assist those with low incomes	Remove (and prevent) monopoly abuses and protect environment (externalities)
Economic theory of regulation	Provide benefits to those able to deliver political support and finance from those offering little political support	Efficiency objective unimportant—more likely to protect industries so as to provide them redistributive benefits

The economic theory of regulation, rather than alternative theories, provides greater understanding of why health policies are enacted and why they have changed over time. The economic theory predicts that government is not concerned with efficiency issues. Redistribution is the main objective of government, but that objective is to redistribute wealth to those who are able to offer political support from those who are unable to do so. Thus, medical licensing boards are inadequately staffed, have never required reexamination for relicensure, and have failed to monitor practicing physicians because organized medicine has been opposed to any approaches for increasing quality that would adversely affect physicians' incomes. Regressive taxes are used to finance programs such as Medicare not because legislators are unaware of their regressive nature, but because the taxes benefit economically those who have a concentrated interest.

The structure and financing of medical services is rational; the participants act according to their calculations of costs and benefits. Viewed in its entirety, however, health policy is uncoordinated and seemingly contradictory. Health policies are inequitable and inefficient; low-income persons end up subsidizing those with higher incomes. These results, however, are the consequences of a rational system. The outcomes were the result of policies intended by the legislators.

DISCUSSION QUESTIONS

1. What were the dissatisfactions with the public-interest view of government?

2. Contrast the benefit-cost calculations of legislators under both the public-interest and economic theories of government.

3. Why are concentrated interests and diffuse costs important in predicting legislative outcomes?

4. Contrast the predictions of the public-interest and economic theories of government with regard to redistributive policies.

5. Evaluate the following policies according to the two differing theories of government:

   a. Medicare and Medicaid beneficiaries, taxation, and generosity of benefits

   b. The performance of state licensing boards in monitoring physician quality

REFERENCES

Feldstein, P. J. 2006. *The Politics of Health Legislation: An Economic Perspective*, 3rd ed. Chicago: Health Administration Press.

Stigler, G. J. 1971. "The Theory of Economic Regulation." *The Bell Journal of Economics* 2 (1): 3–21.

Chapter 31

Medical Research, Medical Education, Alcohol Consumption, and Pollution: Who Should Pay?

AN IMPORTANT ROLE of government is to improve the way markets allocate resources. When markets perform poorly, fewer goods and services are produced, and incomes are lower than they would be otherwise. The usual policy prescription for improving the performance of markets is for the government to eliminate barriers to entry and increase information. Competitive markets, in which no entry barriers are in place and purchasers and producers are fully informed, are likely to produce the correct (or optimal) rate of output. The correct rate occurs if individuals benefiting from the service pay the full costs of producing that service.

Resources are optimally allocated when the additional benefits from consuming the last unit equal the cost of producing that last unit. When still more units are consumed, the costs of those additional units exceed the benefits provided, and the resources would be better used to produce other goods and services whose benefits exceed their costs. As shown in Figure 31.1, when the costs are C_1 and benefits are B_1, the correct rate of output is Q_1. The benefit curve is declining because the more one has of a good, the lower the value of an additional unit will be.

Under certain circumstances, however, even a competitive market may not allocate resources correctly. The optimal rate of output in a market occurs when all costs and benefits are included. Private decision makers consider only their own costs and benefits and exclude the costs or benefits imposed on others, if any. The effect may be that some services are "underproduced," while others are "overproduced."

The quantity of medical and health services may not be optimal because costs and benefits may be imposed on persons other than those who purchase and provide the service. What happens when costs or benefits

447

Figure 31.1: Optimal Rate of Output

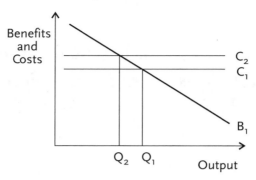

are imposed on someone who is not a voluntary participant in that private transaction? Such "external" costs and benefits must be included; otherwise, either too much or too little of the service is produced and purchased. For example, when external costs are imposed on others, as shown by C_2 in Figure 31.1, the correct rate of output declines from Q_1 to Q_2, where both private (C_1) and external (C_2) costs equal the benefits (B_1) from consuming that good or service.

When such external costs or benefits exist, government should calculate their magnitude and use subsidies and taxes to achieve the "right" rate of output in the affected industry. Subsidies or taxes on the producers in that industry will change the costs of producing a service so producers will adjust their levels of output. The difference between C_1 and C_2, the external cost, is also the size of the tax to be imposed on each unit of the product.

EXTERNAL COSTS AND BENEFITS
Pollution

One reason externalities, such as pollution, occur is that no one owns the resource being exploited. When a resource such as air or water is scarce and no one owns it, a firm may use it as though it were free; it does not become a cost of production as it would if the firm was charged a fee for its use. The lack of property rights over scarce resources is the basis for government intervention. For example, when a firm pollutes a stream in the process of producing its product, those who use the stream for recreational purposes are adversely affected; they bear a cost not included in the firm's calculation of its costs of producing the product. Because the firm has not had to include the external costs of production, it sells the product at a lower price, and the user pays less for that product than the product actually costs society. Because of its lower price, a greater quantity of the product is purchased and produced.

When no property rights over a scarce resource exist and that resource is used by large numbers of people and firms, negotiations among the parties over the use of that resource are likely to be difficult and costly. Government intervention is needed to calculate the external costs and, in the case of pollution, to impose a tax equivalent to the amount of pollution caused on each unit of the product sold. The product's higher price would include both the cost of production and the unit tax; therefore, less of the product would be sold. If all costs and benefits, both private and external, are part of the private decision-making process, the industry will produce the "right" rate of output.

A pollution tax could not be expected to eliminate all pollution, but it will reduce it to the correct level; the tax revenues received by the government would go toward cleaning up the pollution or compensating those who were adversely affected. If the government attempted to eliminate all of the pollution, it would have to stop production of that product completely. Eliminating all pollution could adversely affect a great many people if the total benefits derived from that product outweigh its costs, including the costs of pollution. Consider, for example, the effect of eliminating all air pollution originating from automobiles or electricity production. Clearly, people prefer some quantity of these products to zero air pollution.

Imposing a tax on pollution has another important consequence. The producer of the product will attempt to lower the tax by devising methods to reduce pollution.[1] The firm may move to an area where the costs

---

1. Another approach to reducing pollution that also provides incentives for polluters to search for the most efficient method of reducing pollution is to establish a market for pollution rights. The 1990 Clean Air Act Amendments established the first large-scale use of the tradable permit approach to pollution control. A market for transferable sulfur dioxide emission allowances among electric utilities was established. Along with a cap on annual emissions, electric utilities had an opportunity to trade rights to emit sulfur dioxide. Firms facing high abatement costs had an opportunity to purchase the right to emit pollution from firms with lower costs.

of pollution (hence the tax) are lower, or the firm may innovate in its production process to reduce pollution. The tax creates incentives for producers to lower their production costs, which include the tax.

Imposing a tax directly on pollution is preferable to such indirect methods of controlling pollution as allowing existing firms to continue polluting but not permitting others to enter the market or mandating that all firms use a particular production process to reduce pollution. Such indirect approaches eliminate incentives for producers to search for cheaper ways to reduce pollution.

Based on the example of the external costs of pollution, the role of government seems straightforward: When widespread external costs exist, the government should calculate the size of those costs and assess a tax on each unit of output produced. The purchasers and producers of that product will base their decisions about how much to purchase on all of the costs and benefits (external as well as private) of that product.

Medical Research

The analysis is similar when applied to external benefits. If a university medical researcher develops a new method of performing open-heart surgery that reduces the mortality rate of that procedure, other surgeons will copy the technique to benefit their own patients. An individual researcher/surgeon cannot declare ownership over all possible uses of that technique. If the individual surgeon were not compensated for all those who would eventually benefit, he would not find it feasible or worthwhile to invest time and resources to develop new medical techniques.

Similarly, medical researchers would underproduce the discovery of basic scientific knowledge, as they would not be able to charge all those who would eventually benefit from a cure for cancer, heart disease, and so on. Although difficult, the government should attempt to calculate the potential benefits and subsidize medical research. Unless the external benefits are assessed and the costs shared by potential beneficiaries, the costs of producing medical research will exceed the private benefits.

An alternative to offering a subsidy to private firms is to give them "property" rights or ownership over their discoveries, namely patent protection. Drug companies need incentives to compensate them for risks and investments made in R&D. Patent protection, however, is not possible for all basic research or for new surgical techniques. Unpatented medical research or new drug discoveries can be copied by others who then benefit from the discoveries.

Immunization

Another example of external benefits involves protection from contagious diseases. Individuals who decide to be immunized against contagious diseases base their decisions solely on the costs and benefits to themselves of immunization. However, those who are not immunized also benefit by receiving a "free ride"; their chances of catching that disease are lowered. If immunization were a private decision, not enough individuals would be immunized. The costs of those immunized should be subsidized by imposing a small tax on those who are not immunized but who also benefit. In this manner, the "right" number of people become immunized. The immunization decision thus encompasses private benefits, external benefits, and costs of immunization.

When transaction costs are high, that is, the administrative costs of monitoring, collecting taxes, and subsidizing individuals are substantial, it may be less costly to simply require everyone to be immunized against certain diseases.

Subsidies to the Medically Indigent

Externalities are also the rationale for providing subsidies to the medically indigent. If the only way the poor receive medical care is through voluntary contributions, many people who did not make such contributions would benefit by knowing that the poor are cared for through the contributions of others. Too little would be provided to the medically indigent because those who do not contribute receive a free ride; they benefit without having to pay for that benefit. Government intervention would be appropriate to tax those who benefit by knowing the poor receive medical care.

GOVERNMENT POLICIES WHEN EXTERNALITIES EXIST

In the examples described, the subsidies and taxes are related to the size of the external benefits and costs. Furthermore, the taxes imposed on products that pollute are to be spent for the benefit of those adversely affected. When there are external benefits, the subsidies are financed by taxes on those who receive the external benefit. Patents are an attempt to recover the external benefits from research. In each case, taxes and subsidies are matched according to external costs and benefits.

Recognizing how externalities affect the correct rate of output in an industry is useful for understanding what government policies would be appropriate in a number of additional areas. For example, when a motorcyclist has an accident and receives a head injury as a result of not wearing a helmet, government (society) pays the medical expenses if the cyclist does not have insurance or sufficient personal funds. Fines for not wearing helmets are an attempt to make motorcyclists bear the responsibility for external costs that they would otherwise impose on others. At times, imposing requirements (such as helmet use, immunizations, grade school education) may be the least-costly approach for achieving the correct output.

The same analogy can be used to describe those who can afford to buy health insurance but refuse to do so. When they incur catastrophic medical expenses they cannot pay for, they become a burden on society. Requiring everyone who can afford it to have catastrophic medical coverage is a way of avoiding individuals imposing external costs on others.

Similarly, drunk drivers frequently impose costs on innocent victims. Penalties, such as jail terms, forfeiture of driver's licenses, fines, and higher alcohol taxes, have been used as attempts to shift the responsibility for these external costs back to those who drink and drive. One study concluded that federal and state alcohol taxes should be increased (from an average of 11 cents to 24 cents a drink) to compensate for the external costs imposed on others by excessive drinkers (Manning et al. 1989).

We should be aware, however, that some people might misapply the externalities argument to justify intervention by the government in all markets. For example, if you admire someone's garden, should you be taxed to subsidize the gardener? Should the student who asks a particularly clever question in class be subsidized by a tax on other students? These examples, although simple, illustrate several important points about externalities. First, when only a few individuals are involved, the parties concerned should be able to reach an accommodation among themselves without resorting to government intervention. Second, even when ownership to the property is clear, high transaction costs may make it too costly to charge for external benefits or costs. The owner of the garden can decide whether it is worthwhile to erect a fence and charge a viewing fee. Chances are the cost of doing so will exceed the amount others are willing to pay. Many may thus receive external benefits simply because excluding them or collecting from them is too costly. Only when the external benefits (or costs) become sufficiently large relative to their transaction costs does it pay for the provider of external benefits to either exclude others or charge them for their benefits.

A third point these examples illustrate concerns the relative size of private benefits compared with external benefits. Would the output of the gardener be too small if neighbors did not contribute? Although many goods and services provide external benefits to others, excluding these external benefits does not result in too small a rate of output. In markets in which the external benefits are sufficiently small relative to the total private benefits, excluding external benefits does not affect the optimal rate of output. This type of externality, referred to as an *inframarginal* externality, occurs within the market. Thus, gardeners may receive so much pleasure from their gardens that they put forth the same level of effort with or without their neighbors' admiration.

The concept of inframarginal benefit is important to understanding the issue of financing education for health professionals. We all benefit from knowing that we have access to physicians, dentists, and nurses if we become ill. However, if their educations were not subsidized, would "too few" physicians be available? The education of physicians is heavily subsidized. The average four-year subsidy for a medical education exceeds $500,000. One reason this cost is so high is that medical schools have little incentive for reducing those costs. Given the continual excess demand for a medical education and the lack of a profit motive by non-profit medical schools, the schools have little incentive to be efficient or innovative. For example, some medical educators claim that medical students could be admitted to medical school after two years of college, medical education could be reduced by at least one year, the residency period could be reduced, and innovations in teaching methods and curricula could reduce the cost still more.

Even if physicians had to pay their entire educational costs themselves, however, the economic return on the costs of becoming a physician has been estimated to be sufficiently attractive that we would have had no less than the current number of physicians. Over time, these economic returns on a medical (and dental) education have changed and varied according to specialty status; returns were higher in the 1950s to 1970s than they are currently. Thus, the concept of external benefits in the number of physicians is more likely a case of inframarginal benefits; sufficient private benefits to individuals from becoming a physician would ensure a sufficient supply of physicians even if no subsidies were provided.

A separate issue is whether low-income individuals could afford a medical education if subsidies were removed. Yet making medical and dental education affordable to all qualified individuals could be accomplished more efficiently by targeting subsidies and loan programs than by equally subsidizing everyone who attends medical school regardless of income level. The rationale for large educational subsidies for a health professional education should be reexamined.

DIVERGENCE BETWEEN THEORETIC AND ACTUAL GOVERNMENT POLICY

Correcting for external costs and benefits creates winners and losers. Taxes and subsidies have redistributive effects; taxpayers have lowered incomes, whereas subsidy recipients have increased incomes. Every group affected by external costs and benefits desires favorable treatment and has incentives to influence government policy. For example, an industry that pollutes the air and water has a concentrated interest in forestalling government policy that would increase its production costs. All who benefit from environmental protection must organize and provide legislators with political support if anything more than symbolic legislation is to be directed at imposing external costs on those who pollute. The growth of the environmental movement was an attempt to offset the imbalance between those with "concentrated" interests (polluters) and "diffuse" costs (the public).

The Clean Air Act (1977 amendments) illustrates the divergence between the theoretic approach for resolving external costs and the real-world phenomenon of concentrated and diffuse interests. A greater amount of air pollution is caused when electric utilities burn high-sulfur coal rather than low-sulfur coal. Imposing a tax on the amount of sulfur dioxides (air pollution) emitted would shift the external costs of air pollution to the electric utilities, which would then have an incentive to search for ways to reduce this tax and consequently the amount of air pollution. One alternative would be for the utilities to switch to low-sulfur coal.

Low-sulfur coal, however, is produced only in the West, and it is cheaper to mine than high-sulfur coal. Low-sulfur coal is therefore a competitive threat to the eastern coal interests that produce high-sulfur coal. Faced with taxes based on the amount of air pollution emitted, midwestern and eastern utilities would find it cheaper to pay added transportation costs to have low-sulfur coal shipped from the West. However, the concentrated interests of the eastern coal mines, their heavily unionized employees, and the senate majority leader (who was from West Virginia, which would have been adversely affected) were able to have legislation passed that was directed toward the process of reducing pollution rather than the amount of pollution emitted. Requiring utilities to merely use specified technology ("scrubbers") for reducing pollution eliminated the utilities' incentives to use low-sulfur coal. When specific technology is mandated, the utility loses its incentive to maintain that technology in good operating condition and to search for more efficient approaches to reducing pollution. Western utilities that use low-sulfur coal bear the higher costs of using mandated technology although they could achieve the desired outcomes by less-expensive means (Feldstein 2006).

SUMMARY

Even if medical care markets were competitive, the "right" output might not occur because of external costs and benefits. With regard to personal medical services, externalities are likely to exist related to medical services for the poor and for those who can afford medical insurance but refuse to purchase coverage for catastrophic illness or injury. Why should medical and dental education be so heavily subsidized? Any external benefits are likely to be inframarginal, thereby not affecting the optimal number of health professionals. Imposing taxes on personal behaviors (products), such as excessive alcohol consumption, that may result in external costs will also serve as an incentive to reduce these external costs. Most externalities in health care derive from medical research, medical services for the poor, lack of catastrophic insurance for those who can afford it, alcohol consumption, and pollution.

Implicit in discussions of externalities is the assumption that government regulation can correct these failures of a competitive market. Politicians, however, may at times be even less responsive to correcting external costs and benefits than producers and consumers. When externalities occur, a theoretic framework for determining appropriate government policy provides a basis for evaluating alternative policies. The divergence between theoretic and actual policies can often be explained by a comparison of the amounts of political support offered by those with concentrated and diffuse interests.

DISCUSSION QUESTIONS

1. What is the economist's definition of the correct, or optimal, rate of output?

2. Why do externalities, such as air and water pollution, occur?

3. Why do economists believe there can be an optimal amount of pollution? What would occur if all pollution were eliminated?

4. Explain the rationale for requiring everyone who can afford it to purchase catastrophic health insurance.

5. The number of medical school spaces in this country is limited. Would fewer people become physicians if government subsidies for medical education were reduced?

REFERENCES

Feldstein, P. J. 2006. "The Control of Externalities: Medical Research, Epidemics, and the Environment." In *The Politics of Health Legislation: An Economic Perspective*, 3rd ed. Chicago: Health Administration Press.

Manning, W. G., E. Keeler, J. Newhouse, E. Sloss, and J. Wasserman. 1989. "The Taxes of Sin: Do Smokers and Drinkers Pay Their Way?" *Journal of the American Medical Association* 261 (11): 1604–09.

ADDITIONAL READING

Joskow, P., R. Schmalensee, and E. Bailey. 1998. "The Market for Sulfur Dioxide Emissions." *American Economic Review* 88 (4): 669–85.

Chapter 32

The Canadian Health Care System

THE CANADIAN HEALTH care system, also referred to as a single-payer system, has been suggested as a model for the United States. Starting in the late 1960s, the Canadian government established the basic guidelines for the system, and each province was provided with federal funds contingent on its adherence to the federal guidelines. Under these guidelines everyone has access to hospital and medical services, and they do not have to pay any deductibles or copayments. Patients have free choice of physician and hospital. Private health insurance is not permitted for these basic hospital and medical services.

The basic cost-control mechanism used in Canada is expenditure limits on health providers. Each province sets its own overall health budget and negotiates a total budget, which it cannot exceed, with each hospital. The province also negotiates with the medical association to establish uniform fees for all physicians, who are paid on a fee-for-service basis and must accept the province's fee as payment in full for their services. In some Canadian provinces, physicians' incomes are also subject to controls; once physicians' revenues exceed a certain level, further billings are paid at 25 percent of their fee schedule.

These cost-containment measures have limited the increase in Canadian health expenditures, although providers complain about their budgets and occasionally physicians go on strike. Because each province finances its services through an income tax, receives federal funds, and pays all medical bills, the need for insurance companies is eliminated. The province controls the adoption and financing of high-technology equipment.

According to its proponents, the Canadian system offers universal coverage, comprehensive hospital and medical benefits, no out-of-pocket expenses, and lower administrative costs, while devoting a smaller percentage of the GDP to health care and spending less per capita than the United States. Would the United States be better off if it adopted the Canadian single-payer health system?

UNIVERSAL COVERAGE

According to its proponents, the Canadian system has two major advantages. The first is universal coverage. However, as *adoption of the Canadian system is but one proposal for reform, it should be compared not to the current U.S. system, but to other health care reform proposals to achieve universal coverage* (see Chapter 34). Thus, adopting the Canadian system solely to achieve universal coverage is not necessary. To many the real attractiveness of the Canadian system is based on its presumed ability to control the rising costs of health care.

CONTROLLING HEALTH CARE COSTS IN CANADA

Proponents of a Canadian system point to two cost savings. The first is lower administrative costs; the second is a lower rate of increase in health care costs achieved by imposing expenditure limits on providers. Each approach is discussed.

Administrative Costs

Advocates of the Canadian system claim that if the United States adopted the Canadian system, it could greatly reduce its administrative costs as health insurance companies would no longer be necessary; thereby universal access could be financed at no additional cost (Woolhandler and Himmelstein 1991). Many would agree that administrative costs in the United States could be somewhat lowered with standardization of claims processing and billing.

Simple comparisons of administrative expenses between the two countries, however, are misleading.[1] Administrative and marketing costs

---

1. The administrative savings of moving to a Canadian system are believed to be grossly overstated. For example, in calculating administrative savings the expense of administering self-insured employer plans was included in the expense ratio of insurers. However, the claims payments made on behalf of self-insured employers were not included as part of the insurers' premiums, falsely inflating the expense ratio. Furthermore, included as part of insurers' overhead are premium taxes (a transfer payment to state governments), investment income (essentially a return to employers for advance payment of premiums), and a return on capital (which would also have to be calculated for a public insurer). (See Danzon 1992.)

could be reduced if the United States eliminated choice of health plans and agreed to a standardized set of health benefits. The United States has a wide variety of health plans, such as HMOs, point-of-service plans, and PPOs, that offer different benefits, cost-sharing levels, and access to providers. Competition among health plans offers consumers greater choice at different premiums.

Choice is costly. However, without choice, there would be less innovation in benefit design, patient satisfaction, and competition on health plan premiums. *The diversity of insurance plans reflects differences in enrollees' preferences and how much they are willing to pay for those preferences.*

Lower administrative costs are not synonymous with greater system efficiency. One can imagine very low administrative costs in a system in which physicians and hospitals send their bills to the government and the government simply pays them. These lower administrative costs cause higher health care expenditures because they do not detect or deter inappropriate use or overuse of services. *A trade-off occurs between lower administrative costs and higher health expenditures caused by insufficient monitoring of physician and hospital behavior.* If higher administrative cost resulting from utilization management did not pay for itself by reducing medical expenses and overutilization, managed care plans would not use these measures.

For example, the U.S. Medicare system, which has a similar design as the Canadian system, has much lower administrative costs than private managed care plans. However, the General Accounting Office has criticized Medicare for having administrative costs that are "too low"; billions of dollars could be saved "by adopting the health care management approach of private payers to Medicare's public payer role" (General Accounting Office 1995). Studies have shown that cost-containment approaches, such as preauthorization for hospital admissions, utilization review for hospitalized patients, catastrophic case management, and physician profiling for appropriateness of care, save money.

The health insurance industry in the United States is very competitive and would only increase administrative costs if the benefits from doing so exceeded their costs. Any savings in administrative costs by eliminating cost-containment techniques and patient cost sharing would be more than offset by the increased utilization that would occur. The Canadian system is forgoing substantial savings by not increasing its administrative costs, investing more in cost-containment programs, and developing monitoring mechanisms of physicians' practice patterns.

Rising Health Care Costs

An oft-cited measure of the cost-containment success of the Canadian system is the smaller percentage of Canada's GDP that is devoted to health care. Although correct, this statement can be misleading. At different times GDP may increase faster in one country than another, distorting any conclusion as to which country's health care costs are rising faster.

A more accurate indication of which country's health costs have risen more slowly is a comparison of the rise in per capita health expenditures. Again, one must be careful in making such comparisons, as more than 45 percent of U.S. medical expenditures are by the government for Medicare and Medicaid, which have limited cost controls. Some regions of the United States also have greater managed care penetration than others. This country's medical system has evolved from one that until the 1980s provided limited if any incentives for efficiency to one in which the private sector, in some states more than others, emphasizes managed care delivery systems. Thus, the 1990s performance of the U.S. system, particularly in states with a greater portion of the population in managed care, would be more relevant to compare with the Canadian system.

As shown in Figure 32.1, since the 1980s, per capita health expenditures (adjusted for inflation) have increased at a lower rate in Canada than in the United States. The effect of managed care can be seen by the lower rate of increase in the United States during the 1990s than in prior years. (As a result of the backlash against managed care in the late 1990s, managed care's cost-containment methods were loosened and premiums increased more rapidly.) During the 1990s when managed care was reducing rising premiums in the United States, annual percentage increases (adjusted for inflation) in Canada's per capita health spending were negative. Clearly, therefore, annual percentage increases in per capita health expenditures in Canada have been and continue to be lower than in the United States over an extended period.

Does the Canadian health care system achieve these lower rates of increases in per capita health costs because of greater efficiency?

Differences in Hospital Length of Stay

What are the reasons for the lower rate of increase in per capita health care spending in Canada than the United States? Is Canada more efficient in the way it produces medical services? Although efficiency studies would have to control for many differences between the two countries,

Figure 32.1: Annual Percentage Growth in Real per Capita Health Expenditures in Canada and the United States, 1981–2004

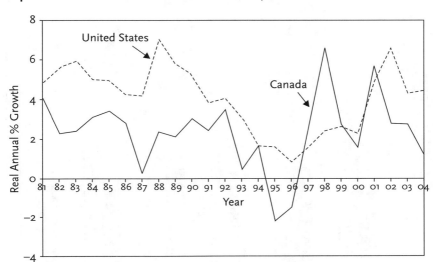

Note: Values are adjusted for inflation using the CPI for each country.

Sources: Health expenditures per capita data from Organisation for Economic Cooperation and Development. 2005. *OECD Health Data, 2005.* Paris: OECD; CPI data from Bureau of Labor Statistics. 2006. [Online information.] http://data.bls.gov, and Statistics Canada. 62-001. [Online information.] http://www.statcan.ca.

such as populations served, distribution of illnesses, outcomes of care, staffing patterns, wage rates, and so on, one simple, although partial, measure of efficiency is differences in lengths of hospital stay.

Managed care systems in the United States have a financial incentive to use the least-costly combination of medical services. Hospitals are the most expensive setting for providing care. Use of the hospital is subject to review; outpatient diagnostics and surgery are used whenever possible, and catastrophic case management may involve renovating a patient's home to make it a lower-cost and more convenient setting in which to care for the patient.

The efficiency gains from managed care are evident in a comparison of utilization data between the United States and Canada. As shown in Figure 32.2, Canadian hospitals have a higher average length of stay than hospitals in the United States, but the difference is becoming smaller. In 1985, the length of stay in Canada was 10.7 days, compared with 7.1 days

Figure 32.2: Average Length of Hospital Stay in Canada and the United States, 1980–2003

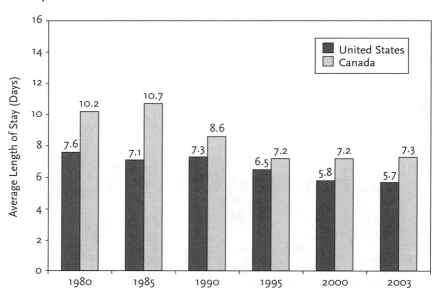

Sources: Data from Organisation for Economic Cooperation and Development. 2005. *OECD Health Data*, 2005. Paris: OECD; 2003 data for Canada from Canadian Institute for Health Information. 2005. *Inpatient Hospitalizations and Average Length of Stay Trends in Canada, 2003–2004 and 2004–2005*, Analysis in Brief, November 30. [Online information.] http://secure.cihi.ca/cihiweb/en/downloads/HMDB_Analysis_in_Brief_FINAL_ENG.pdf.

in the United States. By 2003, the same measure was 7.3 in Canada and 5.7 in the United States. In California, a state with high managed care penetration, it was 4.9 days. The average length of stay for those aged 65 years and older is very high in Canada because few alternative arrangements are available. Canadian hospitals are used inappropriately; many services could be provided in an outpatient setting, the physician's office, or the patient's home.

Annual hospital budgets in Canada also provide administrators with an incentive to fill a portion of their beds with elderly patients who stay many days. If more surgical patients were admitted, hospitals would not receive additional funds to purchase the necessary supplies and nursing personnel to serve them. Thus, as inflation diminishes the real value of

Canadian hospitals' budgets with which to purchase resources, they admit less acutely ill patients and prolong their stays.

If the lower rate of increase in Canada's health expenditures is not a result of greater efficiency, what is it attributable to?

CONSEQUENCES OF STRICT LIMITS ON PER CAPITA COSTS

In the late 1980s, Canada was experiencing rising health care costs and a deep recession. As a result, the federal government reduced its financial commitment to the provinces from its initial 50 percent of each province's health spending to an average of about 20 percent currently. As these federal cash and tax transfers are reduced, the rising cost of the Canadian health system places an increasing financial burden on each province.

The consequence of these rising costs for both the federal and provincial governments has been reduced spending on health care. As shown in Figure 32.1, the annual percentage increase in inflation-adjusted per capita health expenditures fell dramatically between 1990 and 1996. In contrast to the managed care revolution in the United States, this steep decline in Canada was attributable to reduced government funding and not new cost-containment approaches. In the past when such large declines occurred, such as in the early and late 1970s, they were followed by sharp increases in following years. Consequently, between 1998 and 2001, Canada had a more rapid rate of increase in its per capita health expenditures to make up for the very low and negative budgetary allocations in previous years. In more recent years, there were again very low rates of increase in per capita expenditures. This pattern—years of low rates of increase in per capita health expenditures followed by a few years of high expenditures to make up for the resulting severe reductions in access to care—repeats itself.

Government expenditure limits are the inevitable consequence of an unlimited demand for medical services. *No government can fund all of the medical care that is demanded at zero price.* Because expenditure limits result in less care being provided than is demanded at zero price, choices must be made as to how scarce health care resources are to be allocated. Many trade-offs must be made, for example, among preventive care, acute care, access to new technology, and decreasing patient waiting times to receive treatment. With limited dollars, providing more of one choice means less is available to fulfill other choices.

The inevitable consequences of very tight per capita expenditure limits, as has occurred in Canada, are increasing shortages of medical services and decreased access to new technology. Furthermore, as the beneficial effects of preventive care occur in the future, resources are allocated to acute services for patients whose needs are more immediate.

Access to Technology

One of the distinguishing features of the U.S. medical system is the rapid diffusion of technologic innovation. Major advances in diagnostic and treatment procedures have occurred. Imaging equipment has improved diagnostic accuracy and reduced the need for exploratory surgery. New technology has resulted in less-invasive procedures, quicker recovery times, and improved treatment outcomes. Technologic advances have increased the survival rate of low-birth-weight babies and permitted an increasing number and type of organ transplants. *Any comparison of the Canadian and U.S. health systems should consider the rate at which new technology is diffused and made available to patients.*

Managed care, which is characteristic of the U.S. health care system, uses different criteria for adopting and diffusing new technology than does the Canadian system. Two types of technologic advances occur. The first, and simplest to evaluate under managed care, is when new technology reduces costs and increases patient satisfaction. A competitive managed care system will invest the necessary capital to bring about these technologic savings.

The more difficult decision on adopting new technology concerns technology that improves medical outcomes but is much more costly than existing technology. Particularly troublesome is new technology that may have only a low probability of success, for example, 10 percent to 20 percent. In such cases, the patient would like access to the expensive treatment although the MCO may believe it is not worth the expenditure given the low success rate.

Technology that is clearly believed to be beneficial is highly likely to be adopted. If one health plan decided not to adopt the technology when its competitors did, it would lose enrollees. Competition among health plans would force the adoption of highly beneficial technology. The costs of such technology would eventually be passed on to enrollees in the form of higher premiums.

New technology that offers small beneficial effects (e.g., a new method of conducting Pap smears that increases cancer detection by 5 percent or experimental breast cancer treatments for late-stage cancer patients) has caused problems for managed care firms. Several health plans that have denied such treatments have suffered penalties of up to $100 million as a result of lawsuits. To reduce their liability an increasing number of health plans are delegating such decisions to outside firms comprised of ethicists and physicians who have no financial stake in the decision. Thus, the decision by the health plan based on the outside firm's recommendation is divorced from any financial implication.

In Canada the availability of capital to invest in both cost-saving and benefit-increasing technology is determined by the government, not the hospital. Given their budget constraints and reluctance to raise taxes, governments are less likely to provide capital for new technology and for as many units as when firms compete for enrollees. Outpatient diagnostic and surgical services are less available in Canada, denying patients the benefits (and society the cost savings) of such technologic improvements. Costly benefit-increasing technology, such as transplants and experimental treatments, is also less available to Canadians.

A competitive managed care system may adopt technology too soon and have excess technologic capacity. Excess capacity, however, means faster access and lower patient risks. Enrollees may be willing to pay higher premiums to have that excess capacity available. If so, excess technologic capacity is appropriate; the benefits to enrollees of that excess capacity are at least equal to their willingness to pay for it. The adoption of new technology under managed care competition is different from what a government (or quasi-governmental agency) would use, as the government would be concerned with losing political support if it had to raise taxes or incur large budget deficits to increase access to new technology.

Examples of differences in availability of technology between Canada and the United States are shown in Figure 32.3. There are 7 times more lithotriptors available per person in the United States than in Canada, nearly 2 times as many MRI units, and 1.3 times as many computed tomography (CT) scanners per person. In Canada about 59 percent of patients with end-stage renal failure undergo dialysis, compared with 99 percent in the United States (Organisation for Economic Cooperation and Development 2005). Clearly, the likelihood of a patient in the United States receiving any of the services shown in Figure 32.3 is much greater than a similar patient with equal needs who lives in Canada. (How successful would an HMO be in this country if it used access criteria similar to those used in Canada?)

Figure 32.3: Indicators of Medical Technology per Million People, 2002 and 2004

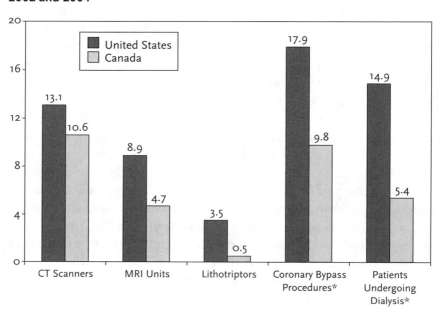

*2002 data.

Sources: Organisation for Economic Cooperation and Development. 2005. *OECD Health Data, 2005.* Paris: OECD; 2004 data for United States from American Hospital Association. 2006. *Hospital Statistics, 2006* ed., Table 7. Chicago: AHA; 2002 data for United States on the number of coronary bypass procedures from National Center for Health Statistics. 2002. *2002 National Hospital Discharge Survey Advance Data* No. 342. [Online information.] http://www.cdc.gov/nchs/data/ad/ad342.pdf.

The Technological Change in Health Care (TECH) Research Network is an international group of researchers who examine differences in technologic change across countries in the treatment, resource costs, and health outcomes for common health problems (TECH 2001). Because knowledge of heart attack treatment has greatly changed in recent years and data from various studies have shown that improvements in outcomes may be the result of differences in medical practices, differences in the adoption of technology are likely to occur between countries in inpatient care for heart attacks.

The researchers found different patterns of technologic change between countries in adopting more intensive cardiac procedures. The United States adopted an "early start and fast growth" pattern, which resulted in relatively high treatment rates in the overall population as well as in the elderly population. Conversely, in Canada the adoption of new technology starts later, its diffusion is slower (as well as lower than in the United States), and the elderly population has lower treatment rates.

The TECH (2001) researchers attribute these differences in the adoption and diffusion of beneficial technology for care of heart attack patients between the United States and Canada to differences in funding and decision making, "such as global budgets for hospitals and central planning of the availability of intensive services" in Canada (p. 37). The researchers further state that, "It is clear that if high-quality care requires rapid innovation and diffusion of valuable high-cost as well as low-cost treatments, quality of care may differ greatly around the world, and national health policy may influence quality in important ways" (p. 38).

Patient Waiting Times

As demand for services exceeds available supply, waiting time is used to ration nonemergency care. For some types of care the quantity of care demanded increases because patients have no copayments. Facing a zero price, patients will demand a high volume of physician visits. Consequently, to see more patients, physicians must spend less time per visit. The physician has the patient return for multiple short visits rather than providing the services previously provided in one visit. Patient time costs are therefore higher under a "free" system with tight fee controls because each visit requires the same patient travel and waiting time regardless of the length of the visit.[2]

Expenditure limits invariably result in high time costs being imposed on patients. However, not all care rationed by waiting time is of low value to the patient. According to a Fraser Institute (Walker and Esmail 2006) report on the Canadian health care system, in 2006 Canadian patients had to wait on average 10.3 weeks for an MRI (the range was 8 to

---

2. The value to the patient of additional physician visits when there are no out-of-pocket payments is low. Generally, the approaches used to limit use of services whose value is worth less than their costs of production are cost-containment techniques and requiring patients to wait longer. Cost containment is included as an explicit administrative expense, whereas implicit patient waiting cost is not.

28 weeks depending on the province), 4.3 weeks for a CT scan (the range was 4 to 9 weeks), and 3.8 weeks for an ultrasound (the range was 2 to 8 weeks). The long waits for first-time mammograms virtually eliminate this screening mechanism as a preventive method.

Acknowledging these long waits and their adverse effects on patients, at least two Canadian provinces pay for heart surgery in the United States. Almost 12 percent of all British Columbians (13.3 percent of those residing in Newfoundland) who require radiation oncology treatment have been sent by the Canadian province to the United States, which is Canada's safety valve. Ontario has contracted with hospitals in Buffalo and Detroit for MRI services. Quebec sent more than 250 cancer patients to the United States for treatment in 1999; 350 cancer patients waited more than eight weeks for radiation or chemotherapy (more than four weeks' waiting time is considered medically risky) (Pearlstein 1999).

The Fraser Institute performs annual surveys on waiting times from referral by the general practitioner to an appointment with a specialist and on the waiting time from appointment with a specialist to treatment. These surveys are done by medical specialty for each Canadian province. Figure 32.4 describes the waiting time for treatment by specialty. For example, for orthopedic surgery (e.g., hips and knees) a person would have to wait on average 40.4 weeks to receive treatment (time from referral by general practitioner to treatment); in some provinces, however, the wait to have the surgery performed may be as short as 31.5 weeks or as long as 70.9 weeks. (In 1991, aged patients in some provinces had to wait up to four years for a hip or knee replacement.) Ophthalmology (e.g., cataract removal) requires an average wait of 27.2 weeks, but this can vary by province from 18.4 to 47.4 weeks. For radiation oncology for prostate cancer, the wait can be as long as 14 weeks or as short as 3 weeks, depending on the province.

The Fraser Institute also asks specialists how long a patient should wait before they receive the recommended treatment. For example, in 2005 (2006 data are unavailable), the actual waiting time for urgent cardiovascular surgery in Prince Edward Island after a patient had seen a specialist was six weeks, whereas specialists believe the reasonable waiting time should not exceed two weeks; for elective cardiovascular surgery the actual waiting time is of course much greater. There have been reports of patients who have died waiting for heart surgery. Clearly, access to care depends on the province in which one lives. Furthermore, the waiting time is not the same for all procedures in a province.

Figure 32.4: Canadian Hospital Waiting Lists: Total Expected Waiting Time from Referral by General Practitioner to Treatment, by Specialty, 2006

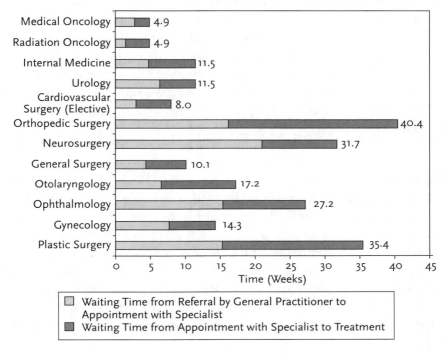

Source: Walker, M., N. Esmail, and D. Wrona. 2006. *Waiting Your Turn: Hospital Waiting Lists in Canada*, 16th ed., The Fraser Institute, October. [Online information.] http://www.fraserinstitute.ca/admin/books/chapterfiles/wyt2006.pdf#.

Canada does not have an egalitarian system. Access to care depends not only on the province in which one lives but also on whether a person can afford to pay for her care in the United States. The failure to consider the higher patient time costs in the Canadian system *understates* health expenditures in Canada. As demand for services exceeds the available supply, *many people would be willing to pay more rather than incur the cost of multiple trips, waiting, or doing without.* Unfortunately, the Canadian system prohibits the purchase of private health insurance for hospital and medical services. Thus, people are legally prohibited from insuring themselves against the risks of not receiving timely care when they require it.

An important consequence of these long waits for medical service is that patients experience pain and discomfort, and some may develop psychological problems . . . The condition of some patients may worsen, making surgery more risky . . . because of the long queue for lithotripsy treatment, many doctors perform surgery to remove kidney stones (also resulting in higher costs), putting the patient at higher risk than with a lithotripsy procedure . . . Often patients experience a financial setback, such as decreased income or loss of a job (while waiting in queues) . . . patients are unable to work because they are physically immobile while they wait for a hip or other joint replacement (General Accounting Office 1991, 59).

Those who are wealthy can afford to skip the queues and purchase medical services in the United States, as did Quebec Premier Robert Bourassa. When he learned that he needed an operation for melanoma in 1990, instead of waiting his turn, at his own expense he went to the United States for his operation (Wood 1990). Similarly, the politically powerful are also able to jump to the head of the queue, as occurred with Canada's health minister, who was able to have his surgery after being diagnosed with prostate cancer in 2001. Other prostate cancer patients were angered by his quick surgery after they had to wait much longer, some as long as a year between diagnosis and surgery (Rupert 2001).

IS CANADA ABANDONING ITS SINGLE-PAYER SYSTEM?
A Quebec patient, forced to wait a year for a hip replacement and prohibited from paying privately for his operation, brought a lawsuit against the government to the Canadian Supreme Court. In a surprise ruling, the Supreme Court concluded that the wait for medical services had become so long that the health system and its ban on private practice violated patients' "life and personal security, inviolability and freedom," which are part of Quebec's Charter of Rights and Freedoms. Furthermore, "The evidence in this case shows that delays in the public health care system are widespread, and that, in some serious cases, patients die as a result of waiting lists for public health care . . . In sum, the prohibition on obtaining private health insurance is not constitutional where the public system fails to deliver reasonable services." Although the ruling applied to Quebec, it is widely believed the court's ruling will affect all of Canada's provinces (Krauss 2005).

As a consequence of the court's ruling, private diagnostic and special surgery clinics have opened in Quebec. The federal government, opposed to the introduction of private medicine, is under great pressure to increase health care spending to reduce waiting times for medical services. To provide quicker access to medical services, Quebec is paying private clinics to serve orthopedic and cataract patients. Supporters of the single-payer system are opposed to a two-tier medical system, believing the private sector will draw physicians and nurses away from the public system, where a severe physician shortage already exists, making waiting times even longer.

The dam may have already broken. The premiers of British Columbia and Alberta are planning to propose legislation to encourage private health insurance and private medical services (Krauss 2006). In anticipation of these changes, private clinics are opening all over Canada and private insurance companies will soon follow.[3] It will be difficult to stop the trend toward privatization and a two-tier medical system that already exists in all other countries.

SHOULD THE UNITED STATES ADOPT THE CANADIAN SYSTEM?

Canada has been the only Westernized country with a single-payer system. Other countries that started with a single-payer system, such as Great Britain, moved to a two-tier system that permitted private medical markets. Canada appears to be moving in the same direction. Governments find that it eventually becomes too expensive to fund all the new technology and medical services its population demands when they do not have to pay any out-of-pocket costs. Inequities develop in a single-payer system; the wealthy can reduce their waiting by traveling to another country, and the politically powerful are able to jump the queue. A two-tier medical system recognizes that there are those who are willing to spend more of their money in return for quicker access to medical services and to the latest medical technology.

Alternative approaches exist to achieve the objectives claimed for a single-payer system. With regard to the equity criterion, namely how

---

3. One physician who is opening private medical clinics said, "This is a country in which dogs can get a hip replacement in under a week and in which humans can wait two to three years" (Krauss 2006). Dogs have also had preferential treatment with regard to diagnostic tests. The government provides funding for hospitals to operate its MRIs only eight hours a day. In 1998, a Canadian hospital offered MRIs to pets in the middle of the night in an effort to make money. After an outcry from angry humans, who at that time were waiting up to a year for nonurgent scans, the hospital was forced to stop this practice (Walkom 2002).

to provide for the uninsured, the Canadian system should be compared not to the current U.S. system, but to one in which the goal is universal coverage. This goal can be achieved in alternative ways, such as by providing income-related subsidies to those with low incomes (see Chapter 34). A single-payer system, as evidenced by the Canadian system, does not provide everyone with equal access to medical care. It should be acknowledged that every health system has multiple tiers; those who can afford it will be able to purchase more medical services or have quicker access to care. Unequal access to care exists in Canada depending on the province in which people live or whether they can afford to pay for their care in the United States.

Arbitrarily limiting the growth in medical expenditures, the cost-containment method used in single-payer systems, will not increase efficiency. Efficiency incentives on the part of patients or medical providers are not used in the Canadian system. Efficiency incentives are important because they affect the cost of any national health insurance plan and the willingness of the public to provide subsidies to those less fortunate than themselves. To whom are government decision makers accountable? What information do they have to make decisions? In a competitive market people can leave a health plan when they are dissatisfied with that plan; in a monopolized system (single payer) they have no similar way in which to express their dissatisfaction with the system. Information is either unavailable or dated in a single-payer system to allow the decision makers to make adjustments based on changes in demand or supply conditions. Also important to which national health insurance plan is adopted are the criteria used for access to and investment in new medical technology. Efficiency, innovation, and capital investment are determined by incentives; a government bureaucracy is highly unlikely to outperform competitive markets in this regard.

Political versus private decision making will result in differences in access to care, technology adoption, efficiency, equity, and even health outcomes. Before the United States places its health care system, comprising almost one-sixth of its economy, under complete government control, single-payer advocates should provide evidence, more than just opinion, showing why a U.S. single-payer system will not suffer the same fate experienced by other countries that have tried and subsequently abandoned their own single-payer systems.

SUMMARY

Proposals for health care reform, such as a single-payer system, should not be evaluated against the current U.S. health system but against other national health insurance proposals to achieve universal coverage and methods to limit rising health care expenditures. Furthermore, single-payer advocates should not dismiss the flaws of the Canadian system by claiming that the United States would be able to devote more money to a U.S. single-payer system. Given rising medical costs, advancements in medical technology, and no limits on patients' access to care, evidence suggests, based on every country that has tried a single-payer system, that a U.S. single-payer system will eventually suffer the same fate as the Canadian system.

Before the United States selects another country's medical system, it should be clear as to both the accuracy of the statements made about the performance of that country's medical system and the criteria by which a system should be evaluated. Controlling the percentage of GDP devoted to medical care or the rise in per capita expenditures should not be the overriding objectives of a medical system; otherwise, the United States should use the British National Health Service, which performs better on these criteria but is clearly unacceptable on other grounds.

The appropriate rate of growth in medical expenditures should be based on how much people are willing to pay (directly and through taxes). There are legitimate reasons for increased medical expenditures, such as an aging population, more chronic illness, new technology that saves lives and improves the quality of life, new diseases, shortages of personnel (thereby requiring wage increases), and so on. Arbitrary expenditure limits, below what would otherwise occur because of these situations, will result in reduced access to medical services and technology.

DISCUSSION QUESTIONS

1. Describe the Canadian health care system and the methods used to control costs.

2. What are the consequences of making medical services free to everyone?

3. Why is the size of administrative expenses (as a percentage of total medical expenditures) a poor indication of a health care system's efficiency?

4. What are the costs (negative effects) of expenditure limits?

5. Contrast the criteria used in Canada and in competitive managed care systems for deciding whether an investment should be made in new technology.

REFERENCES

Danzon, P. M. 1992. "Hidden Overhead Costs: Is Canada's System Really Less Expensive?" *Health Affairs* 11 (1): 21–43.

Krauss, C. 2005. "In Blow to Canada's Health System, Quebec Law Is Voided." *New York Times* June 10, A3.

———. 2006. "Canada's Private Clinics Surge as Public System Falters." *New York Times* February 28, A3.

Organisation for Economic Cooperation and Development. 2005. *OECD Health Data, 2005*. Paris: OECD.

Pearlstein, S. 1999. "Health Care on the Critical List: Canada's Public System Is Overwhelmed, and Under Attack." *The Washington Post* December 18, A20.

Rupert, J. 2001. "Man Protests Rock's Speedy Surgery." *Ottawa Citizen* February 17, D3.

Technological Change in Health Care (TECH) Research Network. 2001. "Technological Change Around the World: Evidence from Heart Attack Care." *Health Affairs* 20 (3): 25–42.

U.S. General Accounting Office. 1991. *Canadian Health Insurance*, GAO/HRD-91-90. Washington, DC: U.S. Government Printing Office.

———. 1995. *Medicare: Rapid Spending Growth Calls for More Prudent Purchasing*, GAO/T-HEHS-95-193. Washington, DC: U.S. Government Printing Office.

Walker, M., and N. Esmail. 2006. *Waiting Your Turn: Hospital Waiting Lists in Canada*, 16th ed. The Fraser Institute. [Online publication; retrieved 1/12/07.] http://www.fraserinstitute.ca/admin/books/chapterfiles/wyt2006.pdf#.

Walkom, T. 2002. "No Pets Ahead of People." *Toronto Star* January 11, A6.

Wood, N. 1990. "Missing But Not Forgotten." *McLean's* December 10, 14.

Woolhandler, S., and D. Himmelstein. 1991. "The Deteriorating Administrative Efficiency of the U.S. Health Care System." *The New England Journal of Medicine* 324 (18): 1253–58.

ADDITIONAL READING

Goodman, J. 2005. *Health Care in a Free Society: Rebutting the Myths of National Health Insurance*, Policy Analysis No. 532, 1–26. Washington, DC: Cato Institute.

Chapter 33

Employer-Mandated
National Health Insurance

AN EMPLOYER MANDATE for health insurance has had a great deal of political support. President Clinton proposed, as part of his national health insurance plan, that employers be required to provide health insurance to their employees and dependents. The Pepper Commission, named after its late chairman, Claude Pepper, endorsed this approach toward national health insurance; Hawaii has instituted it, and many states are currently considering enacting an employer mandate.

In 2004, approximately 48 million people under the age of 65 years were uninsured (an increase from 32 million in 1987). About two-thirds of the uninsured were either employed (full or part time) or in a family with an employed member. Therefore, mandating employers to provide their employees with health insurance would cover a large percentage of the uninsured at small cost to the government. If employers chose not to provide health insurance to their employees, they would have to pay a new payroll tax (either a fixed amount per employee or a percentage of payroll) into a state pool for the uninsured, hence the name "play-or-pay" national health insurance.

Although there are variations on the basic approach, mandated employer proposals generally require the employer to pay 80 percent and the employee 20 percent of the cost of the insurance. (Some states propose requiring employers to spend at least 8 percent of wages for health insurance.) Employees working part time would be eligible for the employer's health insurance. Play-or-pay proposals generally mandate that all employers with more than 100 employees be required to immediately participate; firms with fewer employees would have to participate in subsequent years. Under some proposals small firms would be provided with a tax credit to offset the firm's higher costs, which might ease the transition.

Before analyzing the economic consequences of mandating employers to provide health insurance to the working uninsured, it is useful to examine who the uninsured are and why they do not have insurance.

THE UNINSURED

Of the 253 million persons who were under the age of 65 in 2004 (Medicare eligibility begins at age 65), 19 percent, or 48 million, were without private health insurance (AHRQ 2005).[1] (Medicaid covers about 13 percent, or 34 million, low-income nonelderly.) About 8 percent of those who are working and below the age of 18 years are uninsured (see Table 33.1). The age group with the highest percentage of uninsured employees is 19- to 24-year-olds, who make up 28 percent. These people are generally single adults who are no longer eligible for their parents' health insurance. The percentage of uninsured workers within each age group declines the higher the age group.

When uninsured workers in each age group are examined as a percentage of all uninsured workers, those aged 25 to 34 years represent the greatest portion of all uninsured workers, 29 percent. The second highest numbers of uninsured are those aged 45 to 64 years, 26 percent. The distribution of uninsured workers in the remaining age groups, 19 to 24 and 35 to 44 years of age, are both about 21 percent of the total number of uninsured workers. Thus, the uninsured are predominantly young workers.

When one examines the percentage distribution of the total uninsured population, which includes dependents of workers and those not in the labor force, about 18 percent of the uninsured are children (DeNavas-Walt, Proctor, and Lee 2004). This number has decreased since the 1997 enactment of CHIP, which covers low-income children.

Whites represent 50 percent of the total number of uninsured, although only 12 percent of all whites are uninsured. Twenty percent of

---

1. The Medical Expenditure Panel Survey–Household Component produces estimates of the uninsured for three different periods within a year: at any time during the year, throughout the first half of the year, and the entire year. In 2004, the latest year for which all three measures are available, 25.7 percent of the population under age 65 (nonelderly) was uninsured at some point during the year, 19.0 percent was uninsured throughout the first half of the year, and 13.8 percent was uninsured the entire year (Rhoades 2006).

Table 33.1: Uninsured Workers, by Age Group, 2003

Age (in Years)	Working Population (in Thousands)*	% Distribution of Workers	% Uninsured Within Each Age Group	% Distribution of All Uninsured
16–18	4,734	3.2	7.9	1.7
19–24	17,194	11.8	28.2	21.9
25–34	34,526	23.7	18.8	29.4
35–44	36,855	25.3	12.5	20.9
45–64	52,511	36.0	11.0	26.1

*Excludes persons with unknown self-employment status and does not account for size of establishment.

Source: Agency for Healthcare Research and Quality, Center for Cost and Financing Studies, Medical Expenditure Panel Survey Household Component, personal correspondence with Jeffrey Rhoades, December 8, 2005.

all African Americans are uninsured, and Hispanics have the highest uninsured percentage at 35 percent. Regionally, most of the uninsured (42 percent) are in the South. The West is second with 26 percent; the Midwest has 19 percent, and the Northeast has the fewest (13 percent) (DeNavas-Walt, Proctor, and Lee 2004).

An important characteristic of the employed uninsured is the size of the firm in which they work. The fewer the number of employees, the greater is the likelihood that the employer does not provide health insurance. Thus, 26 percent of employees in small firms (defined as those with fewer than ten employees) are uninsured, compared with only 5 percent in large firms (those with more than 500 employees). Of all of the employed uninsured (including self-employed workers), 72 percent are in firms with fewer than 25 employees, and 17 percent are in firms with 25 to 99 employees. Thus, 88 percent of the total employed uninsured are in firms with fewer than 100 employees (Table 33.2). If self-employed workers are excluded, 53 percent of uninsured workers are in firms with fewer than 25 employees, and 17 percent are in firms with 25 to 99 employees. Thus, 69 percent of the total employed uninsured are in firms with fewer than 100 employees.

A second important work-related characteristic of the employed uninsured is their low wages. As shown in Table 33.3, as of 2003, 59 percent of the employed uninsured earned less than $10 an hour; another

Table 33.2: Uninsured Workers, by Size of Firm, 2003

Characteristic	Working Population (in Thousands)*	% Distribution of Workers	% Uninsured Within Each Group	% Distribution of All Uninsured
Self-employed	17,317	11.2	26.9	18.6
Fewer than 10 workers	35,883	23.1	26.4	38.0
10–24 workers	21,618	13.9	17.4	15.0
25–49 workers	16,275	10.5	14.4	9.4
50–99 workers	16,008	10.3	11.2	7.2
100–499 workers	27,025	17.4	6.9	7.4
500 or more workers	20,924	13.5	5.2	4.3

*Excludes persons with unknown self-employment status and does not account for size of establishment.

Source: Agency for Healthcare Research and Quality, Center for Cost and Financing Studies, Medical Expenditure Panel Survey Household Component, personal correspondence with Jeffrey Rhoades, December 8, 2005.

26 percent earned between $10 and $15 per hour; thus, 85 percent earned less than $15 per hour. With respect to part-time work, 29 percent of uninsured workers work fewer than 35 hours per week. *The picture of the uninsured that emerges is of generally young people who work in small firms and earn low wages.*

WHY THE UNINSURED DO NOT HAVE HEALTH INSURANCE

The employed uninsured do not have health insurance for two important reasons. First, the price of insurance is higher (consequently the demand is lower) for those who are employed in small firms. Smaller firms are unable to take advantage of economies in administering and marketing health insurance, which results in higher insurance costs per employee. Insurance companies also charge small firms higher premiums to make allowance for adverse selection, believing many employees will join just to take advantage of health benefits. Also, for example, an owner might hire a sick relative so her medical costs could be paid. In larger firms with lower turnover rates, employment is less likely primarily for the purpose of receiving health benefits. Finally, many states have mandated

Table 33.3: Percentage Distribution of Uninsured Workers, by Wage Rate and Hours Worked, 2003

Characteristic	Working Population (in Thousands)*	% Distribution of Workers	% Uninsured Within Each Group	% Distribution of All Uninsured
Hours of work				
Fewer than 20	9,975	6.9	16.1	7.5
20–34	20,679	14.3	21.8	21.0
35 or more	113,490	78.7	13.5	71.5
Hourly wage				
Less than $5.00	3,372	2.6	26.4	5.0
$5.00–$9.99	35,990	28.1	26.3	53.7
$10.00–$14.99	33,138	25.9	14.0	26.3
$15.00–$19.99	20,461	16.0	6.3	7.3
$20.00 or more	34,891	27.3	3.9	7.7

*Excludes persons with unknown self-employment status and does not account for size of establishment.

Source: Agency for Healthcare Research and Quality, Center for Cost and Financing Studies, Medical Expenditure Panel Survey Household Component, personal correspondence with Jeffrey Rhoades, December 8, 2005.

various benefits, such as in vitro fertilization and hair transplants, that must be included in any health insurance plan sold in their state. Once included in the insurance policy, employees use these services, increasing the insurance premium. Larger firms, however, are able to self-insure, making them exempt from the costs of these additional mandates. Smaller firms are too small to self-insure and therefore have to pay the higher premium, which lessens their demand for health insurance.

The second reason for the lower demand for health insurance in small firms is the low incomes of their employees. Because 85 percent of the employed uninsured earn less than $15 per hour, health insurance premiums would result in a major reduction in their funds available for other necessities. For example, most uninsured workers earn $10 an hour or less, or roughly $20,000 a year. Requiring them to purchase health insurance would reduce their incomes by 20 percent (insurance cost $4,242 per person per year and $11,480 per year for a family of four in 2006 (The Kaiser Family Foundation and the Health Research and Educational Trust 2006). Instead, when these low-wage employees or their families become ill, they are likely to become eligible for Medicaid, which would not cost them anything. For low-wage workers and their families Medicaid is their health insurance plan.

CONSEQUENCES OF EMPLOYER-MANDATED HEALTH INSURANCE

Failure to Achieve Universal Coverage

Employer-mandated health insurance by itself cannot achieve universal coverage. Even if all working uninsured were covered by an employer mandate, those employed part time and those not employed, together with their dependents, would still not have insurance coverage. This would leave approximately one-third of the uninsured without coverage. To achieve universal coverage an employer mandate must be combined with an insurance subsidy program for these other population groups.

Inequitable Method of Financing

Advocates of an employer mandate have proposed that small firms be given tax credits or subsidies to induce them to offer health insurance to their employees. This approach, however, will likely be inequitable. Although many low-wage employees work in small firms, not everyone employed by small firms earns a low income, such as small legal firms or physician groups. The subsidy could be limited to those small firms with low average incomes. However, some low-wage employees in large firms would not receive subsidies. To eliminate these inequities tax subsidies should be targeted to those in need (i.e., they should be income related) and not according to the size of firm.

Who Pays for Employer Mandates?

Employer mandates require the employer to pay 80 percent and the employee 20 percent of the cost of health insurance. Thus, most of the cost would appear to be borne by the firm. However, whether the employer or the employee actually bears the burden of the tax does not depend on whom the tax is imposed. In competitive industries firms do not make excess profits; otherwise, other firms (including foreign firms) would enter that industry until excess profits no longer exist. When employers are earning a competitive rate of return, they will be unable to bear the burden of the additional tax themselves—or they would eventually go out of business. Instead, faced with a new employee tax, within a short period employers will shift the cost of that tax to others by increasing their prices, decreasing the cash wages paid to their employees, or both.

Imposing a per employee tax on the employer is likely to result in one of three possible outcomes (Blumberg 1999). Exactly which combination occurs will depend on the particular labor and product markets in which the firm competes, because the nature of these markets will determine how much of the higher labor costs is shifted back onto the employee and how much is shifted forward in the form of higher consumer prices. First, to the extent that employees are flexible about the relative portions of their total compensation that go to cash wages and fringe benefits (including health insurance), the cost of labor to the employer is unchanged. An increased employer tax to pay for employees' insurance would result in lower wages, consequently not increasing the cost of labor to the firm. Although employees receive more health insurance, they clearly value the health insurance less than the cash wages it takes to purchase it, because they could have purchased the insurance previously but chose not to. Thus, the first effect of a per employee tax is to make uninsured low-wage employees worse off by forcing a change in how they spend their limited incomes.

The employee tax, however, is unlikely to be shifted entirely back to the employee in the form of lower cash wages. Many employees are at or near the minimum wage; minimum-wage laws prevent the transfer of the health insurance costs to the employee because employees cannot receive cash wages that place them below the minimum wage.

Furthermore, the mix between wages and health insurance is not perfectly flexible, particularly right away; therefore, the cost of labor to the firm will be increased. With higher labor costs the firm will have to increase the prices of its goods and services. These increased prices in turn will lead consumers to purchase fewer goods and services. With a smaller demand for its output the firm will need fewer employees. The firm will also decrease its demand for labor by decreasing the use of part-time employees (if they must be covered by an employer mandate) and increasing overtime work of full-time employees. Thus, a second effect of a health insurance tax per employee is that it raises the cost of these employees, many of whom are teenagers, and causes fewer of them to be employed.

To the extent that labor costs are increased, part of the employee tax is shifted forward in the form of higher consumer prices. This third effect of the tax results in a regressive form of consumer taxation because all consumers, regardless of their income, pay higher prices. Those higher prices represent a greater portion of the incomes of low-income consumers than of high-income consumers. Such a tax is an inequitable method of financing universal health insurance.

Cost to Government

The employer mandate is attractive to government because it shifts the cost of low-wage labor off Medicaid onto the employees and their employers. However, an employer mandate is more costly to the government than it appears. First, because employer-paid health insurance is not considered to be taxable income, the change in compensation from cash wages to health insurance decreases Social Security taxes as well as state and federal income taxes. Second, government welfare expenditures will be higher as a result of the increase in unemployment that would result from layoffs of those near the minimum wage when wages are not flexible downward. Third, additional subsidies and taxes would be necessary to finance care for approximately one-third of the uninsured who are not employed or dependents of an employee if this approach is to achieve universal coverage.

Under pay-or-play proposals many employers will conclude that paying an employee tax is less costly than providing their employees with health insurance. The average annual health insurance premium per employee for a family of four was $11,480 per year in 2006 (The Kaiser Family Foundation and The Health Research and Educational Trust 2006.) (Workers contributed, on average, about 30 percent of that amount. The average annual premium for insured workers, single coverage, was $4,024.) If an employer has to purchase health insurance for its employees or pay 8 percent of payroll into a government pool (a previously specified percentage), it would cost less to pay the 8 percent tax for most of its employees (particularly those with a family). As medical costs continue to increase, more employers are likely to opt for the "pay" rather than the "play" option. One study estimated (at a time when insurance premiums were much lower than today) that 35 percent of employers providing their employees with health insurance would find it cheaper to drop that coverage and pay the tax. Zedlewski, Acs, and Winterbottom (1992) estimate that as many as 40 million employees and their dependents would lose their coverage and be forced into the government pool.

If employers have an option to pay or play, setting the tax too low will make it less costly for employers to pay an employee tax than to provide health insurance. The government will discover that it cannot fund the same set of benefits on the 8 percent tax revenue; estimates place the amount needed to fund the minimum benefits much higher. In addition to employees whose benefits previously cost more than the pay-or-play tax, subsidies would also be required for all those who are eligible for the public pool but cannot afford it. Revenues will be insufficient to finance the expanded public pool.

Just as the cost of other health programs, such as Medicare Parts A and B, increased beyond initial expectations, the necessary tax to finance an employer mandate would have to rise beyond the 8 percent level. As the number of employees (particularly low-wage employees) in the government pool increases, the government will be faced with the choice of raising taxes or limiting payments to hospitals and physicians. The likely result would be a very large Medicaid program for the increasing number of employees shifted to the government pool.

If all firms are required (as the Clinton Administration proposed) to pay a specified percentage of payroll as a tax, the employer's liability for its employees' medical expenses is limited to the size of that percentage tax. The employer no longer has an incentive to use innovative cost-containment measures. The responsibility for managing the medical expenses of all those in the public pool falls to the managers of the pool rather than to each employer for its own employees' medical expenses.

Financing national health insurance through an employer mandate relies on a hidden and inequitable method of financing health insurance for the uninsured. Imposing the tax on the employer makes it appear as though the employer bears the cost of the tax. The tax, however, is shifted to both consumers and employees. In both cases, the tax is regressive. When the tax is borne by labor in the form of lower cash wages, low-wage employees have to pay a higher percentage of their incomes for health insurance. The portion of the tax borne by low-wage consumers represents a higher portion of their incomes.

One of the major concerns with an employer mandate is its effect on firms' demand for labor. As the cost of labor increases, the demand for labor will decrease. The job loss, particularly among those employees near the minimum wage whose wages cannot be reduced to offset the employer tax, is estimated to be 3 million.

This hidden tax on consumers and employees also understates its budgetary effects on the government. Federal and state governments lose tax revenues.

Given the inequities and inefficiencies associated with an employer mandate, why has it received so much political support?

POLITICAL CONSEQUENCES OF EMPLOYER-MANDATED HEALTH INSURANCE
Advantages

The political advantages received by various interest groups outweigh the inequities and inefficiencies that an employer mandate imposes on others. Congress would not have to raise a large amount of tax revenues for an employer-mandated national health insurance plan; such a plan would even reduce Medicaid expenditures. Thus, national health insurance offers the illusion that federal expenditures are little affected. States, whose Medicaid expenditures are increasing faster than any other state expenditure, are reluctant to raise taxes. If the states are able to shift the medical costs of low-wage employees and their dependents from Medicaid onto the employees and their employers, the states' own fiscal problems would be alleviated.

Hospital and physician organizations favor an employer mandate because it would provide insurance to those previously without it, increasing the demand for hospital and physician services. Payment levels to health providers would be higher than Medicaid payment levels. Health insurance companies would similarly benefit because the demand for their services would increase.

Large employers and their unions, who would be unaffected because they already provide health benefits in excess of the mandated minimum, believe they will benefit competitively from mandated employer insurance. Large firms with high labor costs would like to increase the costs of their low-wage competitors, making them less price competitive. Robert Crandall, the chairman of American Airlines, stated that as a result of the difference between the medical costs of American employees and Continental Airlines employees, "Continental's unit cost advantage vs. American's is enormous—and worse yet, is growing! . . . which is why we're supporting . . . legislation mandating minimum [health] benefit levels for all employees" (*The Wall Street Journal* 1987).

Under the Clinton Administration's proposed employer mandate, no employer would have had to pay more than 8 percent of payroll for its employees' health care. The automobile companies and their unions would have benefited greatly under this proposal. Health expenses for auto employees exceed 15 percent of payroll; thus, these companies and their employees would presumably receive the same benefits for less and be able to have higher cash wages. Who will be paying the higher taxes to make this possible?

Opposition

The major political opposition to an employer mandate has been by small business. They are aware of the consequences of an employee tax on the prices they would have to charge, demand for their goods and services, and their demand for labor. Opposition by small business is the major reason this legislation has not been enacted nationally or in the many states where it has been proposed. In an attempt to buy off the political opposition of the powerful small business lobby, legislators have proposed either exempting them from the legislation or offsetting their higher costs by providing them with a subsidy. To date, these approaches have not overcome the skepticism of small businesses toward government eventually increasing their costs.

SUMMARY

An employer-mandated national health insurance plan has numerous political advantages. Although an employer mandate statutorily imposes most of the cost on employers, in reality a large portion of the cost is shifted to the employee in the form of lower wages (or other fringe benefits). An employer mandate would not be equitable, because it would disproportionately affect less-skilled employees. It would increase the cost to employers of low-wage labor and impose a financial burden on those least able to afford it. An important reason for low-wage employees' lack of insurance is that they have more pressing needs for their limited incomes, and Medicaid is available to them as a substitute to buying private health insurance. An employer mandate would also not achieve universal coverage, because not all of the uninsured are employed. Furthermore, an important unintended consequence of this approach would be the displacement of many low-wage employees. Alternative approaches for achieving national health insurance need to be examined.

DISCUSSION QUESTIONS

1. What are the characteristics of the uninsured?

2. Would it be equitable to provide all employees in small firms with a subsidy to purchase health insurance?

3. What is the likely effect of employer-mandated health insurance on the employer's demand for labor?

4. Does an employer-mandated health insurance tax have a regressive, proportional, or progressive effect on the incomes of employees and consumers?

5. Which groups favor and which groups oppose an employer mandate for achieving national health insurance? Why?

REFERENCES

Agency for Healthcare Research and Quality. 2005. *Health Insurance Coverage of the Civilian Noninstitutionalized Population: Health Insurance Coverage* and *Population Characteristic–Population, United States, First Half of 2004*, Table 5. [Online information; retrieved 1/16/07.] http://www.meps.ahrq.gov/mepsweb/data_stats/ summ_tables/hc/hlth_insr/2004/t5_e04.pdf

Blumberg, L. 1999. "Who Pays For Employer-Sponsored Health Insurance?" *Health Affairs* 18 (6): 58–61.

DeNavas-Walt, C., B. D. Proctor, and C. H. Lee, U.S. Census Bureau. 2004. "Income, Poverty, and Health Insurance Coverage in the United States: 2004." In *Current Population Reports*, P60-229. [Online information; retrieved 12/19/06.] http://www. census.gov/prod/2005pubs/p60-229.pdf.

Rhoades, J. A. 2006. "The Uninsured in America, 1996–2005: Estimates for the U.S. Civilian Noninstitutionalized Population Under Age 65." Agency for Healthcare Research and Quality, Medical Expenditure Panel Survey. [Online information; retrieved 12/19/06.] http://www.meps.ahrq.gov/mepsweb/data_files/publications/ st130/stat130.pdf.

The Kaiser Family Foundation and the Health Research and Educational Trust. 2006. *Employer Health Benefits, 2006 Annual Survey*. [Online information; retrieved 12/19/06.] http://www.kff.org/insurance/7527/upload/7527.pdf.

The Wall Street Journal. 1987. "Notable and Quotable." *The Wall Street Journal* August 8, 16.

Zedlewski, S., G. Acs, and C. Winterbottom. 1992. "Play-or-Pay Employer Mandates: Potential Effects." *Health Affairs* 11 (1): 62–83.

ADDITIONAL READINGS

Krueger, A., and U. Reinhardt. 1994. "Economics of Employer Versus Individual Mandates." *Health Affairs* 13 (2, Part II): 34–53.

Steuerle, C. E. 1994. "Implementing Employer and Individual Mandates." *Health Affairs* 13 (2, Part II): 54–68.

Chapter 34

National Health Insurance: Which Approach and Why?

NATIONAL HEALTH INSURANCE is an idea whose time has come and then gone, and it will eventually be back on the political horizon. A variety of national health insurance plans have been proposed, from replicating the Canadian (single-payer) system to expanding existing public programs for the poor, mandating employers to provide coverage for their employees, providing tax credits for the purchase of health insurance, or using HSAs. The proponents of each approach claim different virtues for their plans—one plan is more likely to limit the rise in medical expenditures, another will require a smaller tax increase to implement, one will allow individuals greater choice, and still another may be more politically acceptable. Unless some commonly accepted criteria as to what national health insurance should accomplish are established, evaluating and choosing among these plans will be difficult.

CRITERIA FOR NATIONAL HEALTH INSURANCE
Production Efficiency
Economists are concerned with two issues: efficiency and equity. (When national health insurance proposals are evaluated, the equity criterion is concerned with equitable redistribution.) Efficiency has two parts. The first is *production efficiency*, which determines whether the services (for a given level of quality) are produced at the lowest cost. Efficiency in production not only includes whether the hospital portion of a treatment is produced at lowest cost but also whether the treatment itself is produced at minimum cost. Unless the treatment is provided in the lowest-cost mix of settings, such as hospitals, outpatient care, and home care, the overall cost of providing the treatment will not be as low as is possible.

Ensuring that each component of the treatment (such as hospital services), as well as the entire medical treatment, is produced efficiently requires appropriate financial incentives. These incentives are usually placed on the providers of medical services; however, they could also be placed on consumers, as would occur under an HSA approach. On whom to place the incentives is a controversial issue, but whether the plan includes appropriate incentives for efficiency in production is not.

Efficiency in Consumption

The second aspect of efficiency, referred to as *efficiency in consumption*, is controversial. In other sectors of the economy consumers make choices regarding the amount of income to allocate to different goods and services. Consumers have incentives to consider both the costs and benefits of their choices. Spending their funds on one good means forgoing the benefits of another good or service. When consumers allocate their funds in this manner, resources are directed to their highest-valued uses as perceived by consumers.

Some are opposed to having consumers decide how much should be spent on medical services. They would prefer to have the government decide how much is allocated to medical care, as in the Canadian system. Yet Canadians are unable to purchase additional private health insurance to forgo waits for open-heart surgery, hip replacements, or treatment of other illnesses. Inherent in the concept of efficiency in consumption is that the purpose of national health insurance is to benefit the consumer and that the consumer will be free to purchase more medical services than the minimum level offered in any health insurance plan.

Even if one accepts the concept of consumer decision making, concern has arisen that the costs of consumers' choices may be distorted. If the cost of one choice is subsidized and other choices are not, consumers will demand more of the subsidized choice than if they had to pay its full costs, resulting in inefficiency in consumption. For example, the government does not consider employer-purchased health insurance to be taxable income to the employee. Consumers therefore purchase more health insurance because health insurance is paid with before-tax dollars, whereas other choices such as education and housing must be paid for with after-tax dollars. The tax-free status of employer-paid health insurance, therefore, is a cause of inefficiency because the costs of consumers' other choices are in after-tax dollars.

Thus, a second criterion for national health insurance plans is whether consumers are able to decide how much of their incomes they want to spend on medical services and whether any subsidies distort the costs of their choices.

When production and consumption efficiency are achieved through the use of appropriate incentives, the rate of increase in medical expenditures is considered to be appropriate. Having a national health insurance objective of limiting the rate of increase in medical expenditures would be inappropriate if achieving this objective meant sacrificing the goals of consumption and production efficiency.

Equitable Redistribution

Presumably, an important (some would say the only) objective of national health insurance is to provide additional medical services to the poor. When national health insurance plans are evaluated on how those with low incomes are to be subsidized, one must examine which population groups benefit (are subsidized) and which population groups bear the costs (pay higher taxes). For equitable redistribution to occur those with higher incomes are expected to incur net costs (their taxes are in excess of their benefits), whereas those with low incomes should receive net benefits (benefits in excess of costs). *When an individual's costs are not equal to the benefits he receives, redistribution occurs.* Thus, high-income groups should subsidize the care of those with lower incomes; whether equitable redistribution occurs is the third criterion for evaluating alternative national health insurance plans.

Crucial for determining whether redistribution goes from high- to low-income groups is the definition of beneficiaries and how the plan is financed. Ideally, those with the lowest incomes should receive the largest subsidy (which would decline as income rises), and the subsidy should be financed by a tax that is either proportional or progressive to income. If the tax is proportional to income (e.g., 5 percent), those with the lowest incomes will receive a net benefit because the subsidy they receive (sufficient to purchase a minimum benefit package) will exceed the taxes they pay. When a progressive tax, such as an income tax, is used to finance benefits to those with low incomes, the redistribution from those with high incomes to those with low incomes is even greater.

A regressive payroll tax, such as Social Security (a percentage of earned income up to a maximum income level) or a sales tax, takes a higher portion of income from those who have low incomes than from those with high incomes. Therefore, such taxes are a less-desirable method of financing redistributive programs.

In fact, when a regressive tax is used, the tax paid by many low-income persons may exceed the value of the benefits they receive. For example, if everyone is eligible to receive the same set of benefits but those with higher incomes use more medical services, perhaps because they are located closer to medical providers or their attitudes toward seeking care are different from those with less education (who also have low income), the taxes paid by those with low incomes may exceed the benefits they receive. Perversely, those with low incomes may end up subsidizing the care received by those with higher incomes. (This also occurs when low-income workers subsidize the health benefits of high-income aged.)

An examination of the size of the benefits received by income level in relation to the amount of tax paid is important. Income tax financing is the preferred way to achieve redistribution because it results in greater net benefits to those with low incomes.

Based on the above discussion of efficiency and equitable redistribution, a national health insurance plan should provide incentives for efficiency in production, enable consumers to decide how much of their incomes they want to spend on medical care, and be redistributive—those with lower incomes should receive net benefits, whereas those with higher incomes bear costs in excess of their benefits. All national health insurance proposals should be judged by how well they fulfill these criteria.

An important reason national health insurance plans fail to meet these efficiency and equitable redistribution criteria is that national health insurance proposals have objectives other than improving efficiency or equitable redistribution. These other objectives become obvious when the explicit efficiency and redistributive criteria are used.

NATIONAL HEALTH INSURANCE PROPOSALS

Many different types of national health insurance plans have been proposed. Some proposals are incremental in that they build on the current system and do not propose changes in the delivery of medical services. Others are more radical, and dramatic changes are proposed in the financing and delivery of medical services. In general, however, the types of national health insurance plans proposed can be classified into three broad categories: a single-payer (Canadian) system, employer-mandated heath insurance, and an individual mandate with refundable tax credits. Although separate chapters are devoted to the Canadian approach and an employer mandate, a brief description of each, together with an evaluation of how well they achieve the three criteria, is briefly presented.

Single-Payer National Health Insurance

Under a single-payer system the entire population is covered, benefits are uniform for all, no out-of-pocket expenses are incurred for basic medical services, and, most important, private insurance for hospital and medical services is not permitted (one cannot opt out of the single-payer system). The method of financing may be a combination of income taxes and other sources of funds, such as payroll taxes on the employer and employee, Medicare and Medicaid payments, "sin" taxes (on alcohol and tobacco), or even a sales tax.

The major advantage of a single-payer system is its apparent simplicity in achieving universal coverage. Access to care by those with low incomes and the uninsured is likely to be improved. Single-payer proponents also claim that less would be spent per capita (and a smaller percentage of GDP) on medical services.

The major disadvantages of a single-payer approach concern consumption and production efficiency (see Chapter 32). Global budget caps are used to limit total medical expenditures. Fixed budgets are imposed on hospitals, their capital outlays are controlled by a central authority, and annual limits are placed on the amount each physician can earn. These arbitrarily determined budget levels limit the amount consumers can spend on medical services, forcing them to wait for services or do without. The result is consumer inefficiency. Furthermore, incentives to achieve production efficiency are lacking in a single-payer system, as are incentives for prevention and innovation.

Expansion of Public Programs

Somewhat similar to a single-payer system is the proposal to expand existing public programs, such as Medicaid, by increasing the income limits to allow greater numbers of those with low incomes and the uninsured to become eligible. Medicaid is funded by general income taxes, and its beneficiaries are those with low incomes; thus, the equitable redistribution goal would be appropriate. Advocates of expanding public programs claim that no major changes in the financing or delivery system are required; only changes in the eligibility criteria would be needed. Similarly, more uninsured children could be covered by SCHIP simply by expanding its eligibility levels.

Some have also proposed that uninsured adults aged 55 to 65 years be allowed to "buy into" Medicare. Expanding Medicare to include those under age 65 and increasing Medicaid and SCHIP eligibility to include those with higher incomes would eventually bring greater numbers of the population into a single-payer-type system. Although differences between Medicare and Medicaid exist, both programs have the same characteristics as a single-payer system. Beneficiaries of these programs pay little if anything for use of medical services (when the Medicare patient has Medigap supplementary coverage) and have free choice of provider (except for those enrolled in a Medicaid HMO), providers are paid on a fee-for-service basis, and the government controls expenditures by limiting provider fees. These programs have none of the cost-containment programs, such as utilization management, used by the private sector, nor do they have any incentives for provider efficiency.[1]

Some advocates of expanding public programs view this as an approach to achieve a single-payer system for the United States. Over time, privately insured employees would also prefer to buy into Medicare as their private health insurance premiums and out-of-pocket expenses increase.

The problem with expanding public programs to care for all of the uninsured is that many states cannot afford their share of the matching funds required to include more of the uninsured. Particularly in times of recession, states lack the funds and are reluctant to increase taxes to expand eligibility limits. In fact, many states have been reducing enrollment in SCHIP as their tax revenues have fallen and they face budget deficits. Medicaid and SCHIP do not have a stable source of funding, and states are reluctant to commit themselves to expanding

---

1. Production efficiency could be achieved in Medicaid if the state were to offer Medicaid recipients a choice of competing health plans. Proposals for Medicare reform have similarly proposed providing all the aged with a subsidy to cover the cost of a basic health plan and allowing the aged to choose among different competing health plans, paying a higher out-of-pocket premium if they decide to choose a more expensive health plan, such as traditional Medicare. Such Medicare reform proposals would achieve consumption and production efficiency.

these programs. Allowing the uninsured to buy into Medicare will result in adverse selection; sicker individuals (those without employment-based health insurance) will pay a premium that is below their expected costs. Expanding Medicare to include those under the age of 65 years will merely worsen Medicare's already precarious financial outlook.

Employer-Mandated National Health Insurance

An employer mandate requires employers to either purchase health insurance for their employees or pay a specified amount per employee into a government pool. Although the financial burden for purchasing health insurance is placed on the employer, studies have found that the burden is shifted back to the employee in the form of lower wages. In effect a tax is imposed on low-wage workers (who are typically without health insurance), requiring them to buy health insurance. The amount of health insurance employees would be required to purchase is more than most low-wage workers are willing or able to pay. (Congress is likely to establish a very comprehensive minimum benefit package, as was proposed under President Clinton's health plan. Thus, consumption efficiency is difficult to achieve compared with establishing a catastrophic plan as the minimum benefit level and allowing employees to purchase more than the minimum benefit level.)

To assist low-wage workers it has been proposed that small firms be subsidized rather than low-wage workers themselves. Unfortunately, not all low-wage workers are in small firms, nor are all small-firm employees low-wage workers (e.g., attorneys in small law firms).

The inability to achieve equitable redistribution is the biggest disadvantage of this approach. Furthermore, unless subsidies are provided to those who are not in the work force or who work part time (about 40 percent of the uninsured), an employer mandate will not achieve universal coverage. Production efficiency can be achieved by having health plans compete for employees.

REFUNDABLE TAX CREDITS: AN INCOME-RELATED PROPOSAL

Various tax credits have been proposed over the years. The following proposal attempts to achieve universal coverage in an equitable manner while providing incentives for efficiency in the use and delivery of medical services.

An Individual Mandate

To achieve universal coverage the government must ensure that the two groups without insurance—those who can afford insurance but refuse to purchase it and those who cannot afford insurance—have a minimum level of health insurance. To do so the federal government should, first, require everyone to have a minimum level of health insurance (an "individual mandate"), which could be a catastrophic policy for higher-income persons. Many uninsured are financially able to purchase a high-deductible health insurance plan but choose not to do so. If someone who can afford insurance does not have catastrophic coverage and suffers a large medical expense that has to be subsidized by the community, the person is shifting the risk, hence cost of catastrophic coverage, to the rest of the community.

Proof of insurance would be attached to the person's federal income-tax form. Lack of such evidence would result in the government collecting the appropriate premium as it would if the individual paid insufficient income taxes. The government would then assign the person to a health plan in her area, which the person could change. Thus, everyone who could afford health insurance would not become a burden to others if they suffered a serious illness or accident.

Refundable Tax Credit

The second important role of government in ensuring universal coverage is to provide a refundable tax credit (subsidy) to those with low incomes so they can purchase health insurance. Taxpayers would be allowed to subtract the tax credit to purchase health insurance from their income taxes. Individuals whose tax credit exceeded their tax liabilities would receive a refund for the difference. Thus, if a person's income is too low to pay taxes, the full amount of the credit would be used to provide him with a voucher. As a person's income increased and he had an income-tax liability, the tax credit would offset part of the tax liability, leaving him with part of the tax credit to be used toward purchasing a health insurance voucher. The tax credit must be refundable, or the benefits will go only to those who pay taxes, excluding those with low incomes.

The full tax credit subsidy would be equal to the premium of a managed care plan. (These refundable tax credits are essentially vouchers for a health plan for persons with little or no tax liability.) The tax credit could be an equal dollar amount for all families, such as $6,000, or it could decline with higher incomes. Under a refundable tax credit that declines with higher income, the subsidy would go to those with the lowest incomes. However, providing a tax credit of an absolute dollar amount would be more politically acceptable in that those with middle and higher incomes would also receive some benefit.

The value of the voucher could be determined in several ways. One is for the government to take bids from managed care plans. Alternatively, the voucher could equal the premium of the lowest-cost managed care plan in the market. (This approach is used by an increasing number of employers.) In this manner the preferences of the nonpoor for what they want to purchase from a managed care plan will determine the benefits to be offered to those with low incomes. (Those receiving a full or partial voucher could choose a more expensive health plan by paying the additional cost themselves.)

Consumption efficiency would be achieved by permitting individuals to purchase greater coverage or policies with fewer restrictions on access to providers by paying the additional premium for such plans. Production efficiency would presumably occur as health plans compete for enrollees based on price, quality of services, and access to care. By providing a refundable tax credit, financed from general income taxes, redistributive equity would be achieved.

Health Savings Accounts

A relatively new proposal to financing medical care that places greater responsibility for medical expenses on the individual is the use of HSAs in conjunction with a high-deductible, catastrophic, health insurance policy. HSAs can be an option under the individual-mandate proposal as well as an alternative to be included in Medicare reform proposals.

The basic idea behind an HSA is to combine an inexpensive high-deductible insurance policy with a tax-free savings account. An HSA plan works as follows: A person (or her employer acting on her behalf) purchases a high-deductible health plan and then annually contributes a specified tax-free amount into the HSA. (A high-deductible catastrophic policy has a much lower premium than a comprehensive health insurance policy.) The maximum that can be contributed each year to the HSA account is $2,700 for an individual and $5,450 for a family—or the amount of the deductible of the high-deductible health plan, whichever is lower. (People aged 55 years and older can make additional "catch-up" contributions of $700 each year until they enroll in Medicare.) The maximum out-of-pocket expenses for which the person is liable can be as high as

$5,250 for an individual or $10,500 a year for a family. The person would be at risk for the difference between the out-of-pocket maximum ($5,250) and his annual contribution to his HSA ($2,700), which is $2,550.[2]

HSA proponents claim that an HSA reduces the monthly insurance premium and provides individuals with a financial incentive to be concerned with the prices they pay for medical services and think carefully about which services they really need. (Most high-deductible health plans also include several preventive visits.) Proponents believe that if consumers have a greater financial incentive, medical expenditures will increase at a lower rate. The funds in the HSA account can be invested and grow tax free.

Opponents of HSAs claim that any savings would be relatively small because once the out-of-pocket maximum is reached, the patient has no incentive to spend less. Critics also claim that the adoption and availability of new technology, which is typically used in an inpatient setting, determine expenditure increases, not spending for outpatient services. HSA critics further claim that HSAs would split the insurance risk pools; healthier, lower-risk persons would choose HSAs (thereby gaining financially), and higher-risk persons would remain in more comprehensive plans. HSA proponents disagree, arguing that higher-risk persons would also benefit from and choose HSAs because their total medical out-of-pocket expenses, including prescription drugs, would be subject to a limit. Under Medicare, for example, out-of-pocket expenses are not limited.

HSAs include financial incentives for consumption efficiency to occur. (If consumers are to become informed purchasers, however, more information on provider performance and prices is needed.) Presumably, production efficiency would result as providers compete on price and managed care plans become responsible for providing catastrophic services. Government subsidies would be needed to enable those with low incomes to establish HSAs.

Eliminating the Tax Exclusion for Employer-Purchased Health Insurance

As part of the proposal for an individual mandate, the current exclusion of employer-purchased health insurance from an employee's taxable income would be removed as the tax credit is substituted in its place. The

---

2. Additional information on HSAs may be found at the following web site: http://www.treas.gov/offices/public-affairs/hsa/.

lost revenues from this open-ended subsidy (in 2004 this amounted to $209 billion in lost federal, state, and Social Security taxes each year) would be an important revenue source to offset the new tax credit to those with low incomes (Shields and Haught 2004). (For political reasons the entire tax subsidy for employer-purchased health insurance may not be eliminated; it could be phased out over time, or amounts above a certain limit could be subject to income taxes.)

Replacing Medicare and Medicaid

The refundable tax credit could replace Medicare and Medicaid, using their expenditures to partially offset the cost of the tax credit. Because the tax credit declines with increased incomes, a sharp cut-off of Medicaid benefits (the "notch" effect) and the previous disincentive to work would no longer exist.

Over time, the Medicare system could also become part of this new national health insurance plan. It would be politically difficult to institute an income-related system for those currently on Medicare. Thus, all current Medicare beneficiaries (and those close to the Medicare eligibility age) would receive a fully subsidized voucher in a managed care plan. Those who are perhaps between the ages of 45 and 60 years could receive a partially subsidized voucher related to their Medicare contributions, and the Medicare system could be phased out for those under the age of 45 years.

Effect on Employer-Employee Relationships

The proposed income-related tax credit national health insurance plan should have little effect on current employer and employee relationships. Although the "individual mandate" obligation is on the employee and not the employer, employers would continue to act as a purchaser of health insurance for their employees. Employees would prefer that their employers maintain their current role because of administrative economies in being part of a large group. Employers would also be better able than their employees to evaluate competing health plans. The employer would deduct the employee's premium from wages and indicate that the employee has health insurance on the employee's W-2 form. More employers are likely to offer health coverage to their employees if the obligation is on the employee and not on them.

Currently, individuals and small employers are charged higher premiums than large employer groups because of insurers' fear of adverse selection, that is, people who want to buy insurance because they are ill.

Because everyone would be required to have health insurance, over time insurance companies would be less concerned about adverse selection.[3]

Eliminating State Mandates

State health mandates require private health insurance to cover specific health providers, such as chiropractors, acupuncturists, marriage therapists, and athletic trainers (Arkansas); specific insurance benefits, such as hair transplants, in vitro fertilization, and massage therapy; and specific populations, such as noncustodial children and terminated workers. There are more than 1,800 state mandates across the 50 states. Many states also have regulations requiring AWP laws, which restrict a health plan's ability to exclude hospitals and physicians from its provider networks. Some states have enacted community rating laws, which require insurance premiums to be the same regardless of an individual's (or group's) risk level or claims experience. Furthermore, several states have adopted legislation that requires health insurers to accept anyone who applies, regardless of health status ("guaranteed issue").

These state mandates increase the cost of health insurance, making health insurance too expensive for those with low incomes. Depending on where one lives, mandates can increase the cost of a policy by between 20 percent and 45 percent (Bunce 2006). The high cost of state mandates (as high as several thousand dollars in insurance premiums per person per year) directly affects the number of insured (and uninsured) in a state.

These state regulations would not be needed, and eliminating them would reduce the cost of health insurance. If individuals wished to purchase these services on their own with after-tax dollars, they would be free to do so.

Advantages of Income-Related Refundable Tax Credits

The income-related voucher meets the efficiency and equitable redistribution criteria in the following ways. Everyone is obligated to have a minimum set of health insurance benefits. Those with the lowest incomes would be assured of adequate health insurance and would receive

---

3. People who are uninsured and have a serious health problem would be unable to purchase insurance. These individuals would have to be included in subsidized "high-risk" pools, as occurs in many states. Over time, high-risk pools would become unnecessary as everyone would be required to have insurance and would be included in a health plan before they became ill.

the largest net benefits under the proposed plan. The size of the subsidy would decline as income increases. Employer-purchased health insurance (perhaps above a certain dollar amount) would become part of the employee's taxable income. The resulting increased tax revenues, together with funds from the income-tax system and Medicaid, would provide the funding for the income-related subsidies. Thus, the financing source is based on progressive taxation. Requiring universal coverage means that cost shifting by those who do not purchase insurance to those who do will no longer occur.

The mandate to have insurance is on the *individual,* not on the employer; thus, the individual would be able to change jobs without fear of losing insurance or being denied coverage because of a preexisting condition. Because everyone would be required to have insurance, an employer should be willing to hire someone who is older, is less healthy, or has a preexisting condition because no additional health insurance cost would be incurred by the employer or other employees.

Employees would have incentives to make cost-conscious choices, and a competitive health insurance market would be relied on to achieve efficiency and quality. The greater out-of-pocket liability for employees purchasing more expensive health plans will increase their price sensitivity to different managed care plans. Price (premium) sensitivity by employees (and employers acting on their behalf) will provide price incentives for managed care plans and providers, such as hospitals and physicians, to be as efficient as possible. Unless health plans are responsive to consumers at a premium the consumer is willing to pay, the health plan will not be able to compete in a price-competitive market.

SUMMARY

National health insurance proposals should be judged according to the criteria of efficiency in production, efficiency in consumption, and equitable redistribution, namely whether those with low incomes receive a net benefit. Market-based systems, in contrast to single-payer systems, have demonstrated their ability to achieve the goals of production and consumption efficiency. Subsidies to those with low incomes, as through a refundable tax credit, are a direct method of improving equity and can provide increased choice and result in production efficiency when provided through a market-based system.

A brief description and comparison of the three national health insurance proposals is presented in Table 34.1.

Table 34.1: Comparison of Three National Health Insurance Proposals

Feature	Employer Mandate	Single-Payer System	Individual Mandate with Refundable Tax Credit
How does it work?	Requires all employers to buy health insurance for their employees or pay into a pool.	Provides comprehensive coverage with no out-of-pocket payments. Private insurance is not permitted.	Everyone is required to purchase at least a high-deductible plan and subsidies are provided to those with low incomes.
Does it provide universal coverage?	Excludes those who work part time and those who are not working.	Achieves universal coverage.	Achieves universal coverage.
Is there consumption efficiency?	Partially. Minimum mandated benefits are greater than low-income workers prefer, and employer may not provide choice of health plans.	No. Persons are not permitted to buy medical services or private insurance for services covered by the basic health plan.	Yes. Participants can purchase additional medical services and insurance above minimum required insurance.
Is there production efficiency?	The plan relies on market-based competition to achieve production efficiency.	No consumer or provider incentives are included to encourage efficiency, to minimize the cost of a treatment, or to provide preventive care.	The plan includes consumer and provider incentives for efficiency. It relies on market-based competition to achieve production efficiency.
Is it equitably financed?	Regressive. The plan retains tax-exempt employer coverage and a tax is imposed on employers and employees for typically low-income employees without insurance.	Partially regressive. There is pooling of funds from employers, Medicare, Medicaid, and increased payroll taxes.	Progressive. Income-related subsidies are provided, and there is a limit/phase out of tax-exempt employer-paid insurance.
What are the administrative costs?	High, because of multiple health plans, monitoring, and enforcement of mandate.	Costs are too low to detect fraud and abuse or to institute disease management and other types of programs.	High, because of multiple health plans, monitoring, and enforcement of mandate.
How are health care costs controlled?	The plan relies on the market to achieve appropriate rate of increase in costs.	The plan relies on arbitrary budget caps and regulated fees.	The plan relies on the market to achieve appropriate rate of increase in costs.

An important role of government under national health insurance is to monitor quality and access to care received by those with low incomes. Previously, government has not performed this function well for Medicaid patients. However, allowing those with low incomes to enroll in managed care plans that also serve other population groups will make it likely that employers, unions, and nonprofit organizations will be monitoring care provided in managed care plans. These monitoring activities should benefit all enrollees, including those subsidized by government.

Under a market-based national health insurance system, the rate of increase in medical expenditures would be based on what consumers, balancing cost and use of services, decide is appropriate. The government would not need to set arbitrary limits on total medical expenditures. Instead, the rate of increase in medical expenditures will be the "correct" rate because consumers, through their choices, will make the trade-off between access to care and premiums to pay for that level of access.

DISCUSSION QUESTIONS

1. Discuss the criteria that should be used for evaluating alternative national health insurance proposals.

2. Evaluate the desirability of the following types of taxes for financing national health insurance: payroll, sales, and income tax.

3. What is the justification for requiring everyone (all those who can afford it) to purchase a minimum level of health insurance?

4. Outline (and justify) a proposal for national health insurance. As part of your proposal, discuss the benefit package, beneficiaries, method of financing, delivery of services, and role of government. How well does your proposal meet the criteria discussed earlier?

5. What are alternative ways for treating Medicare under national health insurance?

REFERENCES

Bunce, V. 2006. *Trends in State Mandated Benefits, 2006*. Alexandria, VA: The Council for Affordable Health Insurance. [Online information; retrieved 1/8/07.] http://www.cahi.org/cahi_contents/resources/pdf/TrendsEndsMay2006.pdf.

Sheilds, J., and R. Haught. 2004. "The Cost of Tax-Exempt Health Benefits in 2004." *Health Affairs* Web exclusive, W4-109. [Online information; retrieved 1/8/07.] http://content.healthaffairs.org/cgi/reprint/hlthaff.w4.106v1.pdf.

ADDITIONAL READINGS

Cogan, J., G. Hubbard, and D. Kessler. 2005. "Making Markets Work: Five Steps to a Better Health Care System." *Health Affairs* 24 (6): 1447–57.

Feder, J., L. Levitt, E. O'Brien, and D. Rowland. 2001. "Covering the Low-Income Uninsured: The Case for Expanding Public Programs." *Health Affairs* 20 (1): 27–39.

Fuchs, V., and E. Emanuel. 2005. "Health Care Reform: Why? What? When?" *Health Affairs* 24 (6): 1399–1414.

Hall, M., and C. Havighurst. 2005. "Reviving Managed Care with Health Savings Accounts." *Health Affairs* 24 (6): 1490–1500.

Herzlinger, R. 2004. *Consumer Driven Health Care: Implications for Providers, Payers, and Policymakers*. San Francisco: Jossey-Bass.

Pauly, M., and B. Herring. 2001. "Expanding Coverage via Tax Credits: Trade-offs and Outcomes." *Health Affairs* 20 (1): 9–26.

Chapter 35

Financing Long-Term Care

SPENDING FOR LONG-TERM-CARE services is expected to increase sharply over the next several decades. The population is aging; as shown in Figure 35.1, the number of aged are expected to more than double, from 36.7 million in 2005 (12.4 percent of the population) to 71.5 million in 2030 (19.6 percent of the population), to 86.7 million in 2050 (20.7 percent of the population). The aged are becoming an increasing portion of the population. An aging population that is living longer increases the number at risk for requiring long-term-care services. The fastest-increasing portion of the aged is those aged 85 years and older. As a percentage of all of the aged, this older group is expected to increase from 13.9 percent in 2005 to 24.1 percent in 2050. As the impaired aged increase their demand for services necessary to assist them in those activities necessary for daily living, the cost of providing those services is rising at a rate faster than general inflation.

How long-term-care services should be financed, and by whom, is an important public policy dilemma.

THE NATURE OF LONG-TERM CARE

Long-term care consists of a range of services for those who are unable to function independently, including services that can be provided in the person's home, such as shopping, preparing meals, and housekeeping; in community-based facilities, such as adult day care; and in nursing homes for those who are unable to perform most of the activities necessary for daily living, such as bathing, toileting, dressing, and so on. A nursing home is but the end of a spectrum, in which all of the basic activities are available, for those with the most physical and mental impairments.

Figure 35.1: Percentage of U.S. Population Aged 65 Years and Older, 1980–2050

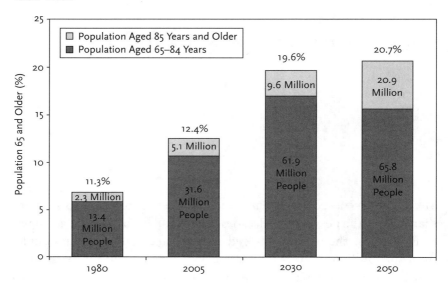

Source: U.S. Census Bureau. 2006. *International Data Base*. [Online information.] http://www.census.gov/cgi-bin/ipc/idbagg.

The need for long-term care increases with age. As shown in Table 35.1, the greatest needs for long-term care are by those aged 85 years and older, 49 percent of whom require long-term-care services. Most long-term care occurs in the home versus an institutional setting.

Informal caregivers are predominantly family members or close relatives. Older men with a long-term-care disability are more likely to have a surviving spouse to provide them with long-term care than are older women. As those requiring long-term-care services age, it becomes increasingly difficult for a spouse to provide the long-term-care services needed by the disabled spouse. In 1999, a wife typically provided 20.5 percent of her husband's long-term-care needs; a husband (because there were fewer husbands) typically provided 14.3 percent of his wife's long-term-care needs. Daughters provided 41.6 percent and sons provided 23.6 percent (Spillman and Black 2005, Table 4). Children are bearing an increasing portion of the informal care needs of their parents. Women more often than men provide the uncompensated care. When the impaired aged is a woman, typically a widow, children and relatives are

Table 35.1: Percentage of People Aged 65 Years and Older with Long-Term-Care Needs, by Age and Place of Residence, 1995

Age Group (in Years)	In Community	In Institutions	Total
65–74	10.9	1.2	12.1
75–84	21.8	5.4	27.2
85 and over	48.8	21.0	69.8

Source: Stone, R. I. 2000, "Long-Term Care for the Elderly with Disabilities: Current Policy, Emerging Trends, and Implications for the 21st Century." *Milbank Memorial Fund.*

the most frequent caregivers. These services by family members, while uncompensated, are costly to the caregivers in terms of added strain on spouses and the need for children to reduce their hours at work or leave their jobs.

The need for nursing home care also increases with age. At any point in time (as of 1999), approximately 4.5 percent of the aged (about 1.5 million) are in a nursing home. An estimated 1 percent of those aged 65 to 74 years are in nursing homes, compared with 4.5 percent of those aged 75 to 84 years and 24.8 percent of those aged 85 years old and older (Centers for Disease Control and Prevention 2006) The main reasons for nursing home use are severe functional deficiencies, mental disabilities (such as Alzheimer's), and lack of a family to provide services in the person's own home.

The fastest-growing portion of the aged is those over 85 years of age, who have the greatest needs for long-term care and nursing homes. Demographic trends will cause a steady increase in the number of very dependent older persons who need long-term care.

CURRENT STATE OF LONG-TERM-CARE FINANCING

Long-term care is very expensive and represents a significant financial risk to the elderly. The national average annual cost for a private room in a nursing home was $75,000 in 2005, and this figure is expected to almost triple by 2025 (MetLife Mature Market Institute 2005). A person turning 65 in 2000 had a 44 percent chance of entering a nursing home at some point in his life. Most of the aged who enter a nursing home will do so for a short period, but 19 percent will stay more than five years and incur 89 percent of all nursing home costs. Because women have a longer life expectancy, a 65-year-old woman has a 51 percent chance of entering a nursing home during her lifetime and, upon entering, has an expected average stay of two years. Furthermore, in-home care is also expensive; the average cost for a home health aide is $19 an hour (MetLife Mature Market Institute 2005). Thus, long-term-care services in a nursing home or an aide to provide care in the home are too costly for most of the aged on fixed incomes with limited assets.

Many aged mistakenly believe Medicare will pay for their long-term-care needs. Medicare protects the aged from acute medical expenses but not from expenses incurred for chronic disability. Included as part of Medicare are home health services for those aged who need part-time skilled nursing care or therapy services and are under the care of a physician. A limited number of postacute care days (100) in a skilled nursing home are covered for those discharged from a hospital. Medicare spending on these services accounted for about 21.9 percent of total long-term-care spending in 2005 (about $37.1 billion). Medicare does not cover the services needed when an aged person has decreased ability to care for herself because of chronic illness, a disability, or normal aging.

In 2005, spending from all public and private sources for long-term care (for all ages) was $169.3 billion, which represents about 8.5 percent of total health care expenditures. The largest component of long-term-care services is for nursing homes, which represent 72.0 percent of such expenditures; home care represents 28.0 percent (Table 35.2). The major sources of long-term-care financing are public programs, primarily Medicaid and Medicare, at 65.7 percent. Individuals provide about 25.4 percent of the costs out of pocket, and the remainder, about 8.8 percent, is covered by private long-term-care insurance. These percentages differ according to whether the long-term-care is provided in a nursing home or in the patient's home. Long-term care insurance covers 8 percent of nursing home costs and 12 percent of home health care. Private long-term-care insurance is beginning to increase; presently only about 10 percent of the aged have such insurance.

The aged or their families pay about 25 percent of all long-term-care expenses out of pocket; on average 30 percent of all nursing home care, a significant financial burden for many, is out of pocket. Although the aged and their families pay about 13 percent of home health costs, these costs do not include the substantial nonfinancial burden imposed on families and relatives who are unpaid caregivers. The Congressional

Table 35.2: Estimated Spending on Long-Term-Care Services, by Type of Service and Payment Source, 2005

Payment Source	Nursing Home Care	Home Health Care	Total
	Billions of Dollars		
Total	$121.9	$47.5	$169.4
Medicare	19.2	17.9	37.1
Medicaid	53.5	15.5	69.0
Other federal	3.0	0.2	3.2
Other state and local	0.3	1.8	2.1
Private insurance	9.1	5.8	14.9
Out-of-pocket and other sources	36.8	6.2	43.0
	% of Total		
Total	72.0%	28.0%	100.0%
Medicare	15.8	37.7	21.9
Medicaid	43.9	32.6	40.7
Other federal	2.5	0.4	1.9
Other state and local	0.2	3.8	1.2
Private insurance	7.5	12.2	8.8
Out-of-pocket and other sources	30.2	13.1	25.4

Source: Data from Centers for Medicare & Medicaid Services, Office of the Actuary, National Health Statistics Group. 2007. [Online information.] http://www.cms.hhs.gov/NationalHealthExpendData/downloads/tables.pdf.

Budget Office (2004) estimates that if the value of donated care were included in the total cost of long-term-care, informal caregivers provide 36 percent of all long-term-care expenses.

Medicaid

Medicaid is a joint federal-state financing program for those with low incomes. The states' share of total Medicaid expenditures was 43 percent in 2005. Total Medicaid expenditures were $313 billion in 2005, of which 22 percent was for payment of long-term-care services; the remainder was for acute care services (Centers for Medicare & Medicaid Services 2007). States vary greatly in their per capita (per person within the state) annual expenditures for long-term care, from $815 in New York to $91 in Nevada (Gibson et al. 2004).

Medicaid is the major payer for nursing home care (44 percent) and pays for a limited amount of in-home coverage (33 percent). Medicaid is the payer of last resort, covering long-term-care expenses only after the impaired aged have exhausted their own financial resources. To qualify for Medicaid, an individual must first spend down his assets and is allowed to keep only $2,000. Current law permits a spouse to retain half of the couple's financial assets, up to a maximum of $95,100 (inflation adjusted) in addition to a private home of any value if it is the principal residence (Social Services Agency 2006).

To limit their Medicaid expenditures, states have restricted the availability of nursing home beds, paid nursing homes low rates, and provided limited in-home services to those eligible for Medicaid. The consequence of these policies has been a continual excess demand for nursing home beds by the impaired aged. Because demand exceeds supply and states set low payment rates, the quality of services provided is often poor. Few states pay nursing homes according to the level of care needed by the patient; thus, nursing homes have an incentive to admit Medicaid patients who have lower care needs and are less costly to care for. When a private-pay patient seeks nursing home care, she will be admitted before the Medicaid patient because her payment exceeds Medicaid reimbursement. As nursing home demand by private patients increases, the excess demand by Medicaid patients will become greater in those states that continue to limit the number of nursing home beds.

The risk of a person entering a nursing home as a private patient and having to spend down his assets was only 6.3 percent in 1985. (The probabilities vary by race and gender.) Most of the aged (59.2 percent) entering a nursing home were private patients; the remainder were those already eligible for Medicaid (17.3 percent) and Medicare or other payers (23.5 percent). Of those private-pay patients who used fewer than three months of nursing home care, 2.7 percent had to spend down their assets to qualify for Medicaid eligibility. For a stay up to six months, a total of 10.5 percent of the aged had to spend down. As the stay increased up to two years, 18.2 percent had to spend down (Spillman and Kemper 1995).

Although the lifetime risk of a person entering a nursing home and having to spend down her assets is relatively low, the fear of incurring this financial burden is the basis of the demand for long-term-care insurance and government subsidies.

Home care expenditures have become a growing share of Medicaid long-term-care expenditures. From 2000 to 2005, Medicaid spending on home care increased from $6 billion to $15.5 billion, an average annual rate of 32 percent, compared with 4 percent on nursing homes. States have also attempted to reduce their nursing home spending by substituting less-costly in-home and community-based long-term-care services (Centers for Medicare & Medicaid Services 2007).[1]

Private Long-Term-Care Insurance

When many people are at risk for a large unexpected expense, but only a few will incur such catastrophic costs, private insurance is a solution for those who can afford it. A private insurance market enables people to reduce their financial risk in exchange for a premium. Given the growing number of aged at risk for financially catastrophic nursing home (and in-home) costs, the potential market for long-term-care insurance is huge. Dependence on Medicaid and the need for government long-term-care subsidies would diminish if more of the aged purchased private long-term-care insurance. Yet fewer than 10 percent of the elderly have private long-term-care insurance.

WHY DO SO FEW AGED BUY LONG-TERM-CARE INSURANCE?

Why has private long-term-care insurance not grown more rapidly? How feasible is it to expect private long-term-care insurance to alleviate the middle-class aged's concerns that their long-term-care needs will be met without burdening their family caregivers or having to spend down their estates?

Characteristics of Long-Term-Care Insurance Policies

Most long-term-care insurance (about 80 percent) is sold to individuals, in contrast to medical insurance, which is mainly sold to groups. Most long-term-care policies cover all forms of long-term-care needs, including nursing homes, home care, and assisted-living facilities. In addition, case management services, medical equipment in the home, and training of caregivers may be included. Most long-term-care plans also have a deductible in the form of days of care the individual must pay (30 to 100

---

1. States cover nonmedical and social support services to allow people to remain in the community. These services include personal care, homemaker assistance, adult day care, chore assistance, and other services shown to be cost effective and necessary to avoid institutionalization. To control costs, however, states limit eligibility and the scope of services covered.

days) before the policy is effective. These deductible provisions ensure that the long-term-care policy is for a chronic condition and does not cover acute medical or rehabilitative services, which is the responsibility of Medicare or private medical insurance.

Long-term-care plans also contain benefit maximums. Policies may limit lifetime benefits to five years in a nursing home. In addition, most policies contain a maximum daily payment for care in a nursing home or for reimbursement for care in the home. These maximum daily benefits are either fixed over time or (for an additional premium) are increased by an annual percentage amount. Furthermore, to qualify for long-term-care benefits, the individual must meet certain criteria, such as requiring substantial assistance in being able to perform several specified activities of daily living for an extended period, such as 90 days.

Long-term-care insurance premiums reflect the cost of providing the services and the risk that the person will need the services as she ages. In 2002, the average annual premium was $2,014 at age 65; if purchased at age 75 it was $4,607, more than double; and at age 85, the average premium was $10,000. If a policy was purchased at age 30, the premium would be only $622 per year, reflecting both the lower risk that a young person would require long-term-care services and that younger people would be paying the premium over a greater number of years than someone who purchased coverage when they were older.

The type of benefits included in a long-term-care policy will greatly affect premiums charged. For example, a policy sold in 2002 for a 70-year-old person will vary as much as five-fold, from a low of about $850 to a high of $4,500 per year depending on benefits included.

Long-term-care insurance premiums are also higher if the purchaser wishes to protect himself against inflation in long-term-care costs. Because most long-term-care policies provide specified cash benefits in the event the purchaser requires long-term care, a long-term-care policy that pays $100 per day for care in a nursing home would not be sufficient if nursing home costs increase at their previous annual growth rate of 6.7 percent; over 20 years the cost per day would be $366. Protection against these additional financial risks increases the premium, making it less affordable to many aged.

Long-term-care policies are guaranteed renewable, and premiums vary by age and risk class, of which there are usually three: preferred, standard, or extra risk. Once a person has purchased a long-term-care plan, she is not charged an additional amount if her health condition changes.

Factors Limiting Demand for Long-Term-Care Insurance

Possible explanations why only 10 percent of the elderly have long-term-care insurance can be classified, first, according to the factors that limit the demand for private long-term-care insurance and, second, according to imperfections on the supply side of the long-term-care insurance market.

The aged's income and ability to pay for long-term-care insurance are quite variable. The oldest old, those most in need of long-term care, generally have lower incomes than the younger aged and are in a higher-risk group; consequently, their insurance premiums are much higher.

A great deal of misinformation exists among the aged—many believe Medicare and Medigap insurance (private insurance that pays Medicare's deductibles and copayments) also cover long-term care (they do not). Also, the elderly may be unaware of their potential long-term-care risks and the financial consequences of those risks. Furthermore, the number of policies, with their differing copayments and benefits, may be confusing to some of the elderly.

An important reason why the elderly may not have long-term-care insurance is the availability of Medicaid. To the extent that the elderly view Medicaid as a low-cost substitute to private long-term-care insurance, they will be less likely to purchase private long-term-care insurance. If the older aged need to enter a nursing home, they have to rely on Medicaid, which is their low-cost long-term-care insurance. To those elderly, however, who wish to bequeath their assets to their children, Medicaid is a poor substitute to privately purchased insurance. Medicaid does not protect an elderly person's financial assets.

Expectations of the elderly that their family will provide financial and nonfinancial support if they require long-term care is another inhibiting factor affecting their demand for insurance. Thus, publicly funded or family-provided long-term care decreases the demand for privately funded insurance.

Possible Market Imperfections in the Supply of Long-Term-Care Insurance

Supply-side concerns relate to whether long-term-care plans are priced significantly above their actuarial fair value ("pure" premium), in which case the premiums would greatly exceed the policy's expected benefits. The greater the difference between the premium and expected benefits (referred to as the loading charge), the lower the demand for such insurance.

Premiums for long-term-care plans may be much higher than the expected benefits for several reasons. There are much greater marketing and administrative costs when long-term-care insurance is sold to individuals than if such insurance were sold to large employer groups. (Individually sold medical insurance contains loading charges as high as 40 percent, compared with loading charges of 10 percent to 15 percent when sold to groups.)

Also increasing the loading charge is insurers' concern about adverse selection.[2] Long-term-care insurance is sold to individuals on a voluntary basis, whereas employer-paid health insurance includes everyone in the group, which eliminates the chance that only sick employees will buy the insurance. Because insurance premiums are based on the average expected claims experience (use rate multiplied by the price of the service) of a particular age group, insurers are concerned that a higher proportion of the impaired aged will buy long-term-care insurance. If the premium is based on a higher expected risk group than exists among the general population of elderly desiring to buy insurance, those elderly of an average risk level will find the premium greatly in excess of their expected benefits. ("Delay of benefits" provisions, indemnity coverage with a large deductible, and copayments are usually included to discourage adverse selection.)

Insurers are also concerned that as insurance becomes available to pay for in-home services, the demand for such services will sharply increase ("moral hazard") beyond the amount believed necessary. To the extent that moral hazard occurs and is not controlled by the insurer, the premium will reflect these higher use rates and greatly exceed the expected benefits for those aged who would not similarly increase their use of services once their insurance started paying for those services.[3]

---

2. Since the late 1980s, insurers have been marketing long-term-care insurance to large employee groups. Group policies have lower loading charges because of their lower administrative and marketing costs. Adverse selection is also less of a concern when everyone in a group participates, particularly when they are at low risk for long-term care. Furthermore, because employees would not be at risk for many years, group long-term-care policies could be sold at very low premiums. Employer-sponsored long-term-care policies may be a useful financing source for future rather than current aged.

3. To lower the cost of providing long-term care, insurers provide comprehensive services, both in-home assistance and nursing home care. In-home services are less expensive (and are preferred by the impaired aged) when they reduce use of the more expensive nursing home. Case managers would ideally be used to evaluate the elderly's needs and determine

Conclusions Regarding the Small Market for Private Long-Term-Care Insurance

The size of the loading charge does not seem to be the determining factor causing the small demand for long-term-care insurance. Such policies charge the same premiums for both men and women of the same age. Brown and Finkelstein (2004a) estimated the loading charge for a 65-year-old man to be 44 percent; he would expect to receive $56 worth of benefits in return for paying a $100 premium. However, because premiums are the same regardless of sex, the loading charge for a 65-year-old woman was estimated to be negative, that is, her expected benefits are greater than the premium paid: $104 in expected benefits in return for paying a $100 premium. Given the very favorable pricing of long-term-care policies for women, still only about 10 percent of elderly women purchase such policies, which is no different from the percentage of men purchasing such policies. These findings suggest that market-supply imperfections, reflected by the loading charge, are insufficient for understanding the limited demand for long-term-care insurance.

Demand factors are therefore more likely explanations for the limited demand for private long-term-care policies. In a second study, the authors conclude that the availability of Medicaid is critical in explaining the limited demand for long-term-care insurance (Brown and Finkelstein 2004b). For an elderly person with median wealth, most of the premiums for a private long-term-care policy pay for the same benefits that would be covered by Medicaid. Furthermore, women are more likely than men to end up on Medicaid, regardless of whether they have private long-term-care insurance, because of their much greater expected lifetime utilization of long-term-care services. Thus, women, even though they might be able to buy private long-term-care insurance with a zero loading charge, would still not buy long-term-care insurance because of the availability of Medicaid.

As long as Medicaid exists in its present form, it will be difficult to increase the demand for private long-term-care insurance.

---

the mix of services to be provided. In-home services could be substituted for nursing home care, and the discretionary use of in-home assistance could be minimized. Controlling adverse selection and discretionary use of services is essential to keeping private long-term-care insurance premiums low. Currently, greater reliance is placed on financial incentives (deductibles and copayments) rather than the use of case managers to control costs.

APPROACHES FOR FINANCING LONG-TERM CARE

The long-term-care needs of the older aged, the aged's fear of having to spend down their assets, and the high cost of private long-term-care insurance form the basis of the aged's demand for government long-term-care subsidies. Providing the aged with a range of long-term-care services, from in-home services to nursing home care, without financially burdening the aged or their children, would require huge government subsidies. Given the rapid increase in both the number and proportion of aged, federal subsidies to all of the aged would be a very large financial burden on the nonaged.

Federal spending on programs benefiting the aged—Medicare, Medicaid, and Social Security—consumed 8.5 percent of GDP as of 2005. By 2035, inflation-adjusted expenditures on these programs will double to 16.4 percent of GDP.[4] Federal spending on the elderly will absorb a larger and, ultimately, an unsustainable share of the federal budget and economic resources. Thanks in part to medical advances, people are living longer and spending more time in retirement, which places greater demands on these three federal programs. The aged are an increasing portion of the total population, and as the baby boomers start retiring in 2011, there will be a declining number of workers per aged to finance the growing costs of Medicaid, Medicare, and Social Security. These demographic, technologic, and economic pressures have profound implications for our economy and the continued funding of these entitlement programs.

Medicaid is also the fastest-growing and second-largest program in state spending. About 69 percent of Medicaid spending is on behalf of the aged and those with disabilities. The growing number of aged will place a greater burden on state budgets in coming years. Expanding public subsidies for long-term care would not only exacerbate federal and state fiscal pressures but would also serve as a disincentive to the purchase of private long-term-care insurance.

Given these trends in both the number and percentage of aged and the likely inability of government to continue financing these benefits, subsidies for financing the long-term-care needs of the aged are likely to be curtailed rather than expanded. The public policy dilemma is what should be the role of government in financing long-term care for the aged?

---

4. The federal share of Medicaid, Medicare, and Social Security is expected to increase, respectively, from 1.5 percent, 2.7 percent, and 4.3 percent of GDP in 2005 to 2.6 percent, 7.5 percent, and 6.3 percent of GDP in 2035.

Given the fiscal pressures on the federal and state governments, it is unlikely a new long-term-care subsidy for all the aged would be enacted in the foreseeable future. Instead, government policy is likely to be, first, a "safety net" for low-income aged and, second, increasing the effectiveness of how those subsidies are spent.

The Government as a Safety Net

When government acts as a safety net, primary responsibility for paying long-term-care expenses would be placed on the individual and the family. The government would fill the gap between the needs of the elderly and what their families and financial resources can provide. Availability of government assistance would be based, as with Medicaid, on the elderly person's income and assets. Similar to Medicaid, such a program would be financed from general taxes; those with higher incomes would bear the financial burden of subsidizing low-income aged. Because states differ in their generosity and financial capacity, resulting in wide variations in long-term-care expenditures per capita, the traditional federal and state roles in financing Medicaid would have to be reevaluated to ensure a more equitable distribution of public support for those with low incomes.

Lengthening the period for asset transfers from three to five years (which is opposed by the American Association of Retired Persons), limiting excludable assets, and enforcing these requirements would reduce Medicaid expenditures, make Medicaid a less-desirable substitute to private long-term-care insurance by middle- and high-income persons, and, consequently, increase the demand for private long-term-care insurance.

Most states now have provisions that prevent people from qualifying for Medicaid within three years of voluntarily impoverishing themselves through bequests of their assets to family members. (States are going after middle- and high-income persons who have adopted estate-planning strategies that permit them to qualify for Medicaid by transferring their assets just before they need nursing home care.) Furthermore, because some assets are excluded for purposes of determining Medicaid eligibility, such as having a house, spending assets on home improvements, having an automobile, and placing assets in certain types of trusts, tightening Medicaid requirements would further reduce eligibility and use public subsidies for those most in need.

Several states have developed innovative long-term-care programs in the expectation that Medicaid's long-term-care expenditures will be reduced while improving patient satisfaction with the care they receive. Several states use "cash and counseling" programs, for example. Under this approach, Medicaid beneficiaries living in the community are provided with funds to purchase long-term-care services rather than rely on Medicaid-provided services. Beneficiaries are given more choice in the type of long-term-care services used and in selecting providers. Medicaid beneficiaries currently have no financial incentive to use long-term care efficiently. Cash and counseling programs give beneficiaries an incentive to shop for lower-priced services and get more care for their budgets. Preliminary evidence from these demonstration projects indicates that participants are more satisfied with the care received and have fewer unmet needs than beneficiaries in traditional Medicaid.

Other innovative programs integrate acute and long-term care. Social HMOs (S/HMOs) receive a monthly premium in return for providing acute and long-term-care services to their enrollees. The S/HMO is at financial risk for the cost of all the medical and long-term-care services its enrollees require. Both healthy and impaired aged are able to enroll in the S/HMO, which has an incentive to improve the efficiency of the care received by its enrollees by both coordinating care and reducing unnecessary services.

The Program for All-Inclusive Care for the Elderly (PACE) model is directed toward Medicare- and Medicaid-eligible beneficiaries who are eligible for nursing home care but want to continue living at home. PACE organizations receive a monthly capitation payment; use a multidisciplinary team of providers, such as physicians, nurses, and case managers; and provide services to enrollees in adult day care centers. Preliminary evaluations indicate less nursing home and hospital use by PACE enrollees. These results may be biased, however, by favorable selection; PACE enrollees may be less impaired than nursing home patients, which is their comparison group.

(Additional innovative approaches for reducing Medicaid's long-term-care expenditures are described in Congressional Budget Office 2006.)

Redistributive Effects of Government Subsidies

Subsidizing the aged's long-term-care expenses has redistributive effects in that some income groups will be taxed to provide benefits to other income groups. Do these redistributive effects improve or worsen equity? Subsidies to the aged result in "intergenerational" redistribution; current workers subsidize the aged. If subsidies are based on income taxes, higher-income workers subsidize the aged. If the subsidy is based on a sales or payroll tax, many persons with low incomes will subsidize the nursing home expenses of middle- and high-income aged. Is it equitable to tax low-income workers to enable the aged to leave their assets to their children? Unless government subsidies are targeted to those aged with the lowest incomes and assets, subsidies to all aged are likely to be inequitable and should be viewed more as asset-protection programs for middle-class aged.

Public long-term-care subsidies affect the demand for private long-term-care insurance. The lower the aged's responsibility for their long-term-care expenses, the lower their likelihood of buying private long-term-care insurance. Appropriate public policy should be to encourage those who can afford it to purchase private long-term-care insurance and use limited public funds for those unable to do so.

SUMMARY

Fewer than 40 percent of the aged will likely be able to afford private long-term-care insurance. Although this percentage indicates that the private insurance market can greatly increase, it also indicates that a sizable number, mainly the older aged, will be unable to purchase insurance or other long-term-care services.

A fundamental issue is whether the elderly should be expected to rely on their own resources for meeting their long-term-care needs, with the government providing a safety net for those unable to do so, or whether subsidies should be provided to all the aged, regardless of their income and assets.

Long-term-care policy requires choices to be made. The aged have greater needs for care, do not wish to be a burden on family members, do not want to spend down their hard-earned assets, and would like to be assured of a high-quality nursing home should they require one. Yet given the projected number of aged, government long-term-care subsidies can be very costly. Such subsidies will require large tax increases at a time when Medicare taxes will also be increased to keep it from going bankrupt. These tax increases will represent a huge financial burden on workers because the number of workers per aged person is declining.

Subsidies also reduce the incentive for many aged to rely on their children or to purchase private long-term-care insurance. To reduce the cost of long-term-care subsidies, subsidies should be targeted to those with the lowest incomes. Estate-planning strategies that enable middle- and high-income aged to transfer their assets shortly before qualifying for Medicaid are inequitable in that they shift their costs to others. To the extent that Medicaid rules are enforced and it becomes a less-desirable substitute to private long-term-care insurance, the demand for private long-term-care insurance will increase. Greater growth in the demand for long-term-care insurance will reduce Medicaid long-term-care expenditures. Educating both workers and the aged about the need to protect themselves against catastrophic long-term-care costs is also important.

DISCUSSION QUESTIONS

1. Describe the demographic and economic trends affecting the outlook for long-term-care.

2. What should be the objectives of a long-term-care policy? How do these objectives differ from the long-term-care goals of the middle class?

3. Evaluate the redistributive effects of income-related refundable tax credits for private long-term-care insurance and medical IRAs.

4. Why has the market for long-term-care insurance grown so slowly?

5. Why does private long-term-care insurance, when sold to the aged, have such a high loading charge relative to the pure premium?

REFERENCES

Brown, J., and A. Finkelstein. 2004a. *Supply or Demand: Why Is the Market for Long-Term Care Insurance So Small?* NBER Working Paper 10782. Cambridge, MA: National Bureau of Economic Research.

———. 2004b. *The Interaction of Public and Private Insurance: Medicaid and the Long Term Insurance Market*, NBER Working Paper No. 10989. Cambridge, MA: National Bureau of Economic Research.

Centers for Disease Control and Prevention. 2006. *Health, United States, 2006.* Calculation based on data in Tables 1 and 102. [Online information; retrieved 12/18/06.] http://www.cdc.gov/nchs/products/pubs/pubd/hus/older.htm.

Centers for Medicare & Medicaid Services. 2007. *National Health Expenditures Tables.* [Online information; retrieved 1/10/07.] http://www.cms.hhs.gov/NationalHealthExpendData/downloads/tables.pdf.

Congressional Budget Office. 2004. *Financing Long-Term Care for the Elderly*, A CBO Paper, April. [Online publication; retrieved 11/15/06.] http://www.cbo.gov/showdoc.cfm?index=5400&sequence=0.

———. 2006. *Medicaid Spending Growth and Options for Controlling Costs*, A CBO Paper, July 13. [Online publication; retrieved 12/18/06.] http://www.cbo.gov/ftpdocs/73xx/doc7387/07-13-Medicaid.pdf.

Gibson, M., S. Gregory, A. Houser, and W. Fox-Grage. 2004. *Across the States: Profiles of Long-Term Care, 2004*, AARP Research Report. [Online publication; retrieved 11/15/06.] http://assets.aarp.org/rgcenter/post-import/d18202_2004 _ats.pdf.

MetLife Mature Market Institute. 2005. *The MetLife Market Survey of Nursing Home & Home Care Costs*, September. [Online publication; retrieved 11/15/06.] http://www. metlife.com/WPSAssets/43838610601138293556V1F2005NHHCSurvey.pdf.

Social Services Agency. 2006. *How Do I Apply for Medi-Cal?* [Online information; retrieved 12/18/06.] http://www.ssa.ocgov.com/Health_Care/Medical_Services/ Skilled_Nursing/default.asp.

Spillman, B., and K. Black. 2005. *Staying the Course: Trends in Family Caregiving*. Washington, DC: AARP Public Policy Institute.

Spillman, B., and P. Kemper. 1995. "Lifetime Patterns of Payment for Nursing Home Care." *Medical Care* 33 (3): 288–96.

Chapter 36

The Politics of Health Care Reform

NATIONAL HEALTH INSURANCE has been a highly visible political issue many times. Each time its proponents have been disappointed, but the issue is unlikely to go away.

Dissatisfaction has been (and still is) evident with this country's health care system. The number of uninsured is increasing, hospitals and physicians are inadequately reimbursed for providing care to the poor, many fear losing their health insurance if they become ill, and the insured find themselves paying higher out-of-pocket payments and still being forced to pay higher insurance premiums. Given public dissatisfaction with the current health system and apparent political support for politicians who favor its reform, why has achieving national health insurance been so difficult?

Advocates for health care reform want to receive benefits in excess of their costs, and the only way they can achieve this is if the government legislates it. However, if most groups are to have net benefits, some group will be stuck paying the costs of those benefits. Which group in society will bear the added costs or taxes? Whichever group has to pay more will oppose legislators who vote to raise their taxes. The major difficulty in health care reform is finding groups that can be taxed to provide net benefits to politically powerful constituencies.

In the past, politically important groups received visible redistributive benefits that less politically powerful groups were taxed to provide. To lessen the opposition of those being taxed, the tax was hidden. For example, splitting the Social Security tax and the Medicare payroll tax between the employer and the employee makes it appear that the employee bears only half of the tax. In reality, economists believe most of the employer share is shifted back to the employee in the form of lower wages, and the rest is shifted forward to consumers as higher prices for goods and services.

To understand the difficulties of health care reform and what compromises are likely to emerge, one must examine the goals of different political constituencies. In doing so, it soon becomes obvious that national health insurance means different things to different groups.

DIFFERING GOALS OF HEALTH CARE REFORM

Many assume that the main purpose of national health insurance is to increase the availability of medical services to those with low incomes. Certainly many individuals support increased services to the poor, but this is not, nor has it ever been, the driving force behind national health insurance—*Medicaid is national health insurance for the poor.* To use the power of government to achieve one's objectives requires political power. The inadequate structure and funding of Medicaid is indicative of the limited political power of the poor and their advocates. These inadequacies are not attributable to the actions of a few miserly bureaucrats or legislators but are instead reflective of the resources that society—the middle class—is willing to devote to the poor. States vary in their generosity and in the criteria used for determining Medicaid eligibility. Few states provide Medicaid eligibility for all those at the federal poverty level, and some states provide benefits only to people at 25 percent of it. How much the nonpoor will spend on charity depends on how much the nonpoor themselves have, how culturally similar the poor are to the nonpoor, and how much it costs to provide for the poor.

Because the nonpoor have the political power to determine the allocation of resources to the poor, one must assume that the inadequacies of Medicaid are reflections of insufficient interest among the nonpoor in improving Medicaid and increasing funding for the poor. If society is unwilling to improve Medicaid, why would it tax itself to enact national health insurance for the poor?

If national health insurance is not primarily for the poor, its broader purpose must be to use the power of government to benefit politically powerful groups. Politically influential groups have a "concentrated" interest in a particular issue and are able to organize themselves to provide political support to legislators by way of campaign contributions, votes, and volunteer time. A group is said to have a concentrated interest if specific regulation or legislation will have a sufficiently large effect to make it worthwhile for the group to invest resources to either forestall or promote that effect. The potential legislative benefits must exceed the group's costs of organizing and providing political support.

This discussion of concentrated interests assumes that legislators will respond to political support because their objective is to be reelected. Legislators are assumed to be similar to the other participants in the policy process and rationally undertake cost-benefit calculations of their actions. However, they weigh the political support gained and lost by their legislative actions, not by the legislation's effect on society.

Initially, physicians and hospitals were the major groups in the health field with a concentrated interest in health legislation. Payment systems under both public and private insurance had a large effect on their revenues, and competitors (such as HMOs, PPOs, outpatient surgery centers, and foreign-trained physicians) also affected hospital and physician revenues. These financial concerns, related to demand for services, methods of pricing, availability of substitutes for their services, and their overall supply, prompted physician and hospital associations to represent (successfully) their concentrated interests before both state and federal legislatures. One demonstration of the American Medical Association's political power was the defeat of President Truman's proposed national health insurance plan. Legislators who had opposed the American Medical Association's economic interests found the association a force to be reckoned with at election time.

These legislative actions by physician and hospital associations were neither very obvious nor initially very costly to the consumers of medical services. Although medical prices rose faster than they would have otherwise, alternatives to the fee-for-service system, such as managed care, were unavailable. These costs to consumers were not sufficiently large to make it worthwhile for them to organize, represent their interests before legislatures, and offer political support to legislators who were favorable to their interests.

The concentrated interests of medical providers and the subsequent diffuse (small) costs imposed on consumers explain much of the legislative history of the financing and delivery of medical services until the early 1960s. The enactment and design of Medicare illustrates *the real purpose of national health insurance: to redistribute wealth, that is, increase benefits to politically powerful groups without their paying the full costs of those benefits by shifting the costs to the less politically powerful.*

Throughout the 1950s and early 1960s, the American Federation of Labor–Congress of Industrial Organizations unions had a concentrated interest in their retirees' medical costs that placed them in opposition to the American Medical Association. Employers had not prefunded union retirees' medical costs but instead paid them as part of current labor expenses. If union retirees' medical expenses could be shifted away from the employer, those funds would be available to be paid as higher wages to union employees.

To ensure that their union retirees would be eligible for Medicare the unions insisted that eligibility be based on those who had paid into the Social Security system while they were working and that the new Medicare program (hospital services) be financed by a separate Medicare payroll tax to be included as part of the Social Security tax. Although the current retirees had not contributed to the proposed Medicare program, they were to become immediately eligible because they had paid Social Security taxes. The use of the Social Security system to determine eligibility became the central issue in the debate over Medicare (Feldstein 2006a).

The American Medical Association was willing to have government assistance go only to those unable to afford medical services, which would have increased the demand for physicians. Thus, the association favored a means-tested program funded by general tax revenues because it was concerned that including the non-poor in the new program would merely substitute government payment for private payment. The American Medical Association believed such a program would cost too much, leading to controls on hospital and physician fees.

With the landslide victory of President Johnson in 1964, the unions achieved their objective. Once Social Security financing was used to determine eligibility for Medicare, Medicare Part B (physician services) was added, financed by general tax revenues.

Although the unions won on the financing mechanism, the Congress acceded to the demands of the medical and hospital associations on all other aspects of the legislation. The system of payment to hospitals and physicians promoted inefficiency (cost-plus payments to hospitals), and restrictions limiting competition were placed on alternative delivery systems.

This historic conflict between opposing concentrated interests in medical care left both sides victorious and illustrates how the power of government can be used to benefit politically important groups. As a result of

Medicare a massive redistribution of wealth occurred in society. The beneficiaries were the aged, union members, and medical providers, and the benefits were financed by a diffuse tax (the Medicare payroll tax) on a large group, the working population, who also paid higher prices for their medical services and more income taxes to finance Medicare Part B. *Medicare was designed to be both inefficient and inequitable simply because it was in the economic interests of those with concentrated interests.*

This brief discussion of Medicare illustrates the real purpose of national health insurance: to redistribute wealth, that is, to increase benefits to politically powerful groups without them having to pay the full costs of those benefits or, similarly, to shift costs from the politically powerful to those who are less so.

GROUPS HAVING A CONCENTRATED INTEREST IN CHANGE

An important reason health policies change is that groups that previously had a diffuse interest develop a concentrated interest in the policy's outcome. For example, the potential benefits to unions of having their retirees' health benefits shifted from the employer to the government (via the taxpayer) under Medicare became sufficiently great as to provide them with a concentrated interest in this issue. Groups with a diffuse interest may develop a concentrated interest as the potential benefits or costs to their members increase.

Today, many more groups have a concentrated interest in health legislation. To understand the conflicting forces pressing for change and national health insurance, however, one has to examine the objectives of several of the more important groups.

Federal and State Governments

Since Medicare and Medicaid were enacted in 1965, every administration has been confronted with rapidly rising Medicare and Medicaid expenditures. As expenditures greatly exceeded projections, what had initially been a diffuse cost became a concentrated cost to successive administrations. Each administration faced choices with potentially high political costs. To prevent the Medicare Trust Fund from going bankrupt the administration could reduce benefits to the aged, increase the Medicare payroll tax (and the wage base to which it applied), or pay hospitals less. No choice was without political costs, but increasing the

Medicare payroll tax and placing limits on how much hospitals were paid were considered less costly than reducing benefits to the aged.

To limit rapidly rising Medicaid expenditures, which are funded from general tax revenues, the states chose to limit Medicaid eligibility and reduce their payments to health providers rather than reduce other politically popular programs or increase taxes. However, the percentage of the poor served by Medicaid declined, as did the participation of physicians and hospitals.

Medicare Part B, funded by general tax revenues, contributes to the federal budget deficit. As these expenditures have risen, each administration's choices have been limited; each choice would be politically costly. The aged's contribution could be increased (they currently pay only 25 percent of the program's cost), but this was seen as the most politically costly option. Instead, less politically costly approaches were used, allowing the program to increase the federal deficit and paying physicians less. (In 1993, total Medicare physician expenditure increases were limited by a volume-expenditure cap, which was changed to an SGR limit in 1997.)

Federal and state administrations developed a concentrated interest in holding down the rise in government expenditures, which placed them in conflict with hospital and physician organizations. Currently, government health policies appear to be concerned primarily with limiting Medicare and Medicaid expenditures. Politically, the least-costly approach has been to pay providers less. Only under Medicaid are the politically weak beneficiaries also adversely affected.

Employers and Unions

Employers, their employees, and unions are interested in reducing the rise in the cost of employees' medical benefits. Rising employee medical expenses became a concern to employers in the 1980s because of more intense import competition. Many employers believe they bear part of the cost of rising insurance premiums. More important, the stimulus for several large corporations, such as GM, to promote national health insurance was a ruling by the Financial Accounting Standards Board requiring employers who provide their retirees with medical benefits to accrue those costs over the working careers of their employees, in the same way corporations account for retirement plans. Companies had to list on their balance sheets and annually expense their (current and future) retiree medical obligations.

Retiree medical benefits were an unfunded liability to those large corporations that provide such benefits. Previously, the employer paid retiree medical costs as they occurred; they were treated as a current expense. Placing the entire liability on the balance sheet reduced the net worth and equity per share of many major corporations, particularly those of union-organized industries located in the Midwest and Northeast, by a significant amount. In addition, corporate earnings are reduced, as a portion of this retiree liability for medical benefits (for both retirees and current employees) has to be expensed annually. For example, GM, which provides health insurance for 1.1 million active and retired workers and their families in the United States, has unfunded retiree medical liabilities of $77 billion and spent $5.6 billion in 2005 (up $800 million from 2003) on medical expenses for its employees, retirees, and dependents (Hawkins 2005; Hawkins and Lundegaard 2005).

Any national health insurance plan that reduces the rate of increase in medical expenditures provides a direct economic benefit to large corporations. The unfunded retiree medical liabilities for these companies would be reduced, and their earnings per share would be increased.

Many large unions, such as the United Auto Workers (UAW), have very generous medical benefits. As the cost of medical care has risen, these unions have had to accept smaller wage increases to maintain their comprehensive medical benefits, which are among the most expensive of all employees. GM spends $14,000 on health care per employee (2005 figures), which, if these costs were shifted to the taxpayer, would be used to increase employee wages.

The economic interests of the major unions, such as the UAW, have not changed since the enactment of Medicare. At that time, they were successful in shifting part of their retirees' medical costs onto the general working population. Since then, the unions' legislative objective has been to maintain their benefits without having to pay the required cost.

To achieve the employers' goal of reducing their unfunded retirees' medical liabilities and the unions' goal of not bearing the full costs of their medical benefits, these costs have to be shifted to others. Through national health insurance, large employers and unions hope to achieve a reduction in the rise of (and their obligation for) their medical expenditures. It would not be surprising if the auto companies and their unions were to support a regulatory system that limits provider price increases and imposes an overall medical expenditure limit.

Physicians and Hospitals

As other groups (particularly federal and state governments) developed a concentrated interest in limiting medical expenditures, the influence of physician and hospital associations declined. A significant portion of their revenues are derived from Medicare and Medicaid, which places them in direct conflict with state and federal efforts to reduce Medicare and Medicaid expenditures.

Hospitals and physicians are striving to limit further deterioration in their financial well-being. Their objective, as opposed to that of other groups with a concentrated interest, is increased medical expenditures. Hospitals represent one of the strongest lobbies for financing medical care to the poor today because it serves their economic interest; they stand to gain additional revenues.

The Aged

The aged have national health insurance for acute care (Medicare). Medicare, however, did not cover outpatient prescription drugs. The aged were at greater financial risk for their outpatient drug costs than for very expensive hospitalizations and physician services, which were covered by Medicare. Thus, an important legislative goal of the aged had been a subsidized Medicare outpatient prescription drug benefit.

Although the long-term financial solvency of Medicare is of great concern, both political parties competed to provide the politically powerful aged with a prescription drug benefit. The 2000 presidential election, which was decided by fewer than 700 votes in Florida, convinced President Bush that the Republicans had to pass a Medicare outpatient prescription drug benefit before the 2004 presidential election to receive the political support of the aged. To compete with the president for the support of the aged, the Democrats proposed a far more expensive drug benefit. To receive support from Democratic senators, while limiting the costs of the new benefit, and trying to ensure that all the aged, even those with relatively small drug costs, would also benefit, the compromise bill included a complicated design with gaps in drug coverage. The new drug benefit, the Medicare Modernization Act, also referred to as Medicare Part D, was enacted in December 2003 (Feldstein 2006b).

The new drug benefit, effective in 2006, enables the aged to shift part of their drug costs to other population groups. However, given the complicated design of the drug benefit and the gaps in drug coverage, the aged will likely want a more comprehensive drug benefit and will want to pay a lower premium for the new benefit. It is also likely that politicians will respond to the demands by the aged to lower their drug costs further. One approach to lowering drug costs being suggested by some legislators is for the government to negotiate with drug companies and thereby control prescription drug prices.

The Middle Class

The middle class (those in the middle income group) has a disproportionate amount of political power, because they are the median voters. It is difficult to form a majority of voters without those in the middle. If national health insurance were a highly visible issue and strongly supported by the middle class, legislators would respond to the political support that would be forthcoming from the middle class. A consideration of why the middle class has not been a strong supporter of national health insurance is therefore instructive.

Rapidly rising medical costs have been a diffuse cost to the middle class. Tax-exempt employer-paid health insurance insulated employees and their families against the rising costs of medical care. Until the advent of managed care, employees had unlimited choice of providers, limited cost sharing, and small (if any) copremiums. *Tax-exempt employer-paid health insurance has been a form of national health insurance for middle- and high-income groups.* The value of this tax subsidy exceeds $190 billion a year in forgone federal, Social Security, and state taxes. Given the significant tax advantages of employer-paid premiums and the fact that increased employer-paid premiums did not visibly lower their wages, middle- and high-income employees were insulated from rising medical costs; thus, national health insurance was not an important financial issue. Employees have probably been at greater financial risk for the long-term-care needs of their aged parents than for their own acute care needs.

Middle-class dissatisfaction with the current system is increasing because they have been forced into more restrictive health plans, are required to pay higher deductibles, and are having to pay higher out-of-pocket health insurance premiums. The public would like unrestricted access to specialists (traditional fee-for-service insurance), low out-of-pocket copayments, and limited monthly health insurance premiums.

Other groups, such as insurance companies, also have a concentrated interest in any national health insurance plan; they do not want to be displaced by a government agency. These conflicting objectives by powerful interest groups explain why no consensus exists as to what national health insurance should attempt to achieve. Federal and state governments, as well as large employers, want to limit the rate of increase in medical expenditures. The previously politically powerful physician and hospital associations want increased medical expenditures. The aged, who have national health insurance, want a more (heavily subsidized) comprehensive prescription drug benefit (and probably subsidies for long-term-care expenses). The unions and the middle class want unrestricted access at no additional cost, presumably by shifting those costs to others, either to different population groups or to providers by paying them less.

The problem with coming to grips with serious reform is not just with special-interest groups but also with the middle class. They are unwilling to have the government increase their taxes to pay for health insurance for the uninsured. Thus, national health insurance is unlikely to occur. Furthermore, the middle class is as yet unwilling to recognize that they must make a trade-off between access to services and the amount they are willing to pay. With respect to this latter concern, politicians have attempted to curry favor with the middle class by making them believe that merely legislating broader access will allow the public increased access without additional cost.

PROSPECTS FOR HEALTH CARE REFORM

The rise of ideology, primarily since the early 1990s, has become another impediment to health care reform. In the latter half of the 1990s, huge federal budget surpluses were projected far into the future. The middle class would not have been required to tax themselves to provide for the uninsured. It was an opportune time to cover the uninsured, without seemingly imposing a financial burden on anyone. And yet Congress was unable to enact national health insurance that would provide universal coverage for all Americans.

Congress could not agree on how the uninsured should be assisted. Republicans favored providing the uninsured with refundable tax credits to buy insurance.[1] Their objective was to strengthen the private health insurance system and allow the insured to have more choice of medical providers and health plans. They also favored placing greater fiscal responsibility on the insured for their health care choices.

---

1. Persons whose tax credit exceeds their tax liabilities would receive a refund for the difference. For those with little or no tax liability the tax credit is essentially a voucher for a health plan.

Conversely, the Democrats supported making the uninsured eligible for (thereby expanding) existing public programs, such as Medicaid, or, as President Clinton proposed, expanding Medicare by allowing those between the ages of 55 and 65 years to buy into Medicare. They also favored expanding eligibility of children (up to age 18) to be covered by Medicaid. Expanding the number of people in public programs makes it easier to convert these programs into a single-payer system, such as the Canadian health care system. The next step would be to include in the single-payer system employer health insurance premiums on behalf of their employees. Accumulating all these funds would not necessitate a huge tax increase to fund such a system.

Proponents of a single-payer system oppose proposals, such as refundable tax credits and Medicare reform (competitive Medicare health plans), because they would strengthen a competitive private health care system. Proposals allowing greater choice of health plans move the medical care system away from the direction they favor. Similarly, these legislators favor proposals that increase the cost of the private system, such as regulating managed care to increase its costs, hence premiums, which will cause the public to demand an alternative system, namely a publicly financed system, such as Medicare (or a single-payer system).

This ideologic divide between proponents of strengthening the private system and those favoring an expanded public (eventually single-payer) system further limits opportunities for assisting the growing number of uninsured.

Now that projections of vast federal budget surpluses have disappeared, the likelihood of legislation providing for the uninsured has similarly faded from the policy agenda. Legislators are unlikely to propose taxing the middle class to cover the uninsured. Instead, health care reform will likely focus on reducing the burden of rising medical expenses on the middle class.

Medical prices, expenditures, and health insurance premiums will continue to increase and consume an even larger portion of GDP. The driving forces behind these increases are, primarily, new medical technology and an aging population. Rising medical prices and higher insurance premiums will become an even greater financial burden to the population and on state and federal budgets to pay for Medicare and Medicaid.

The public, employers, unions, states, and the federal government will seek ways of reducing the burden of these increased premiums and medical expenditures and try to shift their financial burden to others.

The response by legislators to these concerns is likely to be based on those approaches offering the greatest degree of political support rather than solutions that improve efficiency or assist those most affected by these financial burdens.[2] Regulatory responses, such as mandating increased access to care or limiting provider price increases, do not affect the federal budget and offer immediate relief to consumers.

From a legislator's perspective, regulation costs the legislator and the government very little, as he does not have to vote to increase taxes. Instead, a less-visible cost is imposed on the public in terms of higher insurance premiums (when mandating increased access to care) or decreased availability of care and technology (when controls are imposed on prices and profitability). The legislator hopes to receive the political benefits of seeming to respond to the public's concerns without incurring any cost (lost political support). Unfortunately, the indirect long-term consequences of regulation are ignored. As long as the public is led to believe they can have all the care they want without paying for it, serious discussions about the trade-off between access and cost are unlikely to occur.

Trade-offs are inherent in public policy. Arbitrarily reducing the rise in medical expenditures will result in reductions in development of new medical technology, including pharmaceutical discoveries that save lives and reduce suffering, and access to medical services. The trade-off between decreased spending and lower insurance premiums versus less access to medical care and to new discoveries should be explicitly recognized in debates about how much this country should spend on medical services.

SUMMARY

Until national health insurance becomes a visible political issue for which the middle class would be willing to provide its political support, national health insurance is unlikely to be enacted. Given the close division of the Congress and its large ideologic differences, a fundamental disagreement exists on the approach to be used to help the uninsured.

---

2. Enthoven (2004, 27) disappointingly observes, "What is becoming most likely is that the winning candidate in 2008 will make 'Medicare for All' a foundation for his or her platform. And employers, incapable of controlling costs and desperate to get medical expenses off their financial statements, will lead the candidate's campaign finance committee. Labor and small business will join them. The large and growing numbers of uninsured, by then reaching into the middle class, will consider the issue to be of top priority."

Although the number and percentage of the uninsured are increasing, the middle class, and consequently Congress, seems to have little interest in moving quickly and increasing their tax burden to assist those who can offer little political support to enact such a program.

DISCUSSION QUESTIONS

1. What are alternative hypotheses regarding what national health insurance should achieve?

2. Why are groups that have a concentrated interest in particular legislation likely to be more influential in the policy process than groups that have a diffuse interest in the legislation's outcome?

3. How have medical and hospital associations influenced provider payment and delivery systems? Provide specific examples.

4. Discuss the goals of the major groups that have a concentrated interest in health care reform.

5. Why would an employer-mandated national health insurance plan be insufficient by itself to secure the political support of the middle class?

6. Why is the structure and financing of any national health insurance plan likely to be inefficient and inequitable?

REFERENCES

Enthoven, A. 2004. "Market Forces and Efficient Health Care Systems." *Health Affairs* 23 (2): 25–27.

Feldstein, P. 2006a. "Medicare." In *The Politics of Health Legislation: An Economic Perspective*, 3rd ed. Chicago: Health Administration Press.

———. 2006b. "The Medicare Modernization Act, 2003." In *The Politics of Health Legislation: An Economic Perspective*, 3rd ed. Chicago: Health Administration Press.

Hawkins, L., Jr. 2005. "GM Plans to Cut Salaried Staff; Overhaul Looms." *The Wall Street Journal* March 21, A1 and A6.

Hawkins, L., Jr., and K. Lundegaard. 2005. "GM Warns UAW on Health Benefits." *The Wall Street Journal* June 16, A3.

Glossary

actual versus list price—Actual prices are the fees collected or paid for a particular good or service. The difference between actual and list prices are provider discounts, which vary by type of payer.

actuarially fair insurance—Expected insurance payments (benefits) are equivalent to premiums paid by beneficiaries (plus a competitive loading charge).

adverse selection—Occurs when high-risk individuals have more information on their health status than the insurer and are thus able to buy insurance at a premium based on a lower-risk group.

all-payer system—Each payer pays the same charges for hospital and medical services.

American Medical Association (AMA)—A national organization established in 1897 to represent the collective interests of physicians.

antitrust laws—A body of legislation that promotes competition in the U.S. economy.

any-willing-provider (AWP) laws—These laws lessen price competition in that they permit any physician to have access to a health plan's enrollees at the negotiated price. Because physicians cannot be assured of having a greater number of enrollees in return for discounting their prices, physicians have no incentive to compete on price to be included in the health plan's network.

assignment/participation—An agreement whereby the provider accepts the approved fee from the third-party payer and is not permitted to charge the patient more, except for the appropriate copayment fees.

balance billing—When the physician collects from the patient the difference between the third-party payer's approved fee and the physician's fee.

barriers to entry—Barriers, which may be legal (e.g., licensing laws and patents) or economic (e.g., economies of scale), that limit entry into an industry.

benefit–premium ratio—The percentage of the total premium paid out in benefits to each insured group divided by the price of insurance. (Also referred to as the *medical loss ratio*.)

budget neutral—Total payments to providers under the new payment system are set equal to what was spent under the previous payment system.

Canadian-type health system—A form of national health insurance in which medical services are free to everyone and providers are paid by the government. Expenditure limits are used to restrict the growth in medical use and costs.

capitation incentive—When the provider is capitated, he becomes concerned with the coordination of all medical services, providing care in the least-costly manner, monitoring the cost of enrollees' hospital use, increasing physician productivity, prescribing less-costly drugs, and being innovative in the delivery of medical services. Conversely, the provider has an incentive to reduce use of services and decrease patient access.

capitation payment—A risk-sharing arrangement in which the provider group receives a predetermined fixed payment per member per month in return for providing all of the contracted services.

case-mix index—A measure of the relative complexity of the patient mix treated in a given medical care setting.

certificate-of-need (CON) laws—State laws requiring health care providers to receive prior approval from a state agency for capital expenditures exceeding certain predetermined levels. CON laws are an entry barrier.

coinsurance/copayment—A fixed percentage of the medical provider's fee paid by the insurance beneficiary at the point of service.

community rating—The insurance premium is the same to all of the insured, regardless of their claims experience or risk group.

competitive market—The interaction between a large number of buyers and suppliers, where no single seller or buyer can influence the market price.

concentrated interest—When some regulation or legislation has a sufficiently large effect on a group to make it worthwhile for that group to invest resources to either forestall or promote that effect.

consumer-driven health care (CDHC)—Consumers purchase high-deductible health insurance and bear greater responsibility for their use of medical services and the prices they pay health care providers.

consumer sovereignty—Consumers, rather than health professionals or the government, choose the goods and services they can purchase with their incomes.

cost-containment program—Approaches used to reduce health care costs, such as utilization review and patient cost sharing.

cost shifting—The belief that providers charge a higher price to privately insured patients because some payers, such as Medicaid or the uninsured, do not pay their full costs.

declining marginal productivity of health inputs—The additional contribution to output of a health input declines as more of that input is used.

deductible—Consumers pay a flat dollar amount for medical services before their insurance picks up all or part of the remainder of the price of that service.

diagnosis-related group (DRG)—A method of reimbursement established under Medicare to pay hospitals based on a fixed price per admission according to the diagnosis for which the patient is admitted.

diffuse cost—When the burden of a tax or program is spread over a large population and is relatively small per person, so that the per person cost of opposing such a burden exceeds the actual size of the burden on the person.

economic theory of government—A theory of legislative and regulatory outcomes that assumes political markets are no different from economic markets in that organized groups seek to further their self-interests.

economies of scale—The relationship between cost per unit and size of firm. As firm size increases, cost per unit falls, reaches a minimum, and eventually rises. In a competitive market each firm operates at the size that has the lowest per unit costs. For a given size market, the larger the firm size required to achieve the minimum costs of production, the fewer the number of firms that will be able to compete.

economies of scope—Occur when it is less costly for a firm to produce certain services (or products) jointly than if separate firms produced each of the same services independently.

employer-mandated health insurance—Under this health reform plan, all employers are required to purchase medical insurance for their employees or pay a specified amount per employee into a state fund.

experience rating—Insurance premiums are based on the claims experience or risk level, such as age, of each insured group.

externality—Occurs when an action undertaken by an individual (or firm) has secondary effects on others, and these effects are not taken into account by the normal operations of the price system.

fee-for-service payment—A method of payment for medical care services in which payment is made for each unit of service provided.

free choice of provider—This was included in the original Medicare and Medicaid legislation and specified that all beneficiaries had to have access to all providers.

This precluded closed provider panels and capitated HMOs. Economists consider the provision to be anticompetitive in that it limits competition; beneficiaries could not choose a closed provider panel in return for lower prices or increased benefits.

gatekeeper—In many HMOs the primary care physician, or "gatekeeper," is responsible for the administration of the patient's treatment and must coordinate and authorize all medical services, laboratory studies, specialty referrals, and hospitalizations.

geographic market definition—Used in antitrust analysis to determine the relevant market in which a health care provider competes. The broader the geographic market, the greater are the number of substitutes available to the purchaser, and hence the smaller the market share of merging firms.

guaranteed issue—Health insurers have to offer health insurance to those willing to purchase it.

guaranteed renewal—Requires health insurers to renew all health insurance policies within standard rate bands, thereby precluding insurers from dropping individuals or groups who incur high medical costs.

health maintenance organization (HMO)—A type of managed care plan that offers prepaid comprehensive health care coverage for hospital and physician services, relying on its medical providers to minimize the cost of providing medical services. HMOs contract with or directly employ participating health care providers. Enrollees must pay the full cost of receiving services from nonnetwork providers.

health savings account (HSA)—Enacted as part of the Medicare Modernization Act, individuals are permitted to have a high-deductible insurance plan together with a savings account to use toward health care expenses. The unused portion of the savings account can accumulate over time.

horizontal merger—When two or more firms from the same market merge to form one firm.

income elasticity—The percentage change in quantity that occurs with a given percentage change in income. When the percentage change in quantity exceeds the percentage change in income, the service is income "elastic."

indemnity insurance—Medical insurance that pays the provider or the patient a predetermined amount for the medical service provided.

independent practice association (IPA)—A physician-owned and physician-controlled contracting organization comprising solo and small groups of physicians (on a nonexclusive basis) that enables physicians to contract with payers on a unified basis.

individual mandate—A proposed national health insurance plan under which individuals are required to buy a specified minimum level of health insurance (catastrophic insurance). Refundable tax credits are provided to those who have incomes below a certain level.

insurance premium—Consists of two parts: the expected medical expense of the insured group and the loading charge, which includes administrative expenses and profit.

integrated delivery system (IDS)—A health care delivery system that includes or contracts with all of the health care providers to provide coordinated medical services to the patient. An IDS also views itself as being responsible for the health status of its enrolled population.

law of demand—A decrease in price will result in an increase in quantity demanded, other factors affecting demand held constant.

managed care organization (MCO)—An organization that controls medical care costs and quality through provider price discounts, utilization management, drug formularies, and profiling participating providers according to their appropriate use of medical services.

mandated benefits—According to state insurance laws, specific medical services, providers, or population groups must be included in health insurance policies.

marginal benefit—The change in total benefits from purchasing one additional unit.

marginal contribution of medical care to health—The increase in health status resulting from an additional increment of medical services.

marginal cost—The change in total costs from producing one additional unit.

Medicaid—A health insurance program financed by federal and state governments and administered by the states for qualifying segments of the low-income population.

Medicaid risk contract—A Medicaid managed care program in which an HMO contracts to provide medical services in return for a capitation premium.

medical care price index—Calculated by the Bureau of Labor Statistics and included as part of the Consumer Price Index, it is used as a measure of the rate of inflation in medical care prices.

medical group—A group of physicians who coordinate their activities in one or more group facilities and share common overhead expenses, medical records, and professional, technical, and administrative staffs.

medical loss ratio—See benefit–premium ratio.

Medicare—A federally sponsored and supervised health insurance plan for the elderly. *Part A:* Provides hospital insurance for inpatient care, home health agency visits, hospice, and skilled nursing facilities. The aged are responsible for a deductible but do not have to pay an annual premium. *Part B:* Provides payments for physician services, physician-ordered supplies and services, and outpatient hospital services. Part B is voluntary, and the aged pay an annual premium that is 25 percent of the cost of the program in addition to a deductible and copayment. *Part C:* Permits private health plans to compete for serving the aged. *Part D:* A new prescription drug benefit, which includes deductibles and copayments and requires a monthly premium.

Medicare Advantage plans—Enacted as part of the Medicare Modernization Act, private health plans receive a monthly capitation payment from Medicare and accept full financial risk for the cost of all medical benefits (Part A, Part B, and Part D services) to which their enrollees are entitled. Enrollees using nonparticipating providers are responsible for the full charges of such providers. Previously referred to as Medicare+Choice plans.

Medicare risk contract—See *Medicare Advantage plans.*

Medigap insurance policy—Insurance policy privately purchased by the elderly to supplement Medicare coverage by covering deductibles and copayments.

monopoly—A market structure in which there is a single seller of a product that has no close substitutes.

moral hazard—Occurs when a patient can affect the size of his or her loss, as when patients increase their use of medical services when the price of those services is reduced.

multihospital system—A system in which a corporation owns, leases, or manages two or more acute care hospitals.

multipayer system—A system in which reimbursement for medical services is made by multiple third-party payers.

network HMO—A type of HMO that signs contracts with a number of group practices to provide medical services.

nonprice hospital competition—Hospitals compete on the basis of their facilities and services and the latest technology rather than on price.

not-for-profit—An institution that cannot distribute profits to shareholders and is tax exempt.

nurse participation rate—The percentage of trained nurses who are employed.

opportunity cost—Relevant costs for economic decision making; they include explicit and implicit costs. For example, the opportunity costs of a medical education include the forgone income the student could have earned had she not gone to medical school.

out-of-pocket price—The amount that the beneficiary must pay after all other payments have been considered by the health plan.

over-the-counter drug—A drug that is available for public purchase and self-directed use without a prescription.

patient dumping—A situation in which high-cost patients are not admitted to or are discharged early from a hospital because the patient has no insurance or the amount reimbursed by the third-party payer will be less than the cost of caring for that patient.

pay for performance—Higher payments are made to those health care providers who demonstrate that they provide higher-quality services.

per diem payment—A method of payment to institutional providers that is based on a fixed daily amount and does not differ according to the level of service provided.

pharmacy benefit manager (PBM)—Firm that provides administrative services and processes outpatient prescription drug claims for health insurers' prescription drug plans.

physician agency relationship—The physician acts on behalf of the patient. Agency relationships may be perfect or imperfect, and the method of physician payment, fee-for-service or capitation, produces different behavioral responses among imperfect physician agents.

physician hospital organization (PHO)—An organization in which hospitals and their medical staffs develop new types of group practice arrangements that will allow the hospitals to seek contracts from HMOs and other carriers on behalf of the physicians and hospitals together.

play or pay—Under this form of national health insurance (also referred to as an employer mandate), employers are required to provide some basic level of medical insurance to their employees ("play") or pay a certain amount per employee into a government pool that would provide the employee with insurance.

point-of-service plan—A plan that allows the beneficiary to select from participating providers (the health plan) or use nonparticipating providers and pay a high copayment.

portability—Included as part of health insurance reform that enables the insured to change jobs without losing their insurance or being liable for another preexisting exclusion period.

preexisting exclusion—To protect themselves against adverse selection by new enrollees, insurers use a preexisting exclusion clause that excludes treatment for any or specified illnesses that have been diagnosed within the previous (usually) 12 months.

preferred provider organization (PPO)—An arrangement between a panel of health care providers and purchasers of health care services in which a closed panel of providers agrees to supply services to a defined group of patients on a discounted fee-for-service basis. This type of plan offers its members a limited number of physicians and hospitals, negotiated fee schedules, utilization review, and consumer incentives to use PPO-participating providers.

preferred risk selection—Occurs when insurers receive the same premium for everyone in an insured group and try to attract only those with lower risks, whose expected medical costs would be less than the group's average premium.

prescription drug—A drug that can be obtained only with a physician's order.

> *breakthrough (or innovator) drug:* The first brand-name drug to use a particular therapeutic mechanism, that is, to use a particular method of treating a given disease.

> *generic drug:* A copy of a breakthrough drug that the FDA judges to be comparable in terms of such factors as strength, quality, and therapeutic effectiveness. Generic drugs are sold after the patent on a brand-name drug has expired and generally under their chemical names.

> *"me-too" drug:* A brand-name drug that uses the same therapeutic mechanism as a breakthrough drug and thus directly competes with it.

> *multiple-source drug:* A drug available in both brand-name and generic versions from a variety of manufacturers.

> *single-source drug:* A brand-name drug that is still under patent and thus is usually available from only one manufacturer.

price discrimination—An indication of monopoly power by a provider. The provider is able to charge different purchasers different prices according to the purchaser's elasticity of demand (willingness to pay) for the same or a similar service.

price elasticity—The percentage change in quantity divided by the percentage change in price. When the percentage change in quantity exceeds the percentage change in price, the service is price "elastic."

primary care physician—A physician who coordinates all of the routine medical care needs of an individual. Typically, this type of physician specializes in family practice, internal medicine, pediatrics, or obstetrics/gynecology.

process measures of quality—A type of quality assessment that evaluates process of care by measuring the specific way in which care is provided or, with respect to health manpower, the educational requirements.

product market definition—Used in antitrust cases to determine whether the product or service in question has close substitutes, which depends on the willingness of purchasers to use other services if the relative prices change. The closer the substitutes, the smaller is the market share of the product being examined.

prospective payment system (PPS)—A method of payment for medical services in which providers are paid a predetermined rate for the services rendered regardless of the actual costs of care incurred. Medicare uses a PPS for hospital care based on a fixed price per hospital admission (by diagnosis).

public-interest theory of government—Assumes that legislation is enacted to serve the public interest. According to this theory the two basic objectives of government are to improve market efficiency and, based on a societal value judgment, redistribute income.

pure premium—The expected claims experience for an insured group, exclusive of the loading charge. The pure premium for an individual is calculated by multiplying the size of the loss by the probability the loss will occur.

redistribution—When, as a result of public policy, the benefits and costs to a person are not equal, redistribution occurs. For example, based on a societal value judgment that those with higher incomes should be taxed to provide for those with lower incomes, the benefits and costs are not equal for either of the groups affected.

refundable tax credit—A proposal for national health insurance under which individuals are given a tax credit to purchase health insurance. The tax credit may be income related (i.e., declining at higher levels of income). Persons whose tax credit exceeds their tax liabilities would receive a refund for the difference. For those with little or no tax liability the tax credit is essentially a voucher for a health plan.

regressive tax—When those with lower incomes pay a higher portion of their income for a given tax than do those with higher incomes.

report card—Standardized data representing process and outcome measures of quality that are collected by independent organizations to enable purchasers to make more informed choices of health plans and their participating providers.

resource-based relative value scale (RBRVS)—The current Medicare fee-for-service payment system for physicians, initiated in 1992, under which each physician service is assigned a relative value based on the presumed resource costs of performing that service. The relative value for each service is then multiplied by a conversion factor (in dollars) to arrive at the physician's fee.

risk-adjusted premium—The employer adjusts the insurance premium to reflect the risk levels of the employees enrolled with different insurers.

risk pool—Represents a population group that is defined by its expected claim experience.

risk selection—Occurs when insurers attempt to attract a more favorable risk group than the average risk group, which was the basis for the group's premium (preferred risk selection). Similarly, enrollees may seek to join a health plan at a premium that reflects a lower level of risk than their own (adverse selection).

rule of reason—Used in antitrust cases to determine whether the anticompetitive harm caused by a particular activity (e.g., merger) exceeds the procompetitive benefits of not permitting the particular activity.

second opinion—A utilization-review approach in which decisions to initiate a medical intervention are typically reviewed by two physicians.

self-funding self-insurance—A health care program in which employers fund benefit plans from their own resources without purchasing insurance. Self-funded plans may be self-administered, or the employer may contract with an outside administrator for an administrative-service-only arrangement. Employers who self-fund can limit their liability via stop-loss insurance.

single payer—A form of national health insurance in which a single third-party payer, usually the government, pays health care providers and the entire population has free choice of all providers at zero (or little) out-of-pocket expense.

skilled nursing facility—A long-term-care facility that provides inpatient skilled nursing care and rehabilitation services.

specialty PPO—A type of PPO that offers one or more limited health care services or benefits, such as anesthesia, vision, and dental services.

staff-model HMO—A type of HMO that hires salaried physicians to provide health care services on an exclusive basis to the HMO's enrollees.

stop-loss insurance—Insurance coverage providing protection from losses resulting from claims greater than a specific dollar amount (equivalent to a large deductible).

supplier-induced demand—When physicians modify their diagnosis and treatment to favorably affect their own economic well-being.

sustainable growth rate (SGR)—Medicare's expenditure limit on physician payments consists of four elements: the percentage increase in real GDP per capita, a medical inflation rate of physician fee increases, the annual percentage increase in Part B enrollees, and the percentage change in spending for physicians' services resulting from changes in laws and regulations (e.g., expanded Medicare coverage for preventive services).

target income hypothesis—A model of supplier-induced demand that assumes physicians will induce demand only to the extent they will achieve a target income, which is determined by the local income distribution, particularly with respect to the relative incomes of other physicians and professionals in the area.

tax-exempt employer-paid health insurance—Health insurance purchased by the employer on behalf of its employees is not considered to be taxable income to the employee. By lowering the price of insurance the quantity demanded is increased (as is its comprehensiveness). The major beneficiaries are those in higher income-tax brackets.

tertiary care—This type of care includes the most complex services, such as transplantation, open-heart surgery, and burn treatment, provided in inpatient hospital settings.

third-party administrator (TPA)—An independent entity that provides administrative services, such as claims processing, to a company that self-insures. A third-party administrator does not underwrite the risk.

third-party payer—An organization, such as an HMO, insurance company, or government agency, that pays for all or part of the insured's medical services.

triple-option health plan—A type of health plan in which employees may choose from an HMO, a PPO, or an indemnity plan depending on how much they are willing to contribute.

unbundling—Occurs when a provider charges separately for each of the services previously provided together as part of a treatment.

uncompensated care—Services rendered by the provider without reimbursement, as in the case of charity care and bad debts.

universal coverage—When the entire population is eligible for medical services or health insurance.

up-coding—Occurs when the provider bills for a higher-priced diagnosis or service rather than the lower-cost service actually provided.

usual, customary, and reasonable fee—A method of reimbursement in which the fee is "usual" in that physician's office, "customary" in that community, and "reasonable" in terms of the distribution of all physician charges for that service in the community.

vacancy rate—The percentage of a hospital's budgeted RN positions that are unfilled.

vertical integration—The organization of a delivery system that provides an entire range of services to include inpatient care, ambulatory care clinics, outpatient surgery, and home care.

vertical merger—A merger between two firms that have a supplier-buyer relationship.

virtual integration—The organization of a delivery system that relies on contractual relationships rather than complete ownership to provide all medical services required by the patient.

voluntary performance standard—An expenditure target adopted by the Medicare program in 1992 to limit the rate of increase in its expenditures for physicians' services. This was replaced by the SGR formula as part of the Balanced Budget Act of 1997.

Index

Actual premium, 63

Administrative costs: Canadian health care system, 458–59; employer-purchased health insurance, 66; medical group, 165

Adverse selection: in health insurance market, 77–80, 84; long-term care insurance, *512n*, *513n*

Advisory Council on Breakthrough Drugs, 418

Advocacy groups, 381–82

AFDC. *See* Aid to Families with Dependent Children

Aged population: capitation rates, 120; concentrated interest, 528–29; hospital use, 221; increase in, 503, *504f*; Internet and, 312; managed care plans, 267; Medicaid eligibility, 110, 111, 113; medical services utilization, 5–6; physician access issues, 135–36, *136n*, 137; prescription drug use, 357–58

Aid to Families with Dependent Children, 110

AIDS, 375–76

All-payer systems, 235

American Federation of Labor-Congress of Industrial Organizations, 524

American Medical Association: antitrust issues, 288–89; managed care issues, 274; Medicare opposition, *442n*; political power of, 523, 524

Anticompetitive behavior, *375n*

Anticompetitive regulations, 290–92

Antitrust laws: application of, 9, 23

Any-willing-provider laws, 274, 292

Applicant-to-acceptance ratio, 150–52

Association health plans, *293n*

Attorney fees, 186

Average cost pricing, 245

AWP. *See* Any-willing-provider laws

Bad debt, 200

Balance billing: concerns, 127; explanation, 126; limits, 132, 136

Balanced Budget Act: HMO notice, *82n*; Medicaid eligibility provisions, 112; Medicaid waivers, 119; physician fee updates, 131–32

Biased selection, 267

Bioequivalence, 374

Biotechnology firms, 409

Block grants, 115–16

Blue Cross, 42

Bourassa, Premier Robert, 470

British National Health Service, 473

About the Author

PAUL J. FELDSTEIN, Ph.D., has been a professor and the Robert Gumbiner Chair in Health Care Management at the Graduate School of Management, University of California, Irvine, since 1987. His previous position was at the University of Michigan as a professor in both the Department of Economics and the School of Public Health. Before that he was the director of the Division of Research at the American Hospital Association. Professor Feldstein received his Ph.D. from the University of Chicago.

Professor Feldstein has written six books and more than 70 articles on health care. His book *Health Care Economics* is one of the most widely used texts on health economics. His book *The Politics of Health Legislation: An Economic Perspective* uses economic analysis to explain the outcome of health legislation in terms of the interest groups affected.

During leaves from the university, Professor Feldstein worked at the Office of Management and Budget, the Social Security Administration, and the World Health Organization. He has been a consultant to many government and private health agencies, has served as an expert witness on health antitrust issues, and was a board member of Sutter Health, a large not-for-profit health care organization serving Northern California and Province Healthcare, a hospital company serving nonurban populations. He is currently on the board of Odyssey Healthcare, a hospice company.